D0932663

Nursing Professional Development for Clinical Educators

Joan Such Lockhart, PhD, RN, AOCN®, CORLN, CNE, ANEF, FAAN

Oncology Nursing Society
Pittsburgh, Pennsylvania

ONS Publications Department

Publisher and Director of Publications: William A. Tony, BA, CQIA

Managing Editor: Lisa M. George, BA

Assistant Managing Editor: Amy Nicoletti, BA, JD

Acquisitions Editor: John Zaphyr, BA, MEd

Copy Editors: Vanessa Kattouf, BA, Andrew Petyak, BA

Graphic Designer: Dany Sjoen

Editorial Assistant: Judy Holmes

Library of Congress Cataloging-in-Publication Data

Names: Lockhart, Joan Such, author. | Oncology Nursing Society, publisher.

Title: Nursing professional development for clinical educators / by Joan Such Lockhart.

Description: Pittsburgh, Pennsylvania : Oncology Nursing Society, [2016] | Includes bibliographical references and index.

Identifiers: LCCN 2015038354 | ISBN 9781935864776

Subjects: | MESH: Nurse Clinicians–education. | Education, Nursing, Continuing–organization & administration. | Staff Development–methods.

Classification: LCC RT89 | NLM WY 18 | DDC 610.73068–dc23 LC record available at http://lccn.loc.gov/2015038354

Publisher's Note

This book is published by the Oncology Nursing Society (ONS). ONS neither represents nor guarantees that the practices described herein will, if followed, ensure safe and effective patient care. The recommendations contained in this book reflect ONS's judgment regarding the state of general knowledge and practice in the field as of the date of publication. The recommendations may not be appropriate for use in all circumstances. Those who use this book should make their own determinations regarding specific safe and appropriate patient care practices, taking into account the personnel, equipment, and practices available at the hospital or other facility at which they are located. The author and publisher cannot be held responsible for any liability incurred as a consequence from the use or application of any of the contents of this book. Figures and tables are used as examples only. They are not meant to be all-inclusive, nor do they represent endorsement of any particular institution by ONS. Mention of specific products and opinions related to those products do not indicate or imply endorsement by ONS. Websites mentioned are provided for information only; the hosts are responsible for their own content and availability. Unless otherwise indicated, dollar amounts reflect U.S. dollars.

ONS publications are originally published in English. Publishers wishing to translate ONS publications must contact ONS about licensing arrangements. ONS publications cannot be translated without obtaining written permission from ONS. (Individual tables and figures that are reprinted or adapted require additional permission from the original source.) Because translations from English may not always be accurate or precise, ONS disclaims any responsibility for inaccuracies in words or meaning that may occur as a result of the translation. Readers relying on precise information should check the original English version.

Printed in the United States of America

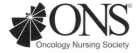

Innovation • Excellence • Advocacy

Dedicated to my sister, Emillie (Mim) Mary Such, and my partner for life, Ray McGill. Your love, patience, and constant faith always kept me moving forward. This book also is in memory of my late parents, Emillie Anne and John T. Such, and my late husband, Edward E. Lockhart.

Disclosure

Editors and authors of books and guidelines provided by the Oncology Nursing Society are expected to disclose to the readers any significant financial interest or other relationships with the manufacturer(s) of any commercial products.

A vested interest may be considered to exist if a contributor is affiliated with or has a financial interest in commercial organizations that may have a direct or indirect interest in the subject matter. A "financial interest" may include, but is not limited to, being a shareholder in the organization; being an employee of the commercial organization; serving on an organization's speakers bureau; or receiving research funding from the organization. An "affiliation" may be holding a position on an advisory board or some other role of benefit to the commercial organization. Vested interest statements appear in the front matter for each publication.

Contributors are expected to disclose any unlabeled or investigational use of products discussed in their content. This information is acknowledged solely for the information of the readers.

The author provided the following disclosure and vested interest information:

The author has no relevant information to disclose.

Contents

Foreword

Nurses have the distinct opportunity to interact with people at their most vulnerable times in life. They, like teachers, shape the future for our global population. What a glorious opportunity to shape nurses' lives—becoming a professional development educator! Two worlds collide and form a new opportunity to affect even more people; this is the intent of being a professional development educator. Just like a clinical specialty, a role specialty helps define what we do as nurses. While many of us say, "I am a nurse," others may say they are a pediatric nurse, obstetric (OB) nurse, or an intensive care nurse. Our attempt is to help others see the kinds of contributions we make as nurses. So, saying that one is a nurse manager, nurse educator, or a professional development educator helps others know more about what we do in this vast field.

Even after just a few years, nurses can identify the large amount of additional information they have learned since graduation. When we add the increasingly rapid changes in health care, we can see that being a professional development educator is a privilege. But, just like how we all do not "do" OB or intensive care, so too we do not all "do" professional development. Having the desire to help others learn, being willing to gain satisfaction indirectly through those we educate, and knowing that we are not directly accountable for those we teach are all factors we must consider when we take on this role. Few graduate degrees prepare nurses for this role. Thus, a book such as this one becomes critical to grasp what the field means and what the breadth and depth of the role entail.

Learning the role is a challenge, but it is one made easier by the presence of this book. Moving from such important influences as the Patient Protection and Affordable Care Act and the issue of patient safety through information technology, Dr. Joan Lockhart helps us to gain the context for this critical role in health care. How do we make certain that newly employed nurses are sufficiently competent to assume a particular role? How do we adapt learning experiences for learners with diverse learning needs and styles? How do we extend our influence beyond our particular designated area? How do we manage our role so that we are effective? How do we deal with the complexity of health care and translate that into a meaningful whole to a team of educators and learners?

Joan's background as a professional development educator (both full and part time) provides her with rich experiences to support the theoretical knowledge needed to perform the role. As has been the case historically, her position was eliminated during a tight financial time. Think about that for a moment. At a time when an organization needs different thinking and fresh ideas, the area that is obligated to facilitate such development is eliminated! Peter Senge, author of the concept of the learning organization, would cringe. That is what makes a book such as this one even more valuable. The wisdom shared is invaluable in gaining insight into a role that must continue to develop and be valued.

Because turnover and growth produce the need for continued orientation efforts, some may forget about the numerous other aspects of the professional development role. This book has taken a broad view so that the importance of transitions for new graduates is highlighted, the aspects of orientation are given their due, and the importance of the rest of the role is explicated through various chapters. For example, we may forget that the educator may be the one responsible for working with staff to advance evidence-based reports or to write about achievements. Thus, those two chapters provide insight into how to work with these growing demands of the role.

Potential is the word that comes to mind as I think about what this book unleashes. It opens the door to broad thinking about a vital role in health care today. Grasping the key messages in this book will place professional development educators in a solid place to advance their careers and, in doing so, advance the health of the nation.

Dr. Patricia S. Yoder-Wise
Professor and Dean Emeritus, Texas Tech University Health Sciences Center
President, The Wise Group

Preface

Background

The specialty practice of nursing professional development (NPD), formerly known as nursing staff development, constantly evolves in response to trends in health care and nursing, advances in technology, and a broad interprofessional perspective to learning and competence. As leaders, NPD specialists (NPDSs) are charged to prepare a competent nursing workforce that can provide care that results in safe and quality patient health outcomes.

In many healthcare settings, clinical nurses assume some NPD responsibilities in addition to their direct patient care duties. Therefore, it is essential that both NPDSs and clinical nurses have access to evidence-based resources to help them perform in their staff educator responsibilities. In addition, educators in both clinical and academic settings must partner to not only facilitate the transition of newly graduated nurses to their first professional nursing roles but also support the lifelong learning of experienced clinical nurses in practice.

The author's experience as a staff development educator in an academic medical center and as an academic educator in a school of nursing offers readers a seamless academic-service perspective to NPD. Promoting the continuing competency and lifelong learning of both new and experienced clinical nurses who care for patients in various practice settings is the primary goal of *Nursing Professional Development for Clinical Educators*.

Target Audiences

This book is an essential resource for NPDSs and clinical nurses who are engaged in NPD activities. Nurses who are new to NPD will find this book extremely helpful in gaining a basic understanding of NPD as a practice specialty and their roles and responsibilities. More experienced NPDSs can rely on this book to strengthen their existing competencies or develop expertise in new areas. Clinical nurses who assume staff educator responsibilities on their clinical units, aspire to become NPDSs, or plan to progress through clinical advancement programs will find this book's content and practical examples essential to their success. Prelicensure RN students or experienced RN to BSN students who are enrolled in their senior-level leadership or professional role transition courses can refer to this book to gain insight into their own professional development and role expectations. Graduate students in master's and clinical- and research-focused doctoral programs can use this book to develop their leadership roles in nursing education and advanced clinical practice. Finally, managers of clinical units and education departments in healthcare organizations can use this book as a resource to orient, prepare, and develop their NPDSs and unit-based staff educators.

Overview

Nursing Professional Development for Clinical Educators is an updated version of the author's previous book titled *Unit-Based Staff Development for Clinical Nurses* (2004) and focuses on the scope and standards for NPDSs set forth by the American Nurses Association and the Association for Nursing Professional Development (formerly the National Nursing Staff Development Organization). Although these standards are currently under revision, the content included in this book will remain vital to their future roles and responsibilities.

Depending on their position and professional experience, NPDSs are responsible for developing healthcare professionals and staff who are employed in various clinical settings across a wide range of specialties. However, to include specific resources for NPDSs across specialties is beyond the scope of this book. Instead, the author used oncology nursing as the primary clinical context throughout the book to enable readers to understand the content presented and use similar avenues and resources specific to their unique clinical practice.

Nursing Professional Development for Clinical Educators offers new and expanded features:
- Personal and conversational writing style that facilitates application to practice
- Review of current nursing and healthcare trends that influence the NPDS role
- Comprehensive content based on current NPDS scope and standards
- Oncology nursing used as a clinical exemplar within the context of NPD
- Integration of content on technology, interprofessional education, and academic partnerships
- Expanded orientation chapter that includes competencies, residency programs, and dedicated education units
- Evidence-based practice and quality improvement included with research
- Helpful websites cited at the end of each chapter.

Nursing Professional Development for Clinical Educators contains 14 chapters that can be used separately to increase understanding on a particular topic or in conjunction with other chapters as they relate to NPDS roles and responsibilities. Chapter 1, Healthcare Trends and Changes in Nursing Professional Development, provides an overview of major healthcare trends and deliveries and ways that the NPD specialty has responded to these changes. Chapter 2, Understanding the Specialty Practice of Nursing Professional Development, elaborates on the professional development of nurses with primary attention to the NPD practice model and as a practice specialty with defined scope and standards. Chapter 3, Getting Prepared for Your Role as a Nursing Professional Development Specialist and Unit-Based Educator, offers strategies that nurses can use to prepare for an NPD role within a healthcare setting, beginning with a self-assessment and realistic plan for prioritizing learning needs and seeking feedback on performance. Chapter 4, Orienting Clinical Nurses to the Organization, Assessing Competence, and Promoting Lifelong Learning, focuses on the orientation component of NPD from the organizational level to a unit-based perspective with particular attention to assessing, developing, and evaluating the competencies of both novice and experienced nurses. The value and progress related to dedicated educational units and residency programs are also discussed in light of student nurses and newly graduated nurses. Chapter 5, Developing a Unit-Based Clinical Preceptorship Program, addresses the key components that NPDSs should consider when designing, implementing, and evaluating the effectiveness of a unit-based preceptor program for student nurses, newly hired graduates, or experienced nurses who are changing their role, position, or specialty focus. Chapter 6, Helping Clinical Nurses Develop Their Educator Role Through Unit-Based In-Service Educational Programs, provides a practical approach and tools that NPDSs can use when developing, conducting, and evaluating the learning outcomes of unit-based in-service educational activities. Chapter 7, Getting Involved in Professional Nursing Organizations and the Community, discusses ways that NPDSs and clinical nurses can share their expertise through their involvement in professional nursing organizations, employer-affiliated community groups, and local neighborhood and religious organizations. Chapter 8, Sharing Your Expertise Through Publishing, uses Lockhart's 10-Step Approach to Publishing to guide NPDSs and other nurse authors in preparing a manuscript for publication in a professional journal. Chapter 9, Sharing Your Expertise Through Abstracts, Oral Presentations, and Posters, guides NPDSs and clinical nurses in ways to share their professional nursing expertise both formally and informally through abstracts, oral presentations, and posters at professional meetings. Chapter 10, Recording Your Professional Nursing Achievements in a Portfolio, walks readers through the steps of creating a professional portfolio to track progress toward career goals and support new job opportunities, promotions, and professional and clinical advancement programs. Chapter 11, Preparing Your Résumé or Curriculum Vitae and Cover Letter, provides helpful strategies for creating the documents needed when applying for a new job, promotion, clinical advancement, or admission to graduate studies. Chapter 12, Promoting Nursing Research and Evidence-Based Practice in the Clinical Setting, explores the educator's roles and responsibilities related to research, evidence-based practice, and quality improvement in the work setting and strategies to develop competencies and the skills of others on a unit-based level. Chapter 13, Meeting the Learning Needs and Marketing the Talents of Clinical Nurses Through Continuing Education Programs, provides NPDSs with a comprehensive review of the steps involved in offering continuing education activities from assessing the learning needs of targeted learners to evaluating and disseminating outcomes. Chapter 14, Developing a Career Plan as a Proactive Approach for the Future, concludes the book by helping NPDSs and clinical nurses develop a professional career plan focused on future goals.

Acknowledgments

Writing this book has been a challenging journey made possible by the understanding and patience of my loving family. Many thanks are extended to my colleagues and doctoral students who helped with literature searches, provided practical clinical examples, and shared their honest feedback: Lisa Whitfield-Harris, Dr. Sally Bennett, Dr. Missy Volino, Debby Lewis, Dr. Anna Vioral, and Sister/Dr. Rosemary Donley. A special appreciation to Dr. Pat Yoder-Wise for her beautiful foreword and constant words of encouragement. A special thanks to Barb Sigler, who began the process for this book, and to the Oncology Nursing Society (ONS) publishing staff: Bill Tony, Lisa George, Amy Nicoletti, John Zaphyr, Dany Sjoen, Judy Holmes, Andrew Petyak, Vanessa Kattouf, and everyone else who assisted in this book's production. Finally, I extend my gratitude to the ONS reviewers for their honest opinions and help in making this book meaningful to clinical educators.

CHAPTER 1

Healthcare Trends and Changes in Nursing Professional Development

THIS chapter provides an overview of healthcare trends that may influence the roles and responsibilities of nurses who lead staff development activities, whether as nursing professional development specialists (NPDSs) or unit-based clinical staff educators. As these trends represent only a sample of changes within the dynamic U.S. healthcare system, further exploration of additional trends is recommended. Nursing professional development (NPD) has also changed in response to these trends in health care. Strategies will be presented to guide nurses in assuming a leadership role and becoming prepared for evolving healthcare trends.

Approximately 2.8 million RNs and 690,000 licensed practical nurses (LPNs) were employed in the U.S. workforce from 2008 to 2010, the largest group of healthcare professionals in the country (U.S. Department of Health and Human Services [U.S. DHHS], 2013b). With this majority in mind, it is imperative that nurses are educated on the strategies that healthcare organizations have developed to manage and survive recent healthcare trends.

It is important for NPDSs and unit-based staff educators to understand how the healthcare delivery system functions, be cognizant of trends and issues that influence these healthcare organizations, and anticipate the future direction of the healthcare delivery system and healthcare organizations.

Overview of Major Healthcare Trends

The implementation of legislative initiatives, such as diagnosis-related groups in the 1980s and managed care in the 1990s, resulted in financial constraints that affected the structure and function of healthcare organizations and the nurses they employed (Shi & Singh, 2015). During those decades, inpatient services shifted to less expensive treatments provided in outpatient care, long-term care, and homecare settings. Today, initiatives are being implemented to strengthen patient safety and improve the quality of healthcare reporting and services.

The Patient Protection and Affordable Care Act

In 2010, a new healthcare reform era began with the Patient Protection and Affordable Care Act (ACA), a federal law designed to provide Americans with affordable health care despite preexisting health conditions (Shi & Singh, 2015; U.S. DHHS, 2014). Under the law, citizens were required (with few exceptions) to enroll in health insurance exchanges by 2013 or purchase some form of public or private health insurance by January 1, 2014 (Shi & Singh, 2015). Those who failed to enroll were taxed (Shi & Singh, 2015). Although many individuals have identified benefits of ACA, others have cited its negative aspects. ACA offers a wealth of information regarding the direction of health care; however, three particular sections provide significant implications to the nursing profession.

Title III, Improving the Quality and Efficiency of Health Care, calls for a transformation of the U.S. healthcare delivery system to improve quality and safety outcomes (U.S. DHHS, 2015). It includes incentives for nurses and physicians who advance quality outcomes and reduce patient errors and harm. It also calls for more attention in designing new patient care models and ensuring quality care for seniors under Medicare.

Title V, Health Care Workforce, aims to increase the number of healthcare providers engaged in primary care and public health services through recruitment and retention strategies, such as scholarships and loan repayment programs for education and training (U.S. DHHS, 2015). It addresses the national nursing shortage by increasing the number of nurses and also increases the number of physicians, physician assistants, mental health workers, and dentists.

Title VI, Transparency and Program Integrity, promotes healthcare environments that embrace the transparent exchange and integrity of information, enabling the public to make informed healthcare decisions (U.S. DHHS, 2015). In particular, it promotes safe, quality care in long-term care settings through the use of employee background checks, continuous quality improvement initiatives, and ongoing staff safety education and training. Attention is paid to research focused on patient-centered outcomes and controlling waste, fraud, and abuse (U.S. DHHS, 2015).

Institute of Medicine Recommendations

The Institute of Medicine (IOM) has played an instrumental role over the past two decades in response to the changes in the U.S. healthcare system, the state of healthcare delivery, and the need to prepare competent healthcare professionals. IOM has issued several landmark reports to guide the future of health care in America. *To Err Is Human: Building a Safer Health System* focused on patient safety and offered healthcare system strategies to decrease the number of preventable medical errors (IOM, 1999). *Crossing the Quality Chasm: A New Health System for the 21st Century* recommended a redesign of the U.S. healthcare system based on an analysis of the quality gap, expectations to support patient and clinician relationships, and ways to foster evidence-based practice (EBP) and stronger information systems (IOM, 2001). The six areas cited as needing improvements were safety, effectiveness, patient-centeredness, timeliness, efficiency, and equity (Berwick, 2012).

In 2004, IOM issued *Keeping Patients Safe: Transforming the Work Environment of Nurses*, which recommended remedies to patient safety threats associated with the working environment. This report also offered an action plan on work issues, such as nurse staffing levels, work hours, and mandatory overtime.

From a collaboration with the Robert Wood Johnson Foundation (RWJF), IOM's 2010 landmark report *The Future of Nursing: Leading Change, Advancing Health* was an effort to "assess and respond to the need to transform the nursing profession" (p. xii) and prepare a nursing workforce suited to meet current and future healthcare changes. The report conveyed four key points (IOM, 2010, p. 4):

- Nurses should practice to the full extent of their education and training.
- Nurses should achieve higher levels of education and training through an improved education system that promotes seamless academic progression.

- Nurses should be full partners, with physicians and other healthcare professionals, in redesigning health care in the United States.
- Effective workforce planning and policy-making require better data collection and an improved information infrastructure.

Figure 1-1 outlines IOM's eight recommendations for preparing nurses for the future and overcoming barriers within work environments.

Consistent with its efforts toward promoting quality health care for Americans, IOM turned its attention to the growing number of cancer survivors and the current state of care available to them (IOM, 2013a). In *Improving the Quality of Cancer Care: Addressing the Challenges of an Aging Population*, IOM noted a substantial increase in the number of older adults being diagnosed with cancer during an era of healthcare workforce shortages (IOM, 2013b). In 2013, IOM published *Delivering High-Quality Cancer Care: Charting a New Course for a System in Crisis*, its comprehensive investigation of cancer care in the United States. IOM made recommendations essential to improving the current cancer care delivery system and quality patient outcomes (IOM, 2013a). Central to these changes, it proposed a conceptual framework of six elements aimed to improve the quality of care across the cancer continuum (IOM, 2013a, pp. 3–5):

- Engaged patients
- An adequately staffed, trained, and coordinated workforce
- Evidence-based cancer care
- A learning healthcare information technology (IT) system for cancer
- Translation of evidence into clinical practice, quality measurement, and performance improvement
- Accessible, affordable cancer care.

IOM's recommendations provide oncology nurses with opportunities to assume leadership roles in changing current and future cancer care services within their work settings (Becze, 2014; Ferrell, McCabe, & Levit, 2013). NPDSs involved in cancer care education should review these recommendations with nurses and develop proactive strategies to positively influence cancer care.

In addition to IOM's cancer care reports, oncology nurses and NPDSs need to understand the national accreditation standards for specialty services, such as those found in the American College of Surgeons Commission on Cancer's (ACS CoC's) *Cancer Program Standards 2012: Ensuring Patient-Centered Care*. According to these standards, "Oncology nursing care is provided by nurses with specialized knowledge and skills" (ACS CoC, 2012, p. 66). Oncology nursing education resources, such as courses available through the Oncology Nursing Society (ONS), are referenced as optimal means for preparing nurses caring for patients with can-

---

Figure 1-1. Institute of Medicine Recommendations on the Future of Nursing

1. Remove scope-of-practice barriers.
2. Expand opportunities for nurses to lead and diffuse collaborative improvement efforts.
3. Implement nurse residency programs.
4. Increase the proportion of nurses with a baccalaureate degree to 80% by 2020.
5. Double the number of nurses with a doctorate by 2020.
6. Ensure that nurses engage in lifelong learning.
7. Prepare and enable nurses to lead change to advance health.
8. Build an infrastructure for the collection and analysis of interprofessional healthcare workforce data.

Note. Based on information from Institute of Medicine, 2010.

cer. Certification in oncology nursing within these organizations is not required but is highly encouraged (ACS CoC, 2012). The credentials and competencies of cancer care nurses must be evaluated on a yearly basis and recorded according to policy (ACS CoC, 2012). Specific criteria for measuring an organization's compliance with these standards are also outlined in the accreditation manual.

Transforming Nursing Education

Another landmark report on the future of nursing, *Educating Nurses: A Call for Radical Transformation* (Benner, Sutphen, Leonard, & Day, 2010), called for a change in how nurses are prepared to meet current and future healthcare demands, claiming that nurses are under-educated to meet the complex challenges in clinical practice and academic settings and are unable to keep up with fast-paced changes in practice, resulting in an education–practice gap. Several recommendations for redesigning nursing education are provided in the report, calling for changes in teaching and learning practices and policy.

Patient Safety in Practice and Education

In addition to IOM and ACA efforts to strengthen patient safety and the quality of health-care reporting and services, other national groups have implemented related initiatives. The Joint Commission, an organization that accredits and certifies healthcare organizations, strives to improve health care for consumers through evaluation of quality and safety standards (Joint Commission, n.d.-a). Nearly two decades ago it created the Sentinel Event Policy, aimed to assist hospitals when they encounter an event that affects a patient (Joint Commission, n.d.-c). A *sentinel event* is a "safety event not primarily related to the natural course of the patient's illness or underlying condition that reaches a patient and results in any of the following: death, permanent harm, or severe temporary harm with an intervention required to sustain life" (Joint Commission, n.d.-c, para. 2).

In 2002, the Joint Commission initiated its National Patient Safety Goals (NPSGs), which focused on solving healthcare safety problems (Joint Commission, n.d.-b). These safety issues included several nursing responsibilities, such as safe medication administration, communication, clinical alarm safety, healthcare-associated infections, and patient identification. Although the Joint Commission identifies new safety priorities each year, prior NPSGs often remain as expectations for successful accreditation (Gorbunoff & Kummeth, 2014).

In an effort to prepare future nurses in meeting national quality and safety standards, the RWJF-funded Quality and Safety Education for Nurses (QSEN) Initiative established compe-tencies expected of students enrolled in prelicensure RN and graduate nursing programs (QSEN Institute, 2012). Created in 2005, QSEN competencies align with those of IOM (2003) and comprise six qualities of knowledge, skills, and attitudes: patient-centered care, teamwork and collaboration, EBP, quality improvement, safety, and informatics (QSEN Institute, 2014). The QSEN Institute also provides teaching resources and ongoing faculty development programs.

Current and Future Nursing Workforce

The nursing shortage (American Association of Colleges of Nursing [AACN], 2014b) has compounded current initiatives and will influence future ones. Although the recent recession led to a slight increase in RN employment within the U.S. (AACN, 2014b), a 2009 study projected that hospitals may expect a "shortfall of RNs developing around 2018 and growing to about 260,000 by 2025" (Buerhaus, Auerbach, & Staiger, 2009, p. w663) unless nursing schools are able to increase their capacity to produce nurses. More recent workforce reports predicted the shortage to continue into 2030, with the greatest need for nurses in the southern and western regions of the country (Juraschek, Zhang, Ranganathan, & Lin, 2012). An aging workforce is among the major reasons for the nursing shortage (Buerhaus et al., 2009; Juraschek et al., 2012). A similar shortage in qualified nursing faculty also has implications for healthcare organizations that need to fill vacant nursing positions, as well as nursing schools, which will need to limit student enrollment (AACN, 2014a). These workforce projections are alarming in an aging, diversifying, and growing U.S. population (U.S. Census Bureau, 2014).

National efforts have been made to increase the number of prepared RNs and the capacity of nursing schools. Attention has been paid to creating a nursing workforce that reflects the demographics of the U.S. population. Since 2008, the RWJF New Careers in Nursing program, a collaboration between RWJF and AACN, has awarded scholarships to underrepresented students who are enrolled in an accelerated nursing program (RWJF, n.d.). It also provides mentoring and leadership development.

Trends in Healthcare Delivery

Healthcare organizations have responded to healthcare trends and managed care in a variety of ways. Unfortunately, some institutions were unable to maintain their financial viability and did not survive decades of economic turmoil. From 1990 to 2000, 208 rural hospitals (7.8% of national rural hospitals) and 296 urban hospitals (10.6% of national urban hospitals) were forced to close (U.S. DHHS, 2003). Many of these closures were attributed to a low census, mergers or relocations, and competition (U.S. DHHS, 2003). According to the American Hospital Association's (AHA's) annual survey of U.S. hospitals, similar shifts in hospital closures continue to occur with a decrease of 37 registered hospitals (5,723 down to 5,686) reported from 2012 to 2013 (AHA, 2014, 2015). Similar declines were noted among rural (1,980 down to 1,971) and urban (3,019 down to 3,003) community hospitals (AHA, 2014, 2015). More recent data from the North Carolina Rural Health Research Program (2015) indicated that 54 U.S rural hospitals have closed their doors between January 2010 and June 2015.

Shi and Singh (2015) reported that the U.S. healthcare delivery has been shifting its focus over the past two decades from individual health within an inpatient, acute care, and illness-oriented context to the health of a community, framed within an outpatient, primary care, and wellness perspective. Hospitals also are transitioning from being independent institutions with fragmented care and duplicated services to integrated systems with managed care and a continuum of services (Shi & Singh, 2015). Health promotion combined with cost reduction has been the impetus for these healthcare changes (Shi & Singh, 2015).

Insightful healthcare organizations have survived these restrictions by reexamining the ways they have internally functioned. These organizations constantly strive to develop cost-effective means to maintain or attain quality and safe patient care outcomes. Numerous changes have occurred within healthcare organizations, but six come to the forefront: financial streamlining, organizational integration and realignment, new models of patient care delivery, work redesign and role changes, safety and quality performance indicators, and health IT.

Financial Streamlining

Past managed care and healthcare reimbursement changes forced many healthcare administrators to review their existing financial policies and procedures. Managers who dealt with patient care services and clinical divisions, such as nursing, were asked to streamline their operating budgets, control unnecessary expenses, seek untapped sources of revenue, and determine return on investments. Major budgetary expenditures, such as salary and other personnel costs associated with healthcare workers, were targeted as expenses that needed to be controlled. Departments were examined based on operating costs and ability to generate additional revenue for the organization.

In addition to reducing direct labor costs, these reimbursement changes forced organizations to closely examine expenses related to patient care services, consumer services, and the approach used to deliver these services. Many low-risk surgeries and treatments and invasive diagnostic procedures that were traditionally inpatient practices were modified using a more cost-effective outpatient approach (Shi & Singh, 2015). In fact, outpatient surgeries increased by nearly 50% from 1980 to 2010 (Shi & Singh, 2015; U.S. DHHS, 2013a).

This shift in healthcare services resulted in a different inpatient profile. For example, individuals admitted to acute care agencies (hospitals) possessed higher acuity levels than in past years, requiring skilled and intensive nursing care. After a shortened length of stay in the hospital, some patients were discharged to other healthcare agencies that offered subacute, intermediate, or extended nursing care. Healthcare workers employed in these transitional units provided much of the nursing care previously performed in the acute care environment. In fact, some organizations added new clinical services, such as transition units, within their own systems to help patients change from acute care to a home setting. Other patients were discharged with or without homecare services. Attention was paid to reducing patient readmission shortly following discharge.

Organizational Integration and Realignment

Beginning in the late 1990s, hospitals underwent organizational integration in an effort to remain viable by becoming cost-effective and diversifying operations with new services or products (Shi & Singh, 2015). Integration strategies included acquisitions, mergers, alliances, joint ventures, and virtual networks (Shi & Singh, 2015).

Many chief operating officers dealt with these financial constraints by focusing on the internal structure of their organizations and the allocation of resources. Some completely reorganized or realigned their structures, whereas others chose to implement minor changes in their existing organizations. Low utilization rates and competition over decades influenced organizational downsizing or rightsizing, often resulting in major changes in or elimination of divisions and departments (U.S. DHHS, 2003). In some instances, services, such as laundry, dietary, and education, were outsourced or contracted through external companies. Many healthcare organizations closed patient units and reduced their number of beds. Some departments that were non–revenue generating or advisory in nature, such as staff education, often faced negative consequences.

Healthcare organizations, confronted by the influence of managed care, focused their efforts on securing their share of the healthcare market. Many agencies diversified services in an attempt to obtain more patients or clients (Shi & Singh, 2015). In an effort to compete with other healthcare organizations for customers, some hospitals expanded or shifted services from inpatient admissions to include outpatient, subacute care, homecare, long-term care, ambulatory care, and community-based efforts.

New Models of Patient Care Delivery

Related to financial and organizational reforms, new models in organizing and delivering care have emerged in an effort to improve primary healthcare services for Americans in settings such as physician offices and community health centers (Agency for Healthcare Research and Quality [AHRQ], n.d.-b). According to AHRQ and the National Committee for Quality Assurance (NCQA), the patient-centered medical home (PCMH) should be viewed as a "model of the organization of primary care that delivers the core functions of primary health care" (AHRQ, n.d.-a, para. 1). In a PCMH, the primary care physician leads a collaborative team of healthcare professionals in providing access to coordinated care services based on the needs and preferences of patients and their families (Caudill, Lofgren, Jennings, & Karpf, 2011).

A PCMH also aims to advance how consumers and healthcare providers perceive their healthcare experience (NCQA, n.d.). A PCMH comprises five elements: comprehensive care, patient-centered (relationship-based) care, coordinated care, accessible services, and quality and safety (AHRQ, n.d.-a). Practices that choose to become PCMHs can apply for NCQA Recognition (NCQA, n.d.).

Similar PCMH models have been created in clinical specialty practices. For example, the Centers for Medicare and Medicaid Services (CMS) (2014c) recently developed an Oncology Care Model (OCM) to address the current state of cancer care in the United States because of the increasing number of older adults diagnosed with or surviving cancer. OCM is a cancer payment model that offers financial incentives to physician practices that increase the quality and coordination of the cancer care services they provide while also decreasing costs. Oncology practices that deliver chemotherapy enter into payment arrangements that include financial and performance accountability for episodes of care (CMS, 2014c) and are evaluated on more than 30 quality measures (Clark, 2015). Practices are expected to offer 24-hour outpatient clinics where patients can receive treatment for their chemotherapy-associated symptoms rather than seek such care at hospital-based emergency departments (Clark, 2015). Scheduled to begin in 2016, OCM is intended to decrease both hospital and pharmacy costs (Clark, 2015).

Work Redesign and Role Changes

Efforts to restructure and downsize in healthcare agencies also compelled healthcare administrators to examine how work was being accomplished. Managers were encouraged to redesign work in a manner that was cost-saving, efficient, and effective. Frequently, all but essential financial and human resources were trimmed from budgets. Employees in these departments were encouraged to rethink their responsibilities and develop innovative ways to perform their jobs. They were asked to "work smarter, not harder" and "do more with less."

New paradigms or models that resulted from these work redesigns often changed the roles and responsibilities previously assumed by employees of these healthcare organizations. Although some workers could easily adjust to their new roles by making minor modifications in their daily activities, others needed to be cross-trained or retrained to gain the knowledge and skills required to function in their new roles.

Safety and Quality Performance Indicators

In concert with cost-effectiveness and efficiency, healthcare organizations focused their efforts on measuring and managing outcomes related to healthcare services, such as patient care (Shi & Singh, 2015). Healthcare workers were challenged on a daily basis to provide quality patient care with fewer resources. Managers were encouraged to make decisions using data-driven outcome measurements (Shi & Singh, 2015). Hospitals focused attention on landmark reports, performance indicators related to patient safety, and ACA-mandated improvements in safety, quality monitoring, and reporting (U.S. DHHS, 2015).

Existing systemwide quality control programs that focused on quality and effectiveness of clinical services were enhanced within healthcare organizations (Shi & Singh, 2015). Managers were encouraged to improve quality and safety goals and reduce associated costs. Outcomes management initiatives, referred to as *total quality management* (TQM), gained popularity (Shi & Singh, 2015). Because the primary focus of TQM is continuous improvement in all organizational processes, managers and employees were encouraged to improve their performance daily.

For example, suppose the nursing staff on your unit wanted to improve their performance related to patient admissions. You would begin by breaking down your existing admissions procedure into its smallest components. While reviewing this process, you decide what steps are essential, who should perform them, and how they can be implemented more efficiently and effectively. During this process, you discover your staff repeated many steps without reason, or perhaps you uncover omissions in other departments that prevented your agency from reaching the best outcome. While working on this problem, you decide to investigate how other healthcare organizations excel in the process, referred to as *benchmarking* (Shi & Singh, 2015). This information is used to refine the admission procedures at your workplace.

The significance of cost-effective, quality patient care has led to the development and implementation of patient-centered and outcome-based tools, such as critical pathways and clinical practice guidelines (Shi & Singh, 2015). These items, developed with input from nurses, are useful in guiding practice and reaching clinical outcomes within prescribed time frames. Innovative patient care delivery models, such as case management, evolved and emphasized meeting patient outcomes within specific time parameters (Shi & Singh, 2015).

Reimbursement for patient care services is negatively affected if a hospital does not adhere to national quality performance standards. Since 2008, CMS has stopped reimbursing to hospitals that experience preventable hospital-acquired conditions (e.g., stage III and IV pressure ulcers, falls and trauma, blood incompatibility) (CMS, 2014a). CMS also includes patient situations referred to as *never events*, such as surgery conducted on the wrong body part, an infant discharged to the wrong individual, and death or disability associated with a medication error (CMS, 2014b).

In an effort to gain national recognition for nursing excellence, some healthcare organizations have sought status in the American Nurses Credentialing Center (ANCC) Magnet Recognition Program®. This program, developed in 1994, is based on national standards of nursing practice and quality indicators and recognizes healthcare organizations that support professional nursing practice in their settings and offer excellent nursing care (ANCC, 2014).

Advancing Information Technology

Hospitals are expected to advance IT initiatives that affect healthcare providers, consumers, and others who engage in healthcare delivery services. To support and expedite this goal, hospitals receive financial incentives to facilitate the adoption of electronic health records (EHRs) within their organizations (Shi & Singh, 2015). These enticements were enabled under the Health Information Technology for Economic and Clinical Health Act in 2009.

In addition to implementing EHRs, Medicare and Medicaid also offer incentives if hospitals demonstrate meaningful use of health IT (Centers for Disease Control and Prevention [CDC], 2012), particularly in quality, safety, efficiency, reduction of health disparities, patient engagement, care coordination, and security of health information (Halamka, 2010; Shi & Singh, 2015). Healthcare organizations are penalized financially if they do not comply with meaningful use expectations (DesRoches, Worzala, & Bates, 2013).

Such IT advances are expected to facilitate daily operations of healthcare organizations and foster information sharing among hospitals for continuity of patient care. Consumer portals offer patients the opportunity to communicate with their clinicians, access health resources and information, and review results of tests and procedures. These advances enable consumers to be active participants in their own care (Shi & Singh, 2015). Further IT advances are still needed, such as comprehensive applications used by providers to manage patient healthcare needs (Conn, 2013).

The use of health-related technology by healthcare providers and consumers has been steadily increasing, as devices and applications used by both groups are becoming increasingly similar (Conn, 2013). Some consumers access their healthcare information from electronic sources, such as the Internet, social media, mobile applications, and patient or survivor portals.

Although healthcare organizations have developed patient portals in response to the meaningful use of health IT, Whitehurst (2014) advised that these organizations rethink their approach and create a comprehensive communication plan to engage patients and consider patient preferences. He offered several suggestions to providers as they revise their technology plan: assess the current state of patient communication, identify the communication needs of specific populations, respect patient preferences, experiment with different methods and tools, be flexible and aware of new technology, and strategically consider the message.

Justice (2014) described several technological sources that chronic cancer survivors can access to stay informed about their healthcare needs and any evolving treatment options. These resources include disease-specific websites, such as the National Cancer Institute (www.cancer.gov); Facebook groups that focus on issues such as myeloproliferative neoplasms; and patient opinion leaders sponsored on social media channels. Justice (2014) also emphasized the value of social media in empowering patients with cancer in managing and understanding their chronic cancer care needs.

Researchers have investigated the influence of technology use on patient outcomes. Gnagnarella et al. (2015) conducted a randomized six-month intervention with social media that aimed to increase the knowledge of healthy eating habits among cancer survivors. Although knowledge levels increased in both the treatment and control groups with no statistically significant differences, studies such as this provide researchers with insight into designing intervention studies to measure patient outcomes related to technology.

Given the technological advances that provide direct access to consumers, patients may find themselves being recipients of direct-to-consumer advertising from businesses, such as pharmaceutical companies (Pharmaceutical Research and Manufacturers of America [PhRMA], 2013). These businesses promote services or products, such as information on diseases and current treatments, directly to consumers (e.g., print advertisements, television spots or commercials, radio spots or commercials) rather than through traditional advertising avenues (e.g., through communication with healthcare providers). PhRMA (2008) has published guiding principles for companies to follow when implementing direct-to-consumer advertisements about prescription medications.

Responding to Changes in Health Care

NPD has also undergone major changes over the past two decades. It was presented as a clinical practice specialty in 2010 by the American Nurses Association (ANA) and the National Nursing Staff Development Organization (NNSDO, now called the Association for Nursing Professional Development [ANPD]) in their publication *Nursing Professional Development: Scope and Standards of Practice* (ANA & NNSDO, 2010). This document presented a system-based NPDS model with inputs, throughputs, and outputs that reflected a major expansion, with changes in the roles, responsibilities, and clinical practices in what was previously known as nursing staff development (ANA, 1992, 1994, 2000, 2015).

Beginning in the 1990s, the restructuring of hospitals brought changes in the structure and function of NPD departments and nurse educators (Lockhart, 2004). These divisions, previously referred to as nursing staff development departments, nursing education and research departments, or NPD departments, were downsized, restructured, or eliminated. Changes also included the redesign of departmental priorities and the shifting and expanding of educator roles (Lockhart, 2004). Whereas a department's core functions were often retained by nurse educators who remained in NPD departments, other services needed to be decentralized and assigned to other nurses, often clinical RNs who worked on patient care units. Some professional development responsibilities were shifted to other nurses within the organization. As the roles assumed by staff development educators changed, so did those of unit-based nurses, as their responsibilities expanded to include direct patient care activities, management duties, and staff education.

Structures were created to facilitate communication between centralized personnel and unit representatives. Shared governance structures provided this opportunity through education councils. Clinical instructors were available to advise and mentor the nurses. Some unit-based nurses mentored and cross-trained RNs who were relocated to different clinical units. Because of their expertise, many unit-based nurses planned and implemented orientation, in-service programs, and competency testing on their units.

Gantz et al. (2012) advised nurse leaders to develop a more global perspective on health systems and workforce issues to gain insight on the best practices of competency development, quality improvement, and financial constraints.

While gaining a broader perspective of health care, it is important that you understand your professional nursing responsibilities. Especially vital is the leadership role you assume as an NPDS in strategically positioning and preparing your team to accomplish organizational and professional goals. The following sections of this chapter will highlight some strategies to consider as you assume a leadership role within your organization, whether it be as an NPDS or unit-based staff educator. In addition to focusing on leadership skills expected of you in the NPDS role, you may also investigate those skills outlined in specialty nursing organizations, such as the Oncology Nursing Society Leadership Competencies (ONS, 2012). These competencies will be discussed further in Chapter 2.

Take Responsibility for Developing Your Competencies

NPDSs need to assume responsibility for developing personal and professional competencies. Begin by reviewing *Nursing Professional Development: Scope and Standards of Practice* (ANA & NNSDO, 2010) and compare these expected competencies with the duties listed in your job description. Discuss any discrepancies between the two sources with your manager and seek clarification as needed. Network with colleagues in professional organizations related to your role, such as ANPD.

Next, conduct a self-inventory of the knowledge, skills, and attitudes expected in your professional role and determine any new skills that you will need to develop. For example, you may need to strengthen your skills in information and educational technology, EBP, or writing for publication. If you are having issues in educational technology, you are not alone. A survey of more than 1,300 ANPD members revealed that educational technology was underused in practice, citing a need for NPDSs to "assume responsibility for personal competence" (Harper, Durkin, Orthoefer, Powers, & Tassinari, 2014, p. 247) related to technology.

As you conduct your assessment, heed the recommendations made in IOM's *The Future of Nursing: Leading Change, Advancing Health* (IOM, 2010). If appropriate, consider pursuing a PhD or DNP and seeking additional learning activities to develop leadership competencies, manage change, and support staff.

Seek experienced NPDSs who can serve as mentors in your professional development. These mentors may be local or accessed through professional organizations.

Assume a Leadership Role Within Your Organization and Profession

Leadership is among the core competencies of an NPDS and encompasses a variety of behaviors, from serving as a change agent and advocate of NPD offerings to being an ethical decision-maker and problem-solver (ANA & NNSDO, 2010). In fact, leadership comprises the largest portion (24%) of the 2014 test content outline designed for NPD board certification (ANCC, 2013). More specifically, the leadership content focuses on topics such as "organizational principles, concepts, and structures; leadership principles and practice; the workplace environment; professional development; and managing resources" (ANCC, 2013, pp. 2–3). Gaining an understanding of these leadership priorities can help you focus your personal development needs and identify appropriate leadership opportunities within your healthcare organization.

Westphal and McNeil (2014) emphasized the important role that nurses who are engaged in continuing education can play by serving in a boardroom. The authors identified nine competencies essential for nurses to be effective in this setting: open communication, planning, active engagement, collaboration, decision-making skills, financial stewardship, organizational skills, advocacy, and visionary skills.

IOM recommendations can guide you in developing a competent staff of nurses and other healthcare professionals that are able to provide safe and quality patient care, lead change, and advance health in your organization. NPDSs are responsible for creating a learning environment that welcomes innovation and supports lifelong learning and continuing competence. NPDSs need to help nurses understand trends, national expectations, and healthcare changes, which will develop them in new roles that align with the current and future directions of healthcare delivery.

Align Priorities With Evidence-Based Sources

Nursing Professional Development: Scope and Standards of Practice (ANA & NNSDO, 2010) details the responsibilities that NPDSs and unit-based educators are expected to assume in their roles. Understanding the mission and goals of your healthcare organization as they correspond to recent and future healthcare trends can help you develop and prioritize goals for the NPD department and educators in alignment with the organization and various evidence-based sources.

The beginning of this chapter described several sources of evidence that NPDSs can use to address educational priorities. As an NPDS, remember that your ultimate goal is the "acquisition of knowledge, skills, and attitudes that support safety and contribute to the protection of the public and provision of quality care" (ANA & NNSDO, 2010, p. 7). Given this charge, various sources of evidence exist to guide you in determining your educational priorities. Especially valuable are the national regulations and standards for quality care and patient safety previously mentioned in this chapter.

For example, NPDSs can use the Joint Commission's sentinel events and NPSGs (Joint Commission, n.d.-b, n.d.-c) and CMS's preventable hospital-acquired conditions and never events (CMS, 2014a, 2014b) to focus educational activities on helping nurses understand these issues, prevent and report incidents, and gain vital competencies. In addition, these sources can help NPDSs and staff educators in conducting a gap analysis to identify essential continuing education programs and support practice initiatives, such as patient hand-off (change-of-shift) reporting; Situation, Background, Assessment, and Recommendation (SBAR) techniques for communication (Narayan, 2013); the use of rapid response teams; and root cause analysis (Connelly, 2012). Also, the "meaningful use" expectation for hospitals provides the rationale for staff education and learning using information technology such as EHRs and other portals. Finally, IOM (2010) recommendations provide support and future direction (see Figure 1-1) for nursing regarding lifelong learning and continuing competence, leadership development, residency programs, continuing education, and practice at the highest level.

Focus on Cost-Effective Results-Oriented Outcomes

Given these educational priorities, you are expected to provide educational activities that lead to "cost-effective, results-oriented outcomes" (Harper et al., 2014, p. 247). Although it is expected that you deliver the throughputs described in the NPDS practice model (ANA & NNSDO, 2010), it is also important that you "evaluate the benefits in relation to costs when both are expressed in dollar terms" (Shi & Singh, 2015, p. 577). Given the current cost-conscience healthcare environment, limited resources, and multiple work priorities, it is important for NPDSs to calculate the return on investment of their professional development efforts and communicate the value of their department and role (Bjørk, Tørstad, Hansen, & Samdal, 2009).

To manage cost-effective, results-oriented outcomes, you need to be familiar with quality improvement, evidence-based projects, and research (see Chapter 12). It is also important to understand the sources of data within an organization and how to collect, manage, analyze, and interpret these data.

NPDSs and staff educators should be able to disseminate the results of their efforts (ANA & NNSDO, 2010). In addition to producing an executive summary of efforts to a manager or other stakeholders within an organization, it is important to share educational efforts through peer-reviewed journal articles and professional oral presentations and posters. This responsibility may require the development of new writing and presentation skills (see Chapter 9).

Anticipate Future Directions and Opportunities for Improvement

Keeping abreast of trends and issues that affect healthcare systems needs to be a priority for NPDSs and unit-based staff educators. Understanding these changes and their potential influence on an employer can help you anticipate the future directions that the healthcare organization needs to take and help position the NPD department or NPD role to support these new initiatives.

For example, you can identify new opportunities to improve educational processes in providing safe, quality patient care. Understanding changes in the preparation of future nurses can help you anticipate changes in how your NPD department will orient and prepare newly hired nurses. A proactive approach can be taken to anticipate and manage potential barriers or threats. Although anticipating change within a dynamic healthcare environment may pose a challenge, it can offer you time to develop new skills and competencies in your nursing staff. To lead change, it is vital that nurses engage in lifelong learning opportunities.

Although predicting the future of health care is a tremendous challenge, Shi and Singh (2015) identified eight forces of future change: social and demographic, political, economic, technological, informational, ecological, global, and anthro-cultural (Shi & Singh, 2015). While the authors advised healthcare leaders to use these forces to guide their strategic planning efforts (Shi & Singh, 2015), gaining insight into these forces may also offer benefits for NPDSs and staff educators.

Summary

Recent healthcare trends have resulted in the restructuring of healthcare organizations. Major changes have also occurred in the scope and standards of NPD. These alterations have resulted in multiple role adjustments for nurses employed in clinical practice settings, such as professional development and unit-based education. Changes in both organizations and NPD departments have also affected the roles and responsibilities of clinical staff nurses. NPDSs and unit-based clinical nurse educators need to take a proactive approach and assume these responsibilities, acquiring the knowledge, skills, and attitudes needed to function effectively in a vital new role.

Helpful Websites

- Association for Nursing Professional Development: www.anpd.org
- Centers for Disease Control and Prevention—Meaningful Use: www.cdc.gov/ehrmeaningfuluse
- Centers for Medicare and Medicaid Services—Hospital-Acquired Infections: www.cms.gov/Medicare/Medicare-Fee-for-Service-Payment/HospitalAcqCond/Hospital-Acquired_Conditions.html
- Centers for Medicare and Medicaid Services—Never Events: www.cms.gov/SMDL/downloads/SMD073108.pdf
- Joint Commission: www.jointcommission.org
- Quality and Safety Education for Nurses Institute—QSEN Competencies: http://qsen.org/competencies

References

Agency for Healthcare Research and Quality. (n.d.-a). Defining the PCMH. Retrieved from http://pcmh.ahrq.gov/page/defining-pcmh

Agency for Healthcare Research and Quality. (n.d.-b). Welcome to the PCMH resource center. Retrieved from http://pcmh.ahrq.gov

American Association of Colleges of Nursing. (2014a). Nursing faculty shortage. Retrieved from http://www.aacn.nche.edu/media-relations/fact-sheets/nursing-faculty-shortage

American Association of Colleges of Nursing. (2014b). Nursing shortage. Retrieved from http://www.aacn.nche.edu/media-relations/fact-sheets/nursing-shortage

American College of Surgeons Commission on Cancer. (2012). *Cancer program standards 2012: Ensuring patient-centered care* [v.1.2.1, released January 2014]. Retrieved from https://www.facs.org/~/media/files/quality%20programs/cancer/coc/programstandards2012.ashx

American Hospital Association. (2014). Fast facts on US hospitals. Retrieved from http://www.aha.org/research/rc/stat-studies/fast-facts1.shtml

American Hospital Association. (2015). Fast facts on US hospitals. Retrieved from http://www.aha.org/research/rc/stat-studies/fast-facts.shtml

American Nurses Association. (1992). *Roles and responsibilities for nursing continuing education and staff development across all settings.* Washington, DC: Author.

American Nurses Association. (1994). *Standards for nursing professional development: Continuing education and staff development.* Washington, DC: Author.

American Nurses Association. (2000). *Scope and standards of practice for nursing professional development.* Washington, DC: Author.

American Nurses Association. (2015). *Nursing: Scope and standards of practice* (3rd ed.). Silver Spring, MD: Author.

American Nurses Association & National Nursing Staff Development Organization. (2010). *Nursing professional development: Scope and standards of practice.* Silver Spring, MD: American Nurses Association.

American Nurses Credentialing Center. (2013). Nursing professional development [Test content outline]. Retrieved from http://www.nursecredentialing.org/NursingProfessionalDevelopment

American Nurses Credentialing Center. (2014). ANCC Magnet Recognition Program®. Retrieved from http://nursecredentialing.org/Magnet.aspx

Becze, E. (2014, January). IOM report on quality cancer care has implications for oncology nurses. *ONS Connect.* Retrieved from http://connect.ons.org/columns/five-minute-in-service/iom-report-on-quality-cancer-care-has-implications-for-oncology-nurses

Benner, P., Sutphen, M., Leonard, V., & Day, L. (2010). *Educating nurses: A call for radical transformation.* San Francisco, CA: Jossey-Bass.

Berwick, D.M. (2012). A user's manual for the IOM's 'quality chasm' report. *Health Affairs, 21,* 80–90. doi:10.1377/hlthaff.21.3.80

Bjørk, I.T., Tørstad, S., Hansen, B.S., & Samdal, G.B. (2009). Estimating the cost of professional activities in health organizations. *Nursing Economics, 27,* 239–244.

Buerhaus, P.I., Auerbach, D.I., & Staiger, D.O. (2009). The recent surge in nurse employment: Causes and implications. *Health Affairs, 28,* w657–w668. doi:10.1377/hlthaff.28.4.w657

Caudill, S., Lofgren, R., Jennings, D., & Karpf, M. (2011). Commentary: Health care reform and primary care: Training physicians for tomorrow's challenges. *Academic Medicine, 86,* 158–160. doi:10.1097/ACM.0b013e3182045f13

Centers for Disease Control and Prevention. (2012). Meaningful use. Retrieved from http://www.cdc.gov/ehrmeaningfuluse

Centers for Medicare and Medicaid Services. (2014a). Hospital-acquired infections. Retrieved from http://www.cms.gov/Medicare/Medicare-Fee-for-Service-Payment/HospitalAcqCond/Hospital-Acquired_Conditions.html

Centers for Medicare and Medicaid Services. (2014b). Never events. Retrieved from https://www.cms.gov/SMDL/downloads/SMD073108.pdf

Centers for Medicare and Medicaid Services. (2014c). Oncology care model. Retrieved from http://innovation.cms.gov/initiatives/Oncology-Care

Clark, C. (2015, February). CMS announces bundled care payments for oncology. *HealthLeaders Media.* Retrieved from http://www.healthleadersmedia.com/content/QUA-313227/CMS-Announces-Bundled-Care-Payments-for-Oncology

Conn, J. (2013). No longer a novelty, medical apps are increasingly valuable to clinicians and patients. *Modern Healthcare.* Retrieved from http://www.modernhealthcare.com/article/20131214/MAGAZINE/312149983

Connelly, L.M. (2012). Root cause analysis. *MEDSURG Nursing, 21,* 316–317.

DesRoches, C.M., Worzala, C., & Bates, S. (2013). Some hospitals are falling behind in meeting 'meaningful use' criteria and could be vulnerable to penalties in 2015. *Health Affairs, 32,* 1355–1360. doi:10.1377/hlthaff.2013.0469

Ferrell, B., McCabe, M.S., & Levit, L. (2013). The Institute of Medicine report on high-quality cancer care: Implications for oncology nursing. *Oncology Nursing Forum, 40,* 603–609.

Gantz, N.R., Sherman, R., Jasper, M., Choo, C.G., Herrin-Griffith, D., & Harris, K. (2012). Global nurse leader perspectives on health systems and workforce challenges. *Journal of Nursing Management, 20,* 433–443. doi:10.1111/j.1365-2834.2012.01393.x

Gnagnarella, P., Misotti, A.M., Santoro, L., Akoumianakis, D., Del Campo, L., De Lorenzo, F., … McVie, J.G. (2015). Nutritional online information for cancer patients: A randomized trial of an Internet communication plus social media intervention. *Journal of Cancer Education.* Advance online publication. doi:10.1007/s13187-015-0820-5

Gorbunoff, E., & Kummeth, P. (2014). *Nursing professional development review manual* (3rd ed.). Silver Spring, MD: American Nurses Credentialing Center.

Halamka, J.D. (2010). Making the most of federal health information technology regulations. *Health Affairs, 29,* 596–600. doi:10.1377/hlthaff.2010.0232

Harper, M.G., Durkin, G., Orthoefer, D.K., Powers, R., & Tassinari, R.M. (2014). ANPD technology survey: The state of NPD practice. *Journal for Nurses in Professional Development, 30,* 242–247. doi:10.1097/NND.0000000000000106

Institute of Medicine. (1999). *To err is human: Building a safer health system.* Washington, DC: National Academies Press.

Institute of Medicine. (2001). *Crossing the quality chasm: A new health system for the 21st century.* Washington, DC: National Academies Press.

Institute of Medicine. (2003). *Health professions education: A bridge to quality.* Washington, DC: National Academies Press.

Institute of Medicine. (2004). *Keeping patients safe: Transforming the work environment of nurses.* Washington, DC: National Academies Press.

Institute of Medicine. (2010). *The future of nursing: Leading change, advancing health.* Washington, DC: National Academies Press.

Institute of Medicine. (2013a). *Delivering high-quality cancer care: Charting a new course for a system in crisis.* Washington, DC: National Academies Press.

Institute of Medicine. (2013b). *Improving the quality of cancer care: Addressing the challenges of an aging population.* Washington, DC: National Academies Press.

Joint Commission. (n.d.-a). About the Joint Commission. Retrieved from http://www.jointcommission.org/about_us/about_the_joint_commission_main.aspx

Joint Commission. (n.d.-b). National Patient Safety Standards. Retrieved from http://www.jointcommission.org/standards_information/npsgs.aspx

Joint Commission. (n.d.-c). Sentinel event policy and procedures. http://www.jointcommission.org/Sentinel_Event_Policy_and_Procedures

Juraschek, S.P., Zhang, X., Ranganathan, V., & Lin, V.W. (2012). United States registered nurse workforce report card and shortage forecast. *American Journal of Medical Quality, 27*(3), 241–249.

Justice, J. (2014). How chronic cancer patients use social media to stay informed. *Social Media Today.* Retrieved from http://www.socialmediatoday.com/content/how-chronic-cancer-patients-use-social-media-stay-informed

Lockhart, J.S. (2004). *Unit-based staff development for clinical nurses.* Pittsburgh, PA: Oncology Nursing Society.

Narayan, M.C. (2013). Using SBAR communications in efforts to prevent patient rehospitalizations. *Home Healthcare Nurse, 31,* 504–515. doi:10.1097/NHH.0b013e3182a87711

National Committee for Quality Assurance. (n.d.). Patient-Centered Medical Home Recognition. Retrieved from http://www.ncqa.org/Programs/Recognition/Practices/PatientCenteredMedicalHomePCMH.aspx

North Carolina Rural Health Research Program. (2015). Rural hospital closures: January 2010–present. Retrieved from https://www.shepscenter.unc.edu/programs-projects/rural-health/rural-hospital-closures

Oncology Nursing Society. (2012). *Oncology Nursing Society leadership competencies.* Retrieved from https://www.ons.org/sites/default/files/leadershipcomps.pdf

Pharmaceutical Research and Manufacturers of America. (2008). *PhRMA guiding principles: Direct to consumer advertisements about prescription medicines.* Retrieved from http://www.phrma.org/sites/default/files/pdf/phrmaguidingprinciplesdec08final.pdf

Pharmaceutical Research and Manufacturers of America. (2013). Direct to consumer pharmaceutical advertising. Retrieved from http://www.phrma.org/direct-to-consumer-advertising

Quality and Safety Education for Nurses Institute. (2012). About. Retrieved from http://qsen.org/about-qsen/V

Quality and Safety Education for Nurses Institute. (2014). QSEN competencies. Retrieved from http://qsen.org/competencies

Robert Wood Johnson Foundation. (n.d.). Robert Wood Johnson Foundation New Careers in Nursing. Retrieved from http://www.newcareersinnursing.org

Shi, L., & Singh, D.A. (2015). *Delivering health care in America: A systems approach* (6th ed.). Burlington, MA: Jones & Bartlett Learning.

U.S. Census Bureau. (2014). State and county quickfacts. Retrieved from http://quickfacts.census.gov/qfd/states/00000.html

U.S. Department of Health and Human Services. (2003). Trends in urban hospital closure 1990–2000. Retrieved from http://oig.hhs.gov/oei/reports/oei-04-02-00611.pdf

U.S. Department of Health and Human Services. (2013a). *Health, United States, 2012 with special feature on emergency care.* Hyattsville, MD: Author.

U.S. Department of Health and Human Services. (2013b). *The US nursing workforce: Trends in supply and education.* Retrieved from http://bhpr.hrsa.gov/healthworkforce/reports/nursingworkforce/nursingworkforcefullreport.pdf

U.S. Department of Health and Human Services. (2014). About the law. Retrieved from http://www.hhs.gov/healthcare/rights/index.html

U.S. Department of Health and Human Services. (2015). The Affordable Care Act. Retrieved from http://www.hhs.gov/healthcare/rights/law/index.html

Westphal, J., & McNeil, P. (2014). Learn to lead in the boardroom. *Journal of Continuing Education in Nursing, 45,* 162–168. doi:10.3928/00220124-20140305-01

Whitehurst, S. (2014). Looking beyond patient portals to engage patients. *Healthcare IT News.* Retrieved from http://www.healthcareitnews.com/blog/looking-beyond-patient-portals-engage-patients

CHAPTER 2

Understanding the Specialty Practice of Nursing Professional Development

C HAPTER 1 described the influence of recent social, political, economic, and legislative changes on both the structure and function of healthcare organizations. It also described how these movements affected the roles and responsibilities of many clinical nurses who, in addition to providing direct patient care, were expected to assist with some of the educational activities previously assumed by NPDSs.

Clinical nurses who assume leadership roles in education may be designated as *unit-based educators*. As a unit-based educator, you will need to develop the knowledge, skills, and attitudes essential to this role, including a thorough understanding of what is involved in developing professional nurses and other healthcare workers. You also must be aware of nursing and healthcare trends, the goals and expectations of your employer, and the roles and responsibilities shifted to you at the unit level.

You will need to know who you are teaching, their particular learning styles and educational needs, and how to meet those needs. For example, helping graduate nurses learn clinical skills may differ from how you might assist experienced RNs or assistive personnel in learning new tasks. You will need to evaluate if your educational activities made a difference in their competencies and revise your teaching strategies accordingly. You must realize when and how learning activities can be accomplished, particularly within a unit-based perspective. This involves using active and creative teaching strategies, self-directed learning activities, flexible programming, and an understanding of the people you teach. This chapter will provide an overview of NPD, describe its standards and model, elaborate on key educational processes contained in the model, and discuss the roles and responsibilities of the NPDS.

Understanding the Professional Development of Nurses

Clinical nurses employed in practice settings must constantly maintain or improve their competencies as direct caregivers. The American Nurses Association (ANA), the organization that establishes standards of practice and professional performance for nurses, views the professional development of nurses as a "lifelong process of active participation by nurses in learning activities to assist in developing and maintaining their continuing competence, enhance their professional practice, and support achievement of career goals" (ANA, 2000, p. 1).

The primary responsibility of the individual nurse is to maintain professional competence through continuing education and lifelong learning (ANA, 2015). However, multiple stakeholders in both service and educational settings are needed to support this goal: licensing bodies and credentialing boards; educational accrediting bodies; administration, faculty, and librarians in academic settings; providers of continuing education programs; specialty and professional organizations; healthcare accreditation systems, hospitals and health systems; and state and federal governments (American Association of Colleges of Nursing [AACN] & Association of American Medical Colleges [AAMC], 2010).

To better understand the NPD process, start by envisioning the profession's big picture. Think about your responsibility to contribute to and develop the nursing profession during your career. Remember that the primary outcome of NPD is safe, quality patient care.

Next, think about being hired in a particular position within a healthcare organization. You have a job description that outlines the behaviors you are expected to perform.

Although these two perspectives appear to be separate entities, the second case is actually part of the big picture. Your daily duties have the potential to make a difference for your patients, other nurses at your workplace, and the profession in general.

Both perspectives involve assuming certain roles and responsibilities. Career landmarks, such as graduating from a nursing program and successfully passing your nursing licensure examination, indicate that you possess the minimum degree of competency as an RN. To maintain and improve your performance and competence, you must continue to participate in learning activities.

As each component of the NPD model is presented, try to remember some of the educational experiences you have had since graduation. Recall your experiences when initially hired. Reflect upon your observations in the clinical setting as a student nurse and try to remember what kind of educational offerings were available to you and the nursing staff in the patient units. Recalling these experiences will help you make sense of the NPD process and gain a holistic perspective of the organization.

Nursing Professional Development as a Practice Specialty

Major changes have occurred in NPD since ANA published its *Scope and Standards of Practice for Nursing Professional Development* in 2000. This document conceptualized NPD as a framework comprising three interrelated educational domains: staff development, continuing education, and academic education (ANA, 2000). Fundamental to this model was the professional development of nurses through continuing competence and lifelong learning with the goal of quality patient care (ANA, 2000).

A decade later, a new and expanded NPD model was published by ANA and the National Nursing Staff Development Organization (NNSDO) titled *Nursing Professional Development: Scope and Standards of Practice* (ANA & NNSDO, 2010). NNSDO changed its name to the Association for Nursing Professional Development (ANPD) shortly after publication to align with changes in NPD and to support the NPDS role (ANPD, n.d.). It is essential that you obtain and carefully read a copy of this publication.

Figure 2-1 employs a systems approach with inputs, throughputs, outputs, and a feedback loop to convey the practice (ANA & NNSDO, 2010). Although designed for the NPD practice specialty, this framework can help all nurses, regardless of specialty, to better understand the abundant opportunities available for professional development.

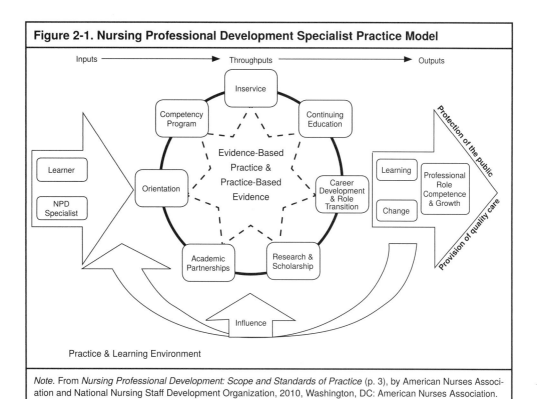

Figure 2-1. Nursing Professional Development Specialist Practice Model

Inputs

Inputs include the NPDS and the learner (ANA & NNSDO, 2010). The NPDS is described as a "registered nurse with expertise in nursing education who influences professional role competencies and professional growth of nurses in a variety of settings" (ANA & NNSDO, 2010, p. 4). The learner is an individual or a group of individuals who engage in the various educational activities within the model to address their learning needs (ANA & NNSDO, 2010).

Within this model, the NPDS and learner have their own environments with boundaries that may overlap during professional development events and are "fluid and evolving" (ANA & NNSDO, 2010, p. 4). While the NPDS's practice environment is defined as the "structural, social, and cultural setting in which nursing occurs," (ANA & NNSDO, 2010, p. 5) the learner's environment is "anywhere learning occurs" (ANA & NNSDO, 2010, p. 5). Therefore, the learner's environment can be anything from virtual learning milieu (e.g., online, social media) to traditional settings, such as the clinical unit, simulation laboratory, or classroom (ANA & NNSDO, 2010).

Throughputs

The NPDS is responsible for promoting eight *throughputs*, or educational processes central to the professional development of nurses: orientation, competency programs, in-service education, continuing education, career development and role transition, research and scholarship, academic partnerships, and evidence-based practice and practice-based evidence (see Figure 2-1) (ANA & NNSDO, 2010). The NPDS's role in each of these activities may vary based on position description and employer expectations. While most throughputs are new or have been expanded, three (orientation, in-service education, and continuing education) continue to exist from the 2000 framework (ANA, 2000).

Orientation

Orientation is the educational process of introducing newly hired nurses or other employees to information they need to function in their assigned roles and carry out their responsibilities (ANA & NNSDO, 2010). Materials included during an employee's orientation are the "philosophy, goals, policies, role expectations, and other factors necessary to function in a specific work setting" (ANA, 2000, p. 6). Orientation is usually implemented by the employer (ANA, 2000).

Nurses participate in an orientation program when they are first hired. They may receive another orientation when their assigned roles, responsibilities, or practice settings change (ANA, 2000). For example, RNs reassigned following organizational restructuring need to be cross-trained to perform competently in their new positions and practice environment. These nurses may engage in a second orientation program, often conducted on the clinical unit, to help them learn how to provide safe, quality nursing care in this new setting. Orientation also is needed when nurses assume a new position that is very different from their previous one. For example, a nurse who shifts roles from a clinical staff nurse on an inpatient unit to a coordinator role in an ambulatory care clinic would benefit from participating in an orientation program.

Orientations help nurses socialize in the organization (ANA, 2000), assisting them in understanding the culture of the organization and becoming a valued member (ANA, 2000). Nurses can focus career planning efforts toward developing these skills.

Orientation programs vary in length, content, and approach. Some organizations sponsor housewide orientation sessions, which are open to all new employees, followed by a special program dedicated to nurses. After attending these general orientation sessions, nurses usually participate in unit-based learning activities aimed at helping them understand expected behaviors related to direct patient care. Orientations (see Chapter 4) that occur in the unit-based setting often are guided by an experienced nurse who serves as a preceptor (see Chapter 5) or mentor to a new nurse, referred to as an *orientee*.

Competency Programs

During the orientation process, it is important for the NPDS to assess and evaluate the performances of new nursing employees through a *competency program* (ANA & NNSDO, 2010). ANA defines *competency* as the "expected level of performance that integrates knowledge, skills, abilities, and judgment" (ANA, 2015, p. 44). Therefore, a competency program refers to an organized testing plan to assess, validate, and develop a nurse's performance level (ANA & NNSDO, 2010). It is often initiated at orientation and repeated at regular, predetermined intervals during the nurse's employment.

According to ANA's position statement on professional role competence, employers are "responsible and accountable to provide an environment conducive to competent practice" (ANA, 2014, para. 1). However, ensuring the competency of nurses and other healthcare workers is also the "shared responsibility of the profession, individual nurses, professional organizations, credentialing and certification entities, regulatory agencies, employers, and other key stakeholders" (ANA, 2014, para. 1).

In-Service Education

In-service education consists of "learning experiences provided in the work setting for the purpose of assisting staff members in performing their assigned functions in that particular agency or institution" (ANA, 2000, p. 24). Similar to orientation, in-service offerings usually are sponsored by employers to help nurses perform according to position descriptions and to "acquire, maintain, or increase their competence" in their environments (ANA, 2000, p. 6). In-service education is warranted not only for nurses who hold current positions, but also for those who have experienced changes in roles and responsibilities.

Although orientation programs may last a few days or even several weeks, in-service programs are usually brief, 15–30-minute sessions. In-service topics are often mandated by the institution or required by external accreditation and regulatory agencies. Regardless of the source, these programs should be based on a thorough assessment that reflects the input and learning needs of staff.

In-service offerings can be presented in a variety of ways depending on organizational preference (see Chapter 6). For instance, some agencies schedule in-service sessions in centralized locations so that all interested staff can attend. Other workplaces integrate in-service offerings into their daily schedules on a unit-based level. It is important that organizations consider active teaching strategies that permit nurses to learn in a self-paced, independent fashion, such as posters, computer-based exercises and simulations, Internet-based programs, programmed instruction modules, and video and audio recordings.

Continuing Education

ANA (2000) defines *continuing education* as the "systematic professional learning experiences designed to augment the knowledge, skills, and attitudes of nurses" (p. 83). Engaging in continuing education activities is intended to influence patient care outcomes and the nurse's professional career plans (ANA, 2000). Unlike orientation and in-service education, which aim at a specific role within a designated healthcare organization, nurses can apply material learned from continuing education to any practice setting or to career needs (ANA & NNSDO, 2010). Many states require nurses to obtain a defined number of contact hours for relicensure.

Nurses can access continuing education activities (see Chapter 13) through a variety of organizations and engage in these activities using a plethora of teaching-learning strategies. The American Nurses Credentialing Center (ANCC) categorizes continuing education activities as being either provider directed, learner directed, or learner paced (ANCC, 2012).

Career Development and Role Transition

In career development and role transition, the NPDS mentors nurses as they develop their career goals, manage their career plans (see Chapter 14), and transition to new roles with different responsibilities. In some instances, the NPDS may be involved in facilitating the organization's succession plan.

Research and Scholarship

The NPDS's participation in research (see Chapter 12) and scholarship activities may vary depending on the specialist's workplace, position description, and level of expertise. Research activities may eventually lead to preparing manuscripts for publication in peer-reviewed nursing journals (see Chapter 8). Scholarship activities may include sharing the staff's practice, research, and service accomplishments through oral or poster presentations or publications (see Chapter 9).

Academic Partnerships

In academic partnerships, NPDSs often serve as liaisons between a hospital and a school of nursing. They may facilitate student orientation and clinical placements, acquire preceptors, collaborate with faculty on various joint initiatives, and share their expertise in a classroom setting. Academic partnerships are intended to be mutually beneficial relationships aimed to support professional development and continuing, lifelong learning (ANA & NNSDO, 2010).

Evidence-Based Practice and Practice-Based Evidence

NPDSs play an integral role in fostering evidence-based practice (EBP) and practice-based evidence (PBE) (ANA & NNSDO, 2010). In fact, these last components are core to the NPD model (ANA & NNSDO, 2010).

According to Melnyk, Fineout-Overholt, Stillwell, and Williamson (2010), *EBP* is a "problem-solving approach to the delivery of health care that integrates the best evidence from studies and patient care data with clinician expertise and patient preferences and values" (p. 51). The ultimate goal of EBP is quality patient care and outcomes.

PBE can be viewed as a "study methodology related more directly to practice effectiveness and improvement that promotes a greater understanding of individual and group differences" (ANA & NNSDO, 2010, p. 45). Evans, Connell, Barkham, Marshall, and Mellor-Clark (2003) described the close association between EBP and PBE as being complementary, with PBE acting as a "bridge for the gap between research and practice" (p. 375) by overcoming some of the limitations associated with EBP. NPDSs engage in EBP and PBE not only in teaching and learning in their specialty practice, but also in the clinical practice specialties of the nurses that they mentor (see Chapter 12).

Outputs, Outcomes, and the Feedback Loop

The primary outcome of the NPDS practice model is the nurse's attainment of appropriate knowledge, skills, and attitudes that will "support safety and contribute to the protection of the public and provision of quality care" (ANA & NNSDO, 2010, p. 7). System outputs related to change, learning, competence, and growth enable this goal to be realized through the help of NPDSs. The model also includes a feedback loop that denotes the "continuous lifelong learning and growth that impacts both professional nursing practice and the professional development of nurses throughout their careers" (p. 8). Through their role, NPDSs can influence "change, behaviors, and the decisions of others" (p. 8).

Clarifying the Roles and Responsibilities of the Nursing Professional Development Specialist

In the current scope and standards, ANA and NNSDO (2010) describe the role of the NPDS as a "registered nurse with expertise in nursing education" (p. 44). NPDSs influence role competence and growth, support lifelong learning of healthcare personnel, and promote an appropriate learning climate (ANA & NNSDO, 2010).

In actual practice, the titles of nurse educators often differ depending on their healthcare organizations. They may be called a nurse educator, clinical educator, professional development specialist, education specialist, education and development specialist, or education clinical specialist. Dorin (2010) described the title of a "staff development specialist" and segmented this role into hospital-based staff development specialists and unit-based specialists. While hospital-based educators provide education to learners, such as hospital employees, unit-based educators serve as unit stabilizers, focusing their teaching efforts to a specific clinical unit. Regardless of title, it is important for you to understand the roles and responsibilities of NPDSs at national and organizational levels.

Responsibility and Accountability

NPDSs have a defined scope of responsibility and accountability in their roles (ANA & NNSDO, 2010):
• Career development
• Education
• Leadership
• Program management
• Compliance initiatives.

Responsibilities may vary depending on the specialist's work setting and position description. Each of these five responsibilities contains several specific activities for clarification. For example, within the "education" responsibility, the specialist may be engaged in continuing education, competency testing, and orientation.

Qualifications and Core Competencies

Currently, ANA and NNSDO (2010) recommend that NPDSs be educated at the graduate level. If nurses have a graduate degree in another related field, then their undergraduate degree must be in nursing. NPDSs should understand adult learning principles and play an active role in their own professional development by participating in continuing education activities, formal academic learning, and certification in professional nursing development or other practice specialties. The executive leader for NPD also needs to be an RN prepared at the doctoral level in nursing or education.

The core competencies of NPDSs include four major areas: career development, education, leadership, and program and project management (Brunt, 2007). Similar to the specialist's responsibilities, each of these competencies contains several measurable behaviors that can be used in the NPDS's annual performance review process. For example, under "education," the specialist may "evaluate the outcomes of staff education or demonstrate proficiency in use of technology" (ANA & NNSDO, 2010, p. 14).

Brunt (2014) recently published an NPD competency tool. Framed using Benner's (1984) novice-to-expert model, this tool can be used by NPDSs to not only assess and validate their competencies but also to help them apply these competencies to daily practice within their healthcare settings (Brunt, 2014).

NPDSs need to obtain additional educational expertise to add to their existing clinical competencies. Formal learning opportunities, such as graduate programs framed in nursing education, are available through academic degree-granting institutions (e.g., schools of nursing). Expertise can also be nurtured and updated through informal avenues, such as continuing education programs offered by professional nursing organizations, experiential learning activities guided by mentors in the workplace, and independent study offerings (e.g., texts, journals, media sources).

Nursing education content recommended by ANA and NNSDO (2010) includes teaching-learning theories, curriculum design, methods for validating learning, research processes, and innovative technology.

Elements of Practice

In its 2000 standards, ANA identified six roles in which staff development educators function: educator, facilitator, change agent, consultant, researcher, and leader. While the latest standards state that these elements still exist as part of the NPDS's role, the difference now is that these elements are intertwined and not separated as they were in the previous model. Figure 2-2 outlines this interconnectedness. Swihart and Johnstone (2010) also emphasized the value of the mentor role for NPDSs who guide newly hired nurses during orientation and throughout their professional careers.

The six elements demand different skill sets from staff educators (ANA, 2000). To function effectively within each of these roles, NPDSs must develop the knowledge, skills, and attitudes required by this specialty.

Educator

An obvious role assumed by NPDSs is that of an educator, especially related to the through-puts of orientation, in-service education, and continuing education (ANA, 2000). This role includes overseeing the entire educational process, from conducting needs assessments to planning, implementing, and evaluating offerings. It is expected that NPDSs understand curriculum design, active teaching-learning strategies, testing and measurement issues, education research, and technology in order to function effectively in this role (ANA, 2000). As educators, nurses need to create an atmosphere conducive to staff learning and incorporate adult learning principles in their offerings (see Chapter 3) (ANA, 2000).

NPDSs can fulfill their educator role in various ways. They can serve as direct providers of learning activities by developing and presenting programs (e.g., a presentation on how to detect abnormal breath sounds in clients with chronic obstructive lung disease). They can implement their roles with nurses in a variety of environments, such as in a classroom or unit conference room, at a patient's bedside, in a client's home, or in an office setting in an ambulatory care clinic. Educators can also use self-directed strategies in their teachings, such as web-based instruction or distance learning, that will provide learners with flexibility and independence.

NPDSs can also contact experts on a chosen topic to fulfill the educator role. For instance, NPDSs may ask a nurse in an IV therapy department to present an in-service offering on changing central venous catheter dressings on patients. In addition to providing staff with an educational offering, the presenter also learns more about the educator role.

Figure 2-2. Elements of Practice for the Nursing Professional Development Specialist

• Educator/facilitator	• Researcher/consultant
• Educator/academic liaison	• Leader/communicator
• Change agent/team member	• Collaborator/adviser/mentor

Note. Based on information from American Nurses Association and National Nursing Staff Development Organization, 2010.

From "Lifelong Learning and Continuing Competence" (p. 409), by J.S. Lockhart and M.M. Gullatte in M.M. Gullatte (Ed.), *Nursing Management: Principles and Practice* (2nd ed.), 2011, Pittsburgh, PA: Oncology Nursing Society. Copyright 2011 by Oncology Nursing Society. Reprinted with permission.

NPDSs can often demonstrate the educator role through informal methods. During their daily interactions with staff, patients, and families on the unit, educators frequently model positive professional behaviors that nurses can imitate.

Clinical instructors can also help other nurses within the organization learn to teach other staff, patients, and families. For example, NPDSs can help staff nurses learn how to present unit-based in-service offerings or participate in orientation and continuing education programs. Nurses can learn to develop a unit-based education plan based on a thorough needs assessment, implement the plan, and evaluate the plan's effectiveness on patient outcomes.

Facilitator

Staff development educators also serve as facilitators within their organizations (ANA, 2000) and traditionally within the context of the teaching-learning process. Facilitators can guide staff to play an active role in identifying and meeting learning needs based on organizational and professional goals. Facilitators also are expected to promote team building among learners within the organization. The current scope and standards have integrated the facilitator role throughout the multiple scope of responsibilities for the NPDS, particularly that of the educator (ANA & NNSDO, 2010). Dickerson (2014) echoed the importance of the facilitator role of the NPDS in guiding the "professional development of learners and the improvement in the quality of care" (p. 289).

Change Agent

Staff development educators are expected to be change agents, a role that includes identifying changes within the organization, helping to implement changes, and supporting clinical staff as they adjust to these changes (ANA, 2000). This role is essential when considering healthcare trends over recent years. For example, NPDSs can help nurses learn new clinical skills after a unit merger or can manage a multipatient assignment during a nursing shortage.

In addition to implementing changes within the organization, staff development educators also are expected to serve as change agents through professional development activities in the local community or on regional, national, or international levels (ANA, 2000).

Consultant

Consultants informally assist individuals to grow as professionals within the organization through activities that can be integrated into daily interactions with individual staff or shared with groups in scheduled educational offerings. Some endeavors include helping nurses learn how to publish in professional journals, developing oral or poster presentations for a conference, and applying research findings on the clinical unit. NPDSs are instrumental in developing staff as unit-based educators, preceptors, and mentors for other nurses. They are expected to be accessible resources for nurses who wish to advance within their workplace and careers.

NPDSs can serve as consultants on a more formal basis by providing professional or expert advice. Although the consultant role can be enacted within the workplace, it often is shared with community and professional organizations (see Chapter 7). For example, a nurse with expertise in NPD might serve as a consultant to another healthcare agency in developing a clinical competency program for nurses or by replicating a successful unit-based clinical research program.

Researcher

Professional development educators function within the role of researcher (see Chapter 12) (ANA, 2000). The role of researcher in staff development is broad and applies to the development of the educator and clinical staff nurses. Depending on work expectations, NPDSs may conduct or assist with research related to their role in education and practice, apply their findings, and evaluate the outcomes (ANA & NNSDO, 2010).

NPDSs may also assist clinical nurses as they both participate in the research process, apply findings to patient care, and share the results of unit-based research efforts through standards, policies, publications, and presentations. NPDSs can foster research participation by providing staff with needs-based educational offerings. An example of this is a unit-based journal club in which staff meet and discuss the findings of research articles on a chosen clinical topic. Educators also can help staff incorporate relevant research findings into practice standards on the clinical unit.

The instructor can coordinate liaisons between staff and research faculty from academic partnerships with schools of nursing, allowing nurses to participate in hands-on research under an experienced mentor. Educators can also encourage staff participation in research by guiding them as they analyze a problem or incident. The educators can model this process within their own departments or on clinical units.

Other methods of supporting research include networking at professional nursing meetings, developing and reading research-based publications, and sharing research projects with the nursing community through oral presentations and posters.

Leader

NPDSs assume a leadership role in their own professional development, including active participation within the organization and in professional nursing and community groups. Within this role, educators coordinate educational experiences and learning activities of nursing staff. For instance, they may organize continuing education programs for the agency and professional community or orchestrate an educational plan for specialty patient units. Professional development educators also design the schedule and content of orientation and competency programs.

NPDSs also participate in various administrative functions associated with either directing a department or being a member of a department, including organizing and preparing documentation related to educational offerings, evaluating staff within the department, and developing and managing departmental resources (human and fiscal) (ANA, 2000). Educators play an important role in seeking outside funding sources, such as education and research grants, to support programs offered by the department. They assume a leadership role in coordinating the clinical placement of nursing students with faculty from affiliated schools of nursing and managing student internship programs.

In addition to the leadership skills outlined by ANA and NNSDO (2010), also consider the competencies emphasized in relevant specialty nursing organizations, such as the Oncology Nursing Society (ONS). ONS leadership competencies cover five domains: personal mastery, vision, knowledge, interpersonal effectiveness, and systems thinking (ONS, 2012). For each competency, oncology nurse leaders may transition among levels of individual, group, or governance. Therefore, an oncology nurse may demonstrate the leadership competency of "lifelong learning" that is housed within the personal mastery domain through individual, group, or governance levels (ONS, 2012).

Supporting the Professional Development of Nurses

Why should healthcare organizations be concerned with the professional development of their nurses and other healthcare workers? Why should they sponsor various professional development and continuing education offerings? Although several sources, such as professional nursing organizations and accreditation agencies, support the need for staff development, it is important to remember that the ultimate goal of NPD is "to support the provision of quality health care within local or global practice environments" (ANA & NNSDO, 2010, p. 9).

Standards of Practice and Professional Performance

ANA serves as the national professional organization for nurses and represents and guides them on a variety of professional nursing and healthcare issues (ANA, 2015). One of ANA's primary functions is to develop scope and standards for professional nursing practice, such as in *Nursing: Scope and Standards of Practice* (ANA, 2015). This document outlines specific examples that describe the "competent level of nursing practice" (p. 15) and "competent level of behavior" (p. 15) expected by professional nurses (ANA, 2015).

As mentioned throughout this chapter, ANA and NNSDO (2010) developed similar standards of practice for NPDSs in *Nursing Professional Development: Scope and Standards*. These standards can serve as valuable resources to develop nurses who are experienced or new to the NPDS role, evaluate their performance within an organization, and prepare them to attain national certification in their specialties (Dickerson, 2014).

To keep pace with current standards and anticipate future needs, nursing standards are constantly being reviewed and revised. Therefore, it is important to stay alert for ongoing revisions and provide feedback when requested. At the time of this writing, ANPD is revising its scope and standards with a publication date anticipated in summer 2016. More information is available at www.anpd.org.

Healthcare organizations that align professional development programs on these standards and criteria maximize their potential success in providing educational offerings tailored to meet specific learning needs. This approach supports positive patient outcomes.

Accreditation of Healthcare Organizations

Similar to schools of nursing, healthcare organizations request review by nonprofit accrediting organizations. Using preestablished standards and criteria related to quality health care, the Joint Commission accredits and certifies U.S. healthcare organizations (Joint Commission, 2014a). The mission of the Joint Commission is "to continuously improve health care for the public, in collaboration with other stakeholders, by evaluating healthcare organizations and inspiring them to excel in providing safe and effective care of the highest quality and value" (Joint Commission, 2014a, para. 1).

To improve patient safety within healthcare organizations, the Joint Commission created the National Patient Safety Goals in 2002 (Joint Commission, 2014b). These continually updated goals target select safety problems in healthcare organizations and provide guidelines to help remedy them. Problem areas noted in these safety goals include accurate patient identification, communication among caregivers, medication safety, and healthcare-related infections (Joint Commission, 2014b).

Because final evaluation results are made readily available to consumers through the Joint Commission website, healthcare organizations that attain a quality rating benefit from standards being made public. A positive evaluation sends a message that the institution strives for excellence in patient care and values consumers.

NPDSs play an important role in ensuring that performance standards are met through the professional development of nurses and other hospital staff. When delivering these educational activities, it is important to track sources of evidence regarding the influence of these offerings on staff performance and patient outcomes.

Recognition of Nursing Practice

Healthcare facilities strive to attain recognition through the ANCC Magnet Recognition Program®. Magnet designation focuses on "quality patient care, nursing excellence, and innovations in nursing practice" (ANCC, n.d.-a, para. 1). As of October 7, 2014, nearly 400 facilities worldwide have received Magnet designation (ANCC, n.d.-c).

According to ANCC, Magnet designation offers a plethora of gains to healthcare organizations, including the ability to attract and retain top talent; improve care, safety, and satisfaction; foster a collaborative culture; advance nursing standards and practice; and grow their business and financial status (ANCC, n.d.-b).

The ANCC Magnet Recognition Program model guides applicants seeking recognition and has five key components: transformational leadership; structural empowerment; exemplary professional practice; new knowledge, innovations, and improvement; and empirical outcomes (ANCC, n.d.-e). Within these components are 14 Forces of Magnetism, or characteristics, that illustrate excellence in nursing practice (ANCC, n.d.-d).

While NPDSs can play a vital role in all of these forces, two appear to relate directly to the current practice model—Force 11: Nurses as Teachers and Force 14: Professional Development (ANA & NNSDO, 2010). These two forces address throughputs, such as academic partnerships, orientation, in-service education, career development, competency programs, preceptors, and mentoring.

Goals of Healthcare Organizations

Healthcare organizations are trying to survive in the current market, constantly competing against other agencies for patients. Faced with this challenge, healthcare organizations have developed goals that focus on providing quality patient care services and attaining positive patient outcomes. Professional development is one way nurses can meet this challenge and reach quality care goals. Education also has the potential to serve as a recruitment and retention strategy for organizations and is often used as a marketing feature.

Consumer Rights to Quality Care

Consumers have a right to receive quality care when they enter a healthcare institution. They deserve to be cared for by nurses and other healthcare professionals who are knowledgeable in their practice, exhibit competent clinical skills, and demonstrate professional behaviors and a caring concern. Providing nurses opportunities for professional development is an essential step in accomplishing this outcome.

Targeting Learners

NPDSs may be involved in orientations, in-service educational offerings, and continuing education programs designed not only for nursing staff but also for individuals who do not provide patient care services. It is important for NPDSs to know their learners. For instance, educators employed in some healthcare organizations are responsible for developing programs that are open to hospital-wide employees, patients, and individuals and groups in the community. This aspect of the NPDS role has important implications for how educators assess, plan, implement, and evaluate educational offerings. Because learners often include healthcare workers, such as clinical nurses and assistive personnel, academic faculty and students, and patients, the needs of these groups will be discussed.

Unit-Based Clinical Staff

Professional development offerings of orientation, in-service education, competency programs, and continuing education may also be extended to assistive personnel or other workers so that they may develop the knowledge, skills, and attitudes needed to provide quality patient care. The educator's responsibility also may extend to training and developing unit secretaries, receptionists, volunteers, and foreign-educated nurses.

Academic Partners: Nursing Students and Faculty

As mentioned earlier, NPDSs are often responsible for coordinating unit placements for nursing students seeking clinical experience. Students may be accompanied to the site by their clinical instructor or require placement with a staff nurse who serves as a preceptor. Just as with new employees, these individuals must be oriented to the organization and clinical unit, informed of clinical policies and procedures, and updated on documentation systems and guidelines. NPDSs also validate the clinical knowledge and skills of faculty through competency testing. Educators need to understand the course objectives and allow students to reach goals with proper clinical placement. All of these measures help to maintain quality patient care.

Assessing When Staff Development Is Needed

In most healthcare organizations, nurses provide patient care 24 hours a day. However, NPDSs are only directly available to nursing staff for, at most, 8–12 hours a day.

Although orientation, in-service educational offerings, and continuing education programs are intended to provide nurses with the knowledge and skills needed to deliver competent care, sometimes nurses encounter unfamiliar patient care situations. These circumstances offer nurses little or no advance notice and deny them the option to delay interventions and wait for guidance from an instructor. It is important for NPDSs to anticipate these critical situations and take a proactive approach.

How can you accommodate meeting the multiple and constant learning needs of the staff? The options that follow, such as determining peak times, setting priorities, ensuring coverage, and providing mentoring, can offer some practical suggestions.

Determine Peak Times for Nursing Professional Development

Start by tracking the peak times that the direct services of NPDSs may be needed on clinical units. Although educators traditionally have worked during daylight hours, organizational changes frequently affect both patient care needs and the availability of resources. NPDSs need to coordinate available assets with peak staff learning times on the clinical units.

For example, suppose you are responsible for meeting the learning needs of staff on a surgical unit. The postoperative patients traditionally returned from postanesthesia recovery (PAR) before 3 pm. Because your unit recently merged with another, there has been an increase in cases during two days of the week. To deal with this increase in patients, surgeons scheduled operating room cases beginning later in the day. This resulted in patients returning from PAR to the clinical unit as late as 8 pm.

Given these changes, it may be wise to reevaluate your accessibility to staff during the evening hours on those two days. This is especially appropriate if you recently acquired new nursing staff who need cross-training or retraining. Once these nurses are comfortable, you may choose to reevaluate your schedule. Therefore, it is important to be flexible and make informed decisions that respond to the staff's learning needs. Or you may consider making more independent learning modules, such as computer simulations, available to nursing staff who need a quick review.

Set Priorities

Another important approach to meeting staff needs with limited resources is to prioritize learning needs and to remain open and flexible. Categorizing needs based on their urgency or criticality will be discussed further in regard to planning in-service offerings in Chapter 6.

Network for 24-Hour Coverage

If your organization has only one nurse who functions as a staff educator for one or more units, try developing a network of experts that can help meet learning needs 24 hours a day (see Chapter 4). Start by developing a group of NPDSs or unit educators. Identify nurses who demonstrate positive behaviors, such as expert clinical skills, excellent interpersonal skills, and strong critical-thinking skills. These nurses should be willing to mentor other staff and act as role models.

In addition to facilitating staff access to human resources, it also is helpful to develop a system through which staff can access reference texts, videos, Internet resources, computer programs, and printed resources as needed.

Mentor Clinical Staff

It is important to select clinical staff who are appropriate candidates for the unit-based clinical educator role. Being an expert practitioner does not mean a nurse can automatically function as an educator. Nurses need to develop educator roles over time, learning what is involved in NPD and how to function within their roles (see Chapter 3).

Summary

Major changes in the scope and standards of practice and performance for nursing professional development have created a new model for this specialty practice, placing emphasis on the qualifications, core competencies, and key elements of the NPDS role. Ultimate outcomes of the model continue to focus on the delivery of quality patient care and safeguarding the public as consumers of healthcare services. These standards also can guide clinical nurses who assume the role of educator within their diverse patient settings.

Helpful Websites

- American Nurses Credentialing Center—ANCC Magnet Recognition Program®: www.nurse credentialing.org/magnet.aspx
- Association for Nursing Professional Development—About ANPD: www.anpd.org
- Joint Commission—Facts About Hospital Accreditation: www.jointcommission.org/accreditation/accreditation_main.aspx
- Joint Commission—For Nurses: www.jointcommission.org/nurses.aspx

References

American Association of Colleges of Nursing & Association of American Medical Colleges. (2010). *Lifelong learning in medicine and nursing: A final conference report.* Washington, DC: Macy Foundation.

American Nurses Association. (2000). *Scope and standards of practice for nursing professional development.* Washington, DC: Author.

American Nurses Association. (2014). Professional role competence [Position statement]. Retrieved from http://www.nursingworld.org/MainMenuCategories/ThePracticeofProfessionalNursing/NursingStandards/Professional-Role-Competence.html

American Nurses Association. (2015). *Nursing: Scope and standards of practice* (3rd ed.). Silver Spring, MD: Author.

American Nurses Association & National Nursing Staff Development Organization. (2010). *Nursing professional development: Scope and standards of practice.* Silver Spring, MD: American Nurses Association.

American Nurses Credentialing Center. (n.d.-a). ANCC Magnet Recognition Program®. Retrieved from http://www.nursecredentialing.org/magnet.aspx

American Nurses Credentialing Center. (n.d.-b). Benefits. Retrieved from http://www.nursecredentialing.org/Magnet/ProgramOverview/WhyBecomeMagnet

American Nurses Credentialing Center. (n.d.-c). Find a magnet hospital. Retrieved from http://www.nursecredentialing.org/Magnet/FindaMagnetFacility.aspx

American Nurses Credentialing Center. (n.d.-d). Forces of magnetism. Retrieved from http://www.nursecredentialing.org/ForcesofMagnetism.aspx

American Nurses Credentialing Center. (n.d.-e). Magnet Recognition Program model. Retrieved from http://www.nursecredentialing.org/Magnet/ProgramOverview/New-Magnet-Model

American Nurses Credentialing Center. (2012). *Educational design process: 2013 mini manual.* Silver Spring, MD: Author.

Association for Nursing Professional Development. (n.d.). A new name, a new foundation for future growth. Retrieved from http://www.anpd.org/?page=WelcometoANPD

Benner, P. (1984). *From novice to expert: Excellence and power in clinical nursing practice.* Menlo Park, CA: Addison-Wesley.

Brunt, B.A. (2007). *Competencies for staff educators.* Marblehead, MA: HCPro, Inc.

Brunt, B.A. (2014). *Nursing professional development competencies: Tools to evaluate and enhance educational development.* Danvers, MA: HCPro, Inc.

Dickerson, P.S. (2014). Grounding our practice in nursing professional development. *Journal of Continuing Education in Nursing, 45,* 288–289. doi:10.3928/00220124-20140625-11

Dorin, M. (2010). Do you want to be a staff-development specialist? *Nursing, 40,* 25. doi:10.1097/01.NURSE.0000387066.37626.98

Evans, C., Connell, J., Barkham, M., Marshall, C., & Mellor-Clark, J. (2003). Practice-based evidence: Benchmarking NHS primary care counselling services at national and local levels. *Journal of Clinical Psychology and Psychotherapy, 10,* 374–388. doi:10.1002/cpp.384

Joint Commission. (2014a). About the Joint Commission. Retrieved from http://www.jointcommission.org/about_us/about_the_joint_commission_main.aspx

Joint Commission. (2014b). National Patient Safety Goals. Retrieved from http://www.jointcommission.org/standards_information/npsgs.aspx

Melnyk, B.M., Fineout-Overholt, E., Stillwell, S.B., & Williamson, K.M. (2010). Evidence-based practice: Step-by-step: The seven steps of evidence-based practice. *American Journal of Nursing, 110*(1), 51–53. doi:10.1097/01.NAJ.0000366056.06605.d2

Oncology Nursing Society. (2012). *Oncology Nursing Society leadership competencies.* Retrieved from https://www.ons.org/sites/default/files/leadershipcomps.pdf

Swihart, D., & Johnstone, D. (2010). What does a nursing professional development specialist (nurse educator) do? *American Nurse Today, 5.* Retrieved from http://www.americannursetoday.com/what-does-a-nursing-professional-development-specialist-nurse-educator-do

Getting Prepared for Your Role as a Nursing Professional Development Specialist and Unit-Based Educator

I N Chapter 2, you learned about the importance of a well-planned orientation program for nurses and other healthcare workers who find themselves assigned to a new role or given additional responsibilities on clinical units. Similarly, this chapter will help you design a personal orientation that will help you succeed in your new role as a NPDS or clinical nurse with educator responsibilities. Information on how to develop an orientation program for newly employed nursing staff, faculty, and nursing students will be discussed in Chapter 4.

Taking on new or added responsibilities as an NPDS may feel overwhelming at first. In a study by Manning and Neville (2009), experienced clinical nurses who transitioned into NPDS roles reported that their new positions were more challenging than they had expected and that they felt stressed and unprepared. Although this study was conducted in New Zealand and was limited to just eight nurses, it serves as a lasting reminder that you must be proactive when assuming your NPDS role.

Before beginning as an NPDS or unit-based educator, it is important to gather key information about your role and responsibilities; analyze, organize, and develop your work plan; and create strategies to evaluate your performance. These steps will require you to review essential materials and documents and meet with key individuals inside and outside your organization. These actions will help you obtain and clarify information regarding your responsibilities and enable you to perform a self-assessment of the knowledge, skills, and attitudes you need to strengthen in your new role.

Gathering Key Information About Your Role and Responsibilities

Gather information about your new position from an organizational perspective, starting with a view of the total organization and then specific divisions and departments. For example, you first might want to review the nursing division, followed by the nursing professional development department (NPDD), and finally your assigned clinical unit(s). Other names for NPDDs include nursing education and professional development, nursing education and research, and nursing practice and professional development. Similarly, the titles of nurse educators also vary by institution.

As you survey your organization, collect data that will enable you to comprehend and clarify your new role and responsibilities. This information will help you understand the beliefs, values, and planned direction or vision of the organization, which will allow you to develop your unit-based educational goals. Because money, personnel, and administrative support are frequently allocated to departments based on organizational goals, it is advantageous to relate your staff educational goals to those of the clinical unit, division or department, and organization.

Understanding the Structure and Function of Your Organization

---

It is important to learn as much as you can about your healthcare organization before beginning your NPDS role. First, research the organization's history, including changes made before and after its recent restructuring. This will give you insight on how to help staff handle these changes and progress into the future. Next, investigate the organization's mission and vision statements, philosophy, strategic goals, and objectives. This will clarify what is valued by the organization and its future direction. Finally, educate yourself on the policies, procedures, and rules that relate to your role as a unit-based educator, as well as the names of key individuals within your organization.

Before you explore your educator role on the clinical unit(s), focus on the division or department level and repeat the same information-gathering process. For example, if your educator position is associated with a centralized NPDD under the direction of the clinical services division or nursing department, investigate both of these divisions. As you learn about these divisions, understand the overall influence that recent restructuring has had on daily operations, such as the manner in which the departments are divided and staffed. Learn the names of key individuals who are responsible for implementing department goals and understand their roles and responsibilities. Meet with them to clarify your alignment with these departments and how you can achieve departmental goals and objectives.

Because you play a significant role in helping the NPDD attain its targeted educational goals, it is important for you to understand the specific aspects of the department. Begin this process by learning about the following components at the organizational and departmental levels: mission and vision statements, philosophy, goals and objectives, and policies and procedures. Other features of the NPDD, such as its educational design, documentation and record-keeping system, and available resources, will also guide you.

Mission and Vision Statements

The mission and vision statements of your organization guide the direction of the NPDD and the manner in which you carry out your role and responsibilities as an educator. This information can shape your position objectives and clarify the boundaries of your role.

An organization's *mission statement* focuses on the reason why it exists, addresses what services it offers, and reveals the demographics of its targeted consumers (Mancini, 2011). It sets the tone for an organization's philosophy, goals, objectives, and policies and procedures. An example of an NPDD mission statement can be found in Figure 3-1.

The *vision statement* describes what the organization ultimately expects to become in the future (Mancini, 2011). Figure 3-2 shows an example NPDD vision statement that you can use

---

Figure 3-1. Sample Mission Statement for a Nursing Professional Development Department

The mission of this department is to provide quality, cost-effective educational offerings and professional development activities that are based on the latest knowledge, foster quality patient care, and support the goals of the nursing profession and this healthcare organization.

Figure 3-2. Sample Vision Statement for a Nursing Professional Development Department

To be a recognized provider of quality and cost-effective educational programs and services for healthcare employees in our healthcare organization and for professionals and laypeople in the regional community

---

as you attempt to blend your aspirations as a unit-based educator with those of the organization and NPDD.

Philosophy

The *philosophy* of an organization should reflect its vision and mission statements and reveal its values and beliefs in the process (Mancini, 2011). Similarly, the NPDD's philosophy should tell you what the department's beliefs are regarding professional nursing development, specifically involving its learners and educators, the teaching-learning process, and its practice and learning environments. It is crucial to understand these philosophies, as they can assist your daily work and help you understand what the organization and department value.

Determine how the department's philosophy compares to your personal philosophy. If you feel uncomfortable with these beliefs or perform your job in opposition to the scope of the department's philosophy, you run the risk of experiencing emotional strain and conflict within yourself, with other educators, or in the NPDD.

The philosophy should clarify who the learners are and to what degree they are involved in the teaching-learning process. Knowing the scope of your learners is especially important if your organization has multiple centers or academic partnerships. Some departments consider all employees within the healthcare organization as learners, while other departments limit learners to nursing staff (e.g., nurses, assistive personnel [AP], unit secretaries). Other employers assume an interprofessional approach, including physical and occupational therapists, nutritionists, and social workers as learners. Patients, families, and the lay community may also be learners in some organizations.

It is significant to determine the role of learners in the teaching-learning process, especially in relation to their professional development. Clarify if learners are expected to assume total responsibility for meeting their learning needs and what role the NPDD plays in their development. You should also establish if the nursing staff plays an active role in educating its peers or if all educational offerings are led and implemented by nurse educators.

Within this philosophy, understand how staff educators perceive and enact the learner and educator roles at your workplace. Although some departmental philosophies depict the nurse educator as a facilitator of learning, actual practice may reflect the educator as the expert or sole bearer of knowledge. Investigate if learning differences based on cultural and ethnic diversities are considered in educational activities.

Goals, Objectives, and the Strategic Plan

A *strategic plan* maps the work of an organization over a period of three to five years and guides the organization's direction and operations to attain future goals (Clyne, 2011). It determines how resources will be distributed and how responsibilities will be delegated, as well as over what time period. You should focus on the specific priorities identified as needs by your department, especially long- and short-term goals.

Ask your unit manager about the defined time span for goals adopted by your organization. In most organizations, a "year" refers to the fiscal year that coincides with the organization's budget period, usually beginning July 1 and ending June 30 the following year. Investigate how the NPDD identifies and prioritizes its goals and allocates departmental resources based on these priorities.

Carefully review the short-term goals developed for the current year. Each goal should be accompanied by observable measurements (outcomes) that indicate successful attainment of the goal, actions needed to help the department meet the goal, and assigned responsibilities for these actions.

The strategic plan of the NPDD has many similarities to a nursing care plan for patients. Both items need to be flexible and accommodate changes as they arise. Goals are developed based on needs identified from a variety of sources, including those you have observed and those expressed by the patient and family. These goals are patient-centered, realistic, measurable, and attainable. Specific interventions are identified to help the patient meet these goals. Specific observable outcomes or measures indicate successful attainment of each goal.

Because goals outlined in the strategic plan guide both the efforts and resources of the NPDD, it is logical for your unit-based goals to align with those of the department. Because your role is an extension of the NPDD, it is also essential that your work is congruent with the department's education plans.

Policies and Procedures

Review the policies and procedures of your organization, division, and NPDD. These statements should be consistent with the organization's mission and vision statements and philosophy, as they help to direct the work of the NPDD. Policies and procedures should also reflect priorities of professional nursing standards published by the American Nurses Association (ANA), accreditation agencies such as the Joint Commission (n.d.), and recognition programs such as the American Nurses Credentialing Center (ANCC) Magnet Recognition Program® (n.d.-a). Similar to its philosophy, an organization's policies and procedures should guide you in your unit-based role and in your communication with other educators. Policies and procedures also enable employees to work together to meet departmental goals.

After reviewing these policies and procedures, note which ones directly apply to your unit-based educator role. In developing your position, decide if new policies and procedures need to be created to guide your activities on the clinical unit. Suggested policies and procedures will be discussed later as they relate to specific staff development components, such as orientation (see Chapter 4), preceptorships (see Chapter 5), and continuing education (see Chapter 13).

Educational Design

Educational design is the department's plan for providing instruction and includes several key features (see Figure 3-3). Consider engaging learners to participate in the educational design. As a unit-based educator, you will need to gain an understanding of the following design components and how they should be reflected in your role.

Description of targeted learners: NPDDs often include the following personnel in educational processes: RNs, licensed practical nurses (LPNs), licensed vocational nurses (LVNs), AP,

---

Figure 3-3. Key Features of an Educational Design for Nursing Professional Development

- Assessment of learning needs
- Description of targeted learners
- Lesson objectives
- Content outline
- Teaching-learning strategies
- Evaluation strategies to assess learning outcomes
- Resources needed for lesson

nursing assistants, and unit secretaries. Faculty and nursing students from affiliating schools of nursing also commonly interface with the NPDD. These schools prepare students at various levels, such as diploma, associate, baccalaureate, master's and doctoral degrees, into the nursing profession.

Although these learners may all be considered adult learners, it is important to pay attention to the educational needs and learning strategies related to the diversity of the learners within your organization (Benedict & Bradley, 2010). For example, it would be paramount to understand the comfort level of various learners in your organization when delivering technology-based educational programs. When developing your unit's educational plan, you would want to include ways to assess learner preferences and strategies. This will enable learning through various delivery methods, such as web-based programs and podcasts. Be sure to take advantage of the talents and experience of learners to facilitate positive outcomes. Avoid making assumptions about preferred learning activities based on age, race, ethnicity, or experience.

Some NPDDs also include interprofessional health-related or non–health-related personnel among their targeted learners (Benedict & Bradley, 2010). For example, your NPDD may provide educational services for coworkers (e.g., social workers, pharmacists), patients and their families, and other individuals living in the community. Perhaps educators in your NPDD teach all agency employees cardiopulmonary resuscitation or offer general classes in conflict management. Find out if this is also part of your unit-based educator role.

Once you know who the NPDD identifies as its learners, clarify who comprises your own learners and learn more about their specific roles and responsibilities within your organization. For example, if you are responsible for meeting the learning needs of LPNs, LVNs, and AP, be sure that you understand their job expectations on the unit. Learn about their role by reviewing their job descriptions.

If you are unfamiliar with staff on your assigned clinical unit(s), spend some time with them to get to know them as professionals. This also will give you an opportunity to clarify your unit-based educator role and understand their needs.

Assessment of learning needs: Now that you know who the learners are, analyze how the NPDD assesses their specific learning needs. Conducting a needs assessment helps nurse educators determine actual competencies of learners related to specific areas (see Chapter 6). Results are compared with competencies that the organization wants its employees to possess in order to provide safe, quality patient care. Educators obtain these desired behaviors using position descriptions, professional nursing standards, healthcare trends, organizational reports, and criteria determined by regulatory and accreditation agencies. The outcomes obtained from a needs assessment are used to help educators plan and implement activities for targeted learners. It is important to understand how staff learning needs are assessed on your clinical unit and how you can access this information. If a needs assessment has not been conducted on your unit, then you will need to do one to develop your plan for unit-based educational activities (see Chapter 13).

To understand how a needs assessment helps employees and how it is used by NPDSs within healthcare organizations, think about the educational processes included in nursing professional development (see Chapter 2) (ANA & National Nursing Staff Development Organization [NNSDO], 2010). NPDSs and staff educators may separate a needs assessment into smaller, more manageable segments. Because learning needs and competencies of nursing staff need to be continually developed and maintained (ANA, 2000), healthcare organizations regularly assess these skills. This is one reason why NPDDs collect, organize, and record employee learning needs, educational activities, and competencies according to NPD processes. The results, although often categorized, still need to be viewed as a whole that is integrated within the continuous process of employee professional development and career planning.

Chapter 2 described how orientation is used to prepare new employees in fulfilling their assigned roles and responsibilities in the workplace. Because orientation focuses on an employee's specific role within the agency, a position description can help determine successful performance or desired competencies. When a group of nurses is hired, their skills are evaluated based on expectations identified in their position descriptions. Assessment of the actual skills of new staff helps determine what competencies need to be developed during orientation. Helping staff develop these desired competencies will enable them to function effectively in their roles. Actual employee competencies are determined through self-assessments, written tests, and skills observations (ANA & NNSDO, 2010). Any differences observed between demonstrated behaviors and desired behaviors should be considered as learning needs (ANA, 2000).

Similarly, Chapter 2 described the purpose of in-service educational activities to "assist nurses as they perform their assigned functions in that particular agency or institution" (ANA, 2000, p. 24). Suppose a physician tells you and your nurse manager that a new chemotherapy drug will be part of a clinical protocol used for patients admitted to your unit. Existing unit staff already are skilled in administering chemotherapy drugs, but they are unfamiliar with this drug and its nursing implications. Use this identified learning need to help existing staff develop their knowledge and skills to safely administer this drug, assess and manage its potential side effects, and provide appropriate patient education. A unit-based in-service program would be an appropriate strategy to accomplish this goal; include a review of this drug as part of the planned educational program.

Chapter 4 will explain ways to assess the learning needs of new staff during orientation, whereas Chapters 6 and 13 will focus on determining learning needs for existing experienced unit staff through in-service education and continuing education, respectively.

While reviewing this information, be sure to learn the process used by your own organization to assess learning needs, how the process prioritizes these needs with limited resources, and the ways in which learners have input into the process. Also, observe what kinds of methods are used to collect this information, such as written surveys, focus groups, or quality improvement reports, and when learning needs are formally assessed. Determine how needs assessment results are used to plan educational activities aimed at correcting any deficiencies and how the influence of educational processes are evaluated. It is also important to understand your responsibilities in this process and how the process affects your role on your clinical unit.

Components of educational offerings: Based on data received from needs assessments, educators develop various educational offerings aimed at strengthening the knowledge, skills, and attitudes of targeted learners. Be sure to review the main components of this process used by educators in the NPDD as they plan each educational activity. These items include objectives, content, teaching strategies, and evaluation methods (see Chapter 6) (ANA, 2000). Use principles of adult learning when designing these educational activities (ANA, 2000), and learn what your role is in this operation. The following example is provided to clarify this process.

Suppose that changing a laryngectomy tube is an expected clinical skill for nurses on your unit. Because only a few nurses can successfully perform this critical task, you identify this as a learning need for select staff nurses. Before you begin to help these nurses develop this competency, you create a plan to teach this skill, identifying a few objectives (outcomes) that describe key behaviors you expect them to demonstrate after receiving instruction. You then outline content that will help these nurses meet these objectives and choose teaching strategies to convey this information. For example, you plan to demonstrate the procedure of changing a tube. You then have the nurses repeat this demonstration as you observe their technique or have them view a video of this procedure. After the program, you evaluate the nurses' ability to meet the objectives and provide them with feedback. You also receive their feedback about the program and your teaching skills.

Ask educators in the NPDD about the strategies that they use to communicate their educational offerings to nursing staff, especially how they identify and inform nurses who urgently need to develop these competencies. Determine if the notification process is conducted in a way that gives nurse managers sufficient time to provide coverage for patient care activities while nurses attend these programs. Find out if staff members are expected to seek out these learning experiences themselves once they obtain permission from their nurse manager or if you are responsible for coordinating this procedure in collaboration with the staff and unit manager.

Resources Available for Educational Activities

Educators need access to various resources, technologies, and facilities for implementing educational activities to meet goals and objectives (ANA, 2000). Managers of NPDDs and clinical units develop a financial plan (budget) each fiscal year that enables their department to meet its goals and objectives. However, managers may ask for your input from a unit-based perspective. Because resources often are limited in most healthcare organizations, you will need to be creative in developing cost-effective educational activities that successfully develop staff competencies.

To provide appropriate advice to managers regarding needed resources, you must learn what the term *resources* means, anticipate the resources you will need to carry out your responsibilities, and know what existing resources are already available.

To better understand resources, think of them as three separate categories: human, fiscal, and material. Human resources consist of people and the services they provide. Fiscal resources are monies that can be allocated for expenditures, such as conference fees, refreshments at receptions, and printing costs for brochures or handouts. Material resources include office supplies, computer hardware and software, and teaching models. Table 3-1 illustrates various resources you may need as a unit-based educator. This table also indicates how each resource can potentially contribute to your unit's educational goals. Because requesting all of these resources may be unrealistic in today's healthcare setting, you will need to prioritize them based on your goals. This task may be easier to accomplish after you have conducted a self-assessment regarding the skills you need in your new role, completed a needs assessment for your clinical unit, and prioritized your goals.

You may have access to resources within your organization (e.g., library, public relations), the NPDD (e.g., teaching models, administrative support), or your clinical unit (e.g., conference rooms, duplication services, Internet access). You also may have access to resources outside your organization through your academic partners at schools of nursing, community agencies, or professional nursing organizations. The Oncology Nursing Society (ONS), for example, offers multiple resources for educators responsible for preparing nurses for oncology practice. In *Standards of Oncology Nursing Education: Generalist and Advanced Practice Levels*, Jacobs and Mayer (2015) outline how oncology nurses need to be prepared in order to provide safe, quality care for cancer survivors as clinical practitioners, researchers, administrators, consultants, and educators.

ONS's subscription-based Educator Resource Center (ERC) contains multiple evidence-based teaching-learning resources (e.g., presentation slides, case studies, journal articles, assessment tools, test questions) that can be used by academic educators and NPDSs (ONS, n.d.-b). You can also access books, journal articles, other publications, and online continuing education courses on cancer care topics, such as chemotherapy, biotherapy, and evidence-based practice.

Table 3-1. Examples of Resources Needed for Unit-Based Educational Activities

Resource	Examples	Purpose Related to Unit-Based Educational Goals
Human	Secretarial support	Assistance with preparing documents, keeping records, duplicating materials, and scheduling rooms
	Audiovisual/technology technicians	Delivery of audiovisual equipment and assistance with operating technology and equipment
	Graphic designers	Helping to prepare slides and posters for teaching and presentations
	Expert presenters	Assistance with presenting educational content
	Expert scholars (research and publication)	Providing consultation with unit-based research and publication efforts of staff
Fiscal	Monies	Registration fees for conferences both internal and external to organization Purchase of unit-based reference books (print or e-books) and teaching models and materials Supporting rewards and incentives for preceptors Funding unit-based celebrations and meetings Assistance with cost of mailings to external agencies
Material	Supplies	Access to teaching models and supplies, audiovisual materials, office supplies, and staff and patient education materials
	Equipment	Access to audiovisual equipment, computer hardware and software, and duplication machines
	Facilities/space	Access to teaching space (e.g., classroom, skills simulation, computer laboratory, computer), storage of teaching materials, and office space for unit-based educator

As an accredited approver of continuing education by ANCC's Commission on Accreditation, ONS can help NPDSs offer CE programs (see Chapter 13) (ONS, n.d.-a).

Other resources may include faculty expertise and access to classrooms; simulation laboratories at affiliated schools; and face-to-face or Internet-based local, regional, or national conferences. Because resources can be found in a variety of places, meet with individuals in these departments to discuss availability.

Documentation, Record-Keeping, and Reports

Familiarize yourself with the documentation system adopted by nurse educators in the NPDD and the overall record-keeping system used to track educational activities. Learn which reports educators need to generate, as well as those issued by other departments. As you obtain this information, think about the implications to your unit-based educator role.

To better understand the documentation and record-keeping system used by nurse educators in your healthcare agency, try contrasting the system with tools you use in patient care. For example, compare a patient's chart (electronic health record [EHR]) with the professional development record of a staff nurse on your unit. Just as the EHR provides you with information about the health status of your patient, the professional development record of staff nurses informs you about their "educational health" in the organization. You also may be involved in helping nurses manage their own professional record or create a professional portfolio (see Chapter 10) for a clinical advancement program.

A patient's EHR contains documents organized in a standard sequence and housed in the clinical unit or within a commercial electronic system. Each form or file within the EHR has its designated purpose. Patient data are documented in an objective manner based on agency policies and professional standards. Information found in the patient's EHR helps nurses plan care and evaluate the effectiveness of that care based on patient outcomes. The EHR is considered confidential and is accessible only by approved healthcare personnel.

Data from the patient records may be accessed to generate various reports used by others in the organization, such as staff who monitor infection rates or handle insurance or government agencies. Others use these reports to make informed decisions that can potentially influence a variety of individuals, such as patients, unit staff, and educators. These reports also can influence the unit, department, and healthcare organization as a whole.

A nurse's professional development record is similar to an EHR in that it contains notations about the nurse's competencies and the effectiveness of the nurse's attendance at educational activities with the main goal of strengthening these abilities. Educators or preceptors document the nurse's performance and progress at time intervals determined by departmental policies and procedures. Staff records are private documents accessed only by individuals who are granted permission by the nurse or organization.

Similar to patient records, various reports are generated based on the data obtained from the professional records of staff nurses. These reports can be used for program evaluation and decision-making purposes and can influence individual, departmental, and organizational goals. It is important to understand your organization's policy related to accessing these data and disseminating them in aggregate forms. Although some reports focus on individual staff, others may reflect data based on groups of workers or staff on particular clinical units. For example, staff nurses may need access to continuing education programs they attended and the contact hours they earned to apply for recertification in a clinical specialty, develop their résumé, or create a portfolio for their promotion. A manager might ask the nurse for information about competency testing or evaluation as a unit-based preceptor or presenter in a unit-based in-service as documentation for an annual performance review. Administrators may also need reports related to program outcomes for accreditation or recognition purposes.

NPDDs use different record-keeping systems; be sure to find out what methods are used at your organization. Some organizations maintain records using hard copies and self-designed computer databases, whereas others use commercial learning management systems. In addition to keeping data organized, the department also may develop records that reflect the work (programs) of educators in the NPDD. For example, the NPDD may document the number of orientations, in-service educational offerings, and continuing education programs implemented within a fiscal year, along with the number and type of healthcare workers who attended each educational activity. This type of information can be useful in creating reports for the administrator in the nursing division or develop a fiscal plan for the department.

Regardless of the type of documentation, record-keeping system, or reports the NPDD generates, it is important to know about each process and the individuals responsible for the process. Ask where records are stored, how they can be retrieved, and who has permission to access them. In some organizations, staff records are maintained in the unit manager's office, whereas others archive records in the NPDD. As mentioned earlier, some departments maintain the professional development data in a computerized database or software system that allows for easy storage and retrieval.

Now that you understand the documentation and record-keeping system from an NPDD perspective, clarify what your role is at the unit-based level. Find out which aspects of the professional development process you will be responsible for documenting and your role in the overall record-keeping system. Ask what reports you need to generate, for whom, and how often. Additional guidance regarding documentation and record-keeping will be discussed in Chapter 4 on orientation, Chapter 6 on unit-based in-service education, and Chapter 13 on continuing education programs.

Clarifying Your Role as a Unit-Based Educator in the Clinical Setting

After you gain an understanding of the organization, nursing division, and NPDD, you can focus on your educator role on the clinical unit. If you are responsible for more than one clinical unit, be sure to examine each of them. Clarify your role with your immediate supervisor and review the performance standards and expectations listed in your position description. Depending on your organization, your supervisor might be the nurse manager of your unit or the manager or educator in the NPDD.

Start by learning about what organizational changes the unit has experienced over recent years and what the plan and strategic goals are for the unit. Obtain this information from the nurse manager of the clinical unit and the NPDS, as appropriate. Spend time on the unit observing the nursing care and talking with the staff about their understanding and interests regarding their professional development.

Gain knowledge about how the unit is structured and how it functions. Ask how staff on the clinical unit implement the vision, mission, philosophy, and goals of the organization and nursing department. Focus on any unit-specific policies and procedures and learn more information about the unit's staff members, including their names, positions, and strengths. Try to determine which staff members might be considered the unit's "star," or "champion," as they will undoubtedly help you meet the unit's goals.

Try to understand both the unit manager's and staff's philosophy of professional nursing development. Compare their philosophies with your own and those of the NPDD. Determine the staff's past and current learning needs. Ask questions about the available unit-based resources that will help maximize your role as educator.

How do the nurses perceive the importance of lifelong professional development? Do they feel they already have attained the competencies they will need to care for patients? How do staff members view their role in the teaching-learning process? Is their role one of personal responsibility and active participation, or do they view their role in education as a passive one directed by the educator?

Clarify your role and responsibilities as a unit-based staff educator. Start by finding your position on the department's organizational chart and noting the authority and communication lines between you and others. Determine the people you are responsible and accountable for as an educator. Locate individuals who hold similar positions as yourself; you are responsible for helping them meet their learning needs. Set time aside to meet with these individuals and ask questions.

Using your job description, determine your superiors, such as the nurse manager or NPDS. Check if you report to more than one manager, especially if you are the educator for more than one unit or if you also perform direct patient care activities. If you report to more than one person, know what aspects of your job description are related to each supervisor.

Closely examine your job description and the specific performance standards and expectations listed for the unit-based educator and other assumed roles. Seek clarification from your supervisor about each expectation and discuss realistic ways to manage multiple roles. Note whether your staff educator responsibilities include all aspects of professional development for staff or if they are confined to designated educational processes (throughputs), such as orientation or in-service educational offerings. Discuss additional department or organization committees to which you may be assigned. Be sure to clarify any vague statements with your supervisor, especially if you have multiple roles composed of a combination of advisory and line authority. Understand how you are evaluated and the procedures and expectations that you should follow.

Conducting a Self-Assessment for Your Role as Unit-Based Educator

Once you have investigated the organization, nursing division, NPDD, and clinical unit, spend some time reflecting on your own beliefs about education. Uncover what you value in the teaching-learning process and how you envision your role as unit-based educator. Compare your philosophy of NPD and lifelong learning with that of the NPDD and your clinical unit.

Next, conduct a self-assessment of your qualities so that you can compare them with those needed in your new role. Make a list of your personal and professional strengths, such as knowledge you have on special topics, your expertise in performing certain skills, and your attitudes or beliefs. Figure 3-4 lists some examples of desired qualities of unit-based educators.

Remember to include direct patient care abilities such as coordination, interpersonal, and critical-thinking skills that are also valued as a unit-based educator. Consider your personal qualities, like your flexibility, creativity, and optimism. For example, you might be a good listener or a strong group leader. Perhaps you excel at handling medical technology needed to care for patients on your unit. Maybe you are skilled at providing homecare instructions to patients and families. All of these should be included as strengths.

Figure 3-4. Possible Desired Qualities of Nursing Professional Development Specialists as Unit-Based Educators

Knowledge
- Teaching-learning process
- Adult learning principles and learning styles
- Clinical skills
- Implementing change
- Understanding of professional activities (e.g., research, publication)

Skills
- Negotiation
- Conflict management
- Problem solving
- Ability to develop an agenda and run a meeting
- Communication and interpersonal relationships
- Organization and effective time management
- Leadership management
- Technology

Attitudes
- Seeks learning experiences
- Self-directed and dependable
- Treats all staff fairly and respectfully
- Creates a positive work environment
- Possesses an optimistic perspective

Use your new position description as a guide to create a second list that contains knowledge, skills, and attitudes you perceive as essential to achieve success as a unit-based educator. Arrange this list in order of importance, starting with the most important quality and ending with the least important. Obtain this information from others in your organization, such as nurse managers, NPDSs, and other unit-based educators. Ask coworkers to give feedback about your skills. Seek help from publications on this topic, your colleagues who work at other agencies, and academic partners. Note how the abilities that you need to function as a unit-based educator parallel with skills required in your clinical staff nurse role.

Given the multiple and diverse responsibilities included in the NPDS or unit-based educator role, Shellenbarger (2009) suggested using time and project management techniques to help attain work goals. The first step involves tracking your daily activities over a period of time, which will allow you to analyze and modify your work patterns and interruptions. Next, use these assessment data to prioritize your tasks, focusing on the most important tasks first and scheduling them during a time when you have the most energy to be effective. Also, use daily to-do lists based on small, manageable, and incremental steps. Finally, Shellenbarger (2009) suggested creating an organized work space that will facilitate your time and project management goals.

Determining Unit-Based Staff Development Needs

To carry out your role as unit-based educator, it is essential that you have information regarding the educational and professional needs of the nursing staff on your unit. These needs will guide you in developing educational plans and goals for the unit staff. You also will need to evaluate the effectiveness of your unit-based education plan.

Educational Needs

Learn how your organization determines the learning needs of staff on your unit. This duty may be your responsibility, the responsibility of a specialist in your centralized NPDD, or the responsibility of your unit's nurse manager.

The learning needs of staff are determined using a variety of approaches and will be described in later chapters that discuss orientation (see Chapter 4), in-service education (see Chapter 6), and continuing education (see Chapter 13). However, it is helpful to compile an ongoing master list of learning needs. As learning needs become evident on a daily basis, add them to the list, upgrading their urgency as needed. In addition to conducting formal needs assessment surveys or group sessions, be sure to use feedback from meeting key individuals in your agency, such as the educator in the NPDD, your nurse manager, and other unit-based educators. Consider current professional nursing and healthcare trends and issues and how they can affect nurses within your organization. Spend some time meeting with unit staff to understand their perspective of their learning needs.

Professional Development Needs

In addition to your role as educator, you may be asked to assist staff development educators in activities that reflect their multiple roles (see Chapter 2). This information may be available from the NPDS or nurse manager and should reflect the direction of the organization and should guide your professional development plan.

For example, your department may need you to help staff members develop formal presentations or prepare manuscripts for publication, or you may be advised to encourage staff participation in clinical research projects or in continuing education programs for the local community. If your nursing department has a clinical advancement program, you may need to assist clinical nurses in developing their résumés and portfolios. If you have never performed some of these activities, include them as part of your own professional development plan.

Analyzing, Organizing, and Planning Your Work

Once you have gathered information about your own learning needs and those of the staff on your clinical unit(s), spend some time analyzing and organizing them. Start by focusing on your needs first before diving into the needs for the unit.

Creating a Plan for Self-Development

After you have collected data about yourself and your role, compare both lists of qualities. Determine the qualities that are desired, the ones you already demonstrate, and those you do not yet have. Label those you already possess as being excellent (3), adequate (2), or not adequate (1). Although you probably have excellent clinical skills, it is likely that your new unit-based educator skills are not as fully developed.

Use this information to develop a professional career plan (see Chapter 14) that will help you strengthen the qualities you listed as being adequate (2) or inadequate (1). Because it is unrealistic to develop all these competencies immediately, use a priority approach to determine which skills to develop first. Investigate various resources both inside and outside your healthcare organization that can help you attain these goals, including mentors, professional nursing organizations, formal and informal educational offerings, and other colleagues.

Mentors

Mentors can help you improve your skills as a unit-based educator. You may choose individuals you admire and are comfortable with, such as an educator in the NPDD, your unit manager, or a more experienced unit-based educator. Also consider mentors outside of your agency, such as a nurse faculty member from the school of nursing you attended or a colleague you met at a conference.

Professional Nursing Organizations

Join one or more professional nursing organizations related to your learning needs and career plan. Clinically oriented nursing organizations, such as the American Association of Critical-Care Nurses (www.aacn.org) or ONS (www.ons.org), offer educational programs focused on topics related to clinical nursing practice and may also sponsor educational activities that target educator needs. Other organizations, such as Sigma Theta Tau International Honor Society of Nursing (www.nursingsociety.org), offer professional development programs for nurses in diverse roles (e.g., clinical practice, education, research, administration). Some nursing organizations, such as the Association for Nursing Professional Development (www.anpd.org), are entirely dedicated to meeting the needs of nurses who function as NPDSs and staff educators. The Professional Nurse Educators Group (PNEG) (www.pneg.org), a virtual network composed of nurse educators who work in academic, professional nursing development, commercial, and other educational settings across the United States, sponsors an annual conference and various opportunities to network with other educators through an email list, face-to-face sessions, and social media (PNEG, n.d.).

In addition to these programs, take advantage of the many networking opportunities these organizations provide, especially through conferences or special interest groups (SIGs). Explore organizational products, such as books, journals, newsletters, and Internet-based resources like ONS's ERC (ONS, n.d.-b). Many national organizations have local chapters and SIGs or communities that enable active participation for nurses at an affordable cost.

Investigate nursing journals that focus on your unit-based educator role, such as *Journal for Nurses in Professional Development* (http://journals.lww.com/jnsdonline/pages/default. aspx) and *Journal of Continuing Education in Nursing* (www.healio.com/nursing/journals/ jcen/2014-8-45-8). Consider accessing other nursing education journals that target academic educators for more helpful information.

Standards, Accreditation, and Recognition Programs

Become familiar with the national professional standards that guide the specialty nursing practice and professional performance of NPDS, such as *Nursing Professional Development: Scope and Standards of Practice* (ANA & NNSDO, 2010). This document was introduced in Chapter 2.

In addition to NPD standards, review other publications that can direct you in your nursing practice role, particularly with regard to professional issues, social policy, and ethics: *Nursing: Scope and Standards of Practice* (ANA, 2015), *Nursing's Social Policy Statement: The Essence of the Profession* (ANA, 2010), and the *Guide to the Code of Ethics for Nurses With Interpretive Statements: Development, Interpretation, and Application* (Fowler, 2015).

After reflecting on the mission and vision statements of your employer, nursing division, and NPDD, examine how they compare with the elements contained in the NPDS practice model. Ask yourself the following questions pertaining to the model, the department, and your specific role and responsibilities:

- How do department functions align with the NPDS practice model?
- According to my department's mission and goals, who are the targeted learners?
- What is expected of me in relation to the model's developmental and educational processes addressed by my department? For example:
  - What role do I play related to academic partnerships with affiliated school of nursing faculty and students?
  - What are my responsibilities regarding orientation, in-service education, and continuing education activities?
  - What role do I play in developing staff related to research and scholarship?
  - What resources are available to me to facilitate these processes?
- What resources are available to me for my own career development and role transition?

In addition to standards, familiarize yourself with the current expectations of accreditation agencies, such as the Joint Commission. Your nurse manager, nurse educator, or agency librarian can help you locate relevant portions of Joint Commission guidelines. Clarify the role that you play in this process, especially in nursing practice and education standards.

Investigate if your healthcare organization needs to comply with any additional specialty-based national accreditation standards, such as the American College of Surgeons Commission on Cancer's (ACS CoC's) *Cancer Program Standards 2012: Ensuring Patient-Centered Care* (ACS CoC, 2012). It is essential to familiarize yourself with these standards, as they address the educational preparation needed for nurses who provide cancer care to patients within your organization and the evidence that needs to be assessed and documented to confirm compliance with these standards.

Discover if your healthcare organization plans on seeking Magnet designation. Or perhaps it already holds this outstanding recognition and is seeking renewal. If so, acquaint yourself with the application, its requirements, and your role and responsibilities.

Formal and Informal Educational Offerings

In addition to educational offerings sponsored by professional nursing organizations, consider attending continuing education programs presented by your workplace or academic partners. Enroll in formal academic courses that focus on the educator role. Ask nursing faculty from affiliated schools of nursing to share their expertise during in-service educational sessions for unit-based educators in return for serving as preceptors for their students. Also, seek informal educational activities, such as books, journals, videos, and Internet-based sources.

Consider seeking certification as an NPDS through ANCC (www.nursecredentialing.org/NPD-Eligibility.aspx) as well as through various specialty organizations (see Chapter 7) that match your expertise and career plan. Investigating the eligibility criteria for certification in advance will give you time to prepare for the examination, especially related to formal academic preparation, clinical hours as an RN and in professional development, and continuing education in professional development (ANCC, n.d.-b).

Peer Support Groups

Along with these various resources, remember that colleagues in similar positions also can provide support. Think about developing a unit-based educator support group in your organization or establishing communication pathways through email.

Consider implementing a journal club as a strategy to develop your educator skills and network with NPDSs and clinical nurses who assume educator functions on patient units. Journal clubs can be conducted face-to-face or online using a unit-based approach at your healthcare organization or even externally with colleagues at a local or regional level. Typically, journal clubs target clinical nurses and offer a forum where they can review and discuss research articles on topics of interest in order to strengthen their research or evidence-based skills (Polit & Beck, 2012). In this case, try using the journal club format to review articles that pertain to your educator role and responsibilities.

Ravin (2012) described a successful journal club that focused on adult learning and NPD. It implemented seven nurse educators employed within a continuing education provider unit at a national nursing specialty organization. Participants identified a need to "increase their knowledge about adult learning to enhance development of educational activities" (Ravin, 2012, p. 452). The journal club (see Chapter 12) also provided the nurses with experience in searching, reviewing, and critiquing the evidence provided in educational research articles and recognizing the value of sponsoring evidence-based continuing education programs on clinical topics of interest. Outcomes tracked over a five-year period were quite positive, with attention paid to observing participants' application of learning in their nurse planner responsibilities. Ravin (2012) recommended eight key elements essential for successful journal clubs: leadership, goals and objectives, target audience, scheduling, adaptability, process, meeting, and evaluation.

Establishing a Plan for Unit-Based Staff Development

After you develop a plan to strengthen your competencies as a unit-based educator, prepare another plan to meet the professional development needs of clinical staff on your unit. Start by organizing and analyzing the data you obtained about the staff's learning needs from various sources. Develop several goals or objectives (outcomes) you hope to accomplish within the year.

Although you want a holistic perspective of each staff member's competencies related to patient care needs on the clinical unit, this may be an overwhelming task. To make your work more manageable, try organizing it into smaller, more realistic components. Select a method that facilitates your unit-based record-keeping and reporting systems and matches your work with any centralized educational efforts. Your method also should be cost-effective.

One approach is to categorize the unit's education plan into the developmental and educational throughputs addressed in the NPDS practice model: orientation, competency programs, in-service, continuing education, career development and role transition, research and scholarship, and academic partnerships (ANA & NNSDO, 2010). Begin by sorting individual learning needs (competencies), included in your master list, into similar categories. Because you have limited resources, organize these needs in order of their priority. Develop goals and objectives (outcomes) that will enable staff to meet these needs. Sort each category, along with its goals, into the educational process (e.g., orientation, in-service education, continuing education) that might best meet these goals. Because staff learning needs are constant and changing, try to visualize your efforts as an educational plan in progress.

Suppose all nurses on your unit will need to perform venipunctures on patients to obtain blood specimens during the unit's evening shift. This need was brought to your attention by the unit's nurse manager as a recent departmental decision and policy change. Because of organizational restructuring, the staff who routinely provided this service from a centralized location were transferred to an ambulatory patient setting. The responsibility for drawing blood samples must be assumed by nurses on your clinical unit three months from now.

You decide that a unit-based in-service educational program is the best way for staff to master this skill. None of the existing staff know how to perform venipunctures, but they have prior knowledge concerning its complications. This brief in-service session will be sufficient time to review the procedure, discuss key issues, and provide a demonstration on a model arm. There also will be time for you to guide staff as they provide a return demonstration. This unit-based session will be easier for staff to attend while they are providing patient care. To help staff master their venipuncture skills, you later team each nurse with a phlebotomist for a brief, intensive practicum. Because it is unrealistic to expect all staff to attend these sessions at one time, you initially target nurses who need to master this skill first, such as those who work the evening shift. After demonstrating competence in venipunctures, these nurses can become the "experts" responsible for teaching remaining staff. This cost-effective approach will not only meet the learning needs of the staff but also enable staff to develop their unit-based presentation and preceptor skills.

Consider using a similar approach in preparing oncology nurses at your organization to manage neutropenia and an increased risk for infection, a symptom experienced by many patients who have received chemotherapy. For example, you decide to offer a one-hour continuing education program for nurses on this topic, exploring the available teaching-learning resources housed in the ERC database (ONS, n.d.-b). From this database, you download a customizable slide presentation on infection and some case studies that will help learners apply evidence-based principles of managing infection to their clinical practice. You also review ONS's Putting Evidence Into Practice website (see Chapter 12), which contains evidence-based interventions for preventing infection in patients with cancer (ONS, 2015). You then look over the information noted on the ONS website for approver units (ONS, n.d.-a) in order to seek continuing nursing education (CNE) to successfully complete the program, as oncology nurses need these CNE credits to maintain RN licenses or certifications.

Developing a Communication System

As a unit-based educator, it is imperative that you communicate with various individuals both inside and outside the organization. This will not only help you meet your goals but also will provide all staff with a sense of commitment to the educational activities of the unit. Consider key individuals you will need to communicate with on a regular basis and available strategies to accomplish this line of communication.

Start by making a list of these individuals and the communication methods available in your organization, such as emails, email distribution lists, or an intranet system. Try meeting with these individuals to determine the most effective approach. For example, you may want to have monthly meetings with your nurse manager or staff educator to update them on the progress of unit-based activities. Perhaps you can rely on email to share changes between meetings. If all staff have access to email, consider regular updates about the unit's educational activities. Also, consider traditional methods, such as face-to-face meetings, posters, signs, written memos, and printed or electronic newsletters. You will need to decide what the most effective approach will be based on your organization.

In addition to these communication systems, let staff know the best way to contact you if you are not on the clinical unit (e.g., voicemail message, cell phone, pager, email, text). Keep them abreast of your schedule and who will handle your responsibilities when you are away.

Capitalizing on the Strengths of the Unit Staff

Meeting the educational needs of staff on the clinical unit is a 24/7 responsibility. Because of this, you will need to develop creative strategies that will deal with this time frame and contribute to staff professional development. For example, think of including staff in the development of an education committee to meet departmental goals on your unit. Or perhaps your healthcare organization has a shared governance structure with councils, like the Nursing Professional Development Council or Professional Practice and Education Council, composed of nurses who can help with professional development decisions.

This committee can consist of interested staff or staff you previously selected to assist with the planning and implementation of educational activities on the unit. When meeting oncology-related learning needs, consider asking experienced oncology nurses to join you in planning, implementing, and evaluating the unit-based educational session. Nurse experts may include experienced oncology nurses who already work on the clinical unit, advanced practice nurses employed within your hospital, or academic partners, such as faculty with oncology experience who affiliate with your hospital. Including other experts when planning educational programs has the potential to increase the staff's participation and interest in the program, help you meet the staff's learning needs, develop the leadership skills of colleagues, and obtain recognition for colleagues' expertise in oncology. The development of a preceptorship program is another example.

In developing these approaches, match staff with tasks based on their strengths and interests, if possible. This is another reason why it is important for you to be familiar with unit staff, including their strengths, needs for improvement, motivation, and professional goals.

Evaluating Your Effectiveness in Meeting Goals

Similar to a patient's plan of care and consistent with the outputs mentioned in the NPDS practice model, you will need to develop a plan to evaluate how effective your interventions were in meeting both your personal goals and the unit's staff development goals. Evaluate your progress at the end of the fiscal year prior to developing a new plan for the following year. However, tracking your progress on an ongoing basis (i.e., monthly) will enable you to revise your plan if it is not on target. This feedback process is also consistent with the professional development model (ANA & NNSDO, 2010).

Evaluation of Personal Goals as a Unit-Based Educator

Earlier in this chapter you inventoried your personal and professional qualities and compared them with those needed to be an effective unit-based educator. Using your prioritized list as a guide, you developed realistic career goals to accomplish during the year along with strategies.

Spend time each month reviewing your personal career plan and assessing your progress. Take this opportunity to revise your plan if it is unrealistic or if unexpected opportunities to develop other skills arise. You may decide that competencies other than the ones you had previously identified should be a priority to develop.

In addition to your self-evaluation, obtain feedback from others about your performance. Other NPDSs in the NPDD, your unit manager, and other experienced unit-based educators may be the most helpful. Incorporate feedback you receive during your formal performance evaluation and make changes as needed.

Evaluation of Unit-Based Staff Development Goals

In addition to your personal goals, evaluate goals created for the professional development needs of the unit personnel. Track your progress monthly and revise. Likewise, conduct a summary evaluation before you design a plan for the following year.

For example, suppose one of your goals was to develop a preceptor preparation program for your unit. Evaluate your progress on this project each month based on the specific measurements you outlined from the start. If you find that you are off course one month, revise your approach as needed to get back on track.

In addition to collecting objective data about unit-based educational activities, obtain input from others on the unit, such as the staff and nurse manager. Staff members can share their perspectives about your ability to help them meet their learning needs. The unit manager can give you feedback based on unit reports, such as patient satisfaction surveys, patient outcomes, performance indicators, competencies, and incident reports.

Summary

In preparing for an NPDS or unit-based educator role, you will need to gather information about your organization, nursing division, the NPDD, and your assigned clinical unit(s). You also need to conduct a self-assessment based on your performance expectations and develop a realistic plan for ongoing professional and career development. Prioritize your learning needs and develop a plan based on these data and implement the plan. Obtain feedback about your performance as an educator and the effectiveness of the educational offerings to strengthen the competency of targeted learners.

Helpful Websites

- American Nurses Credentialing Center—ANCC Magnet Recognition Program®: www
.nursecredentialing.org/magnet.aspx
- Association for Nursing Professional Development—About ANPD: www.anpd.org
- Joint Commission—What is Accreditation?: www.jointcommission.org/accreditation/
accreditation_main.aspx
- Professional Nurse Educators Group—About: http://pneg.org

References

American College of Surgeons Commission on Cancer Care. (2012). *Cancer program standards 2012: Ensuring patient-centered care* [v.1.2.1, released January 2014]. Retrieved from https://www.facs.org/~/media/files/quality%20 programs/cancer/coc/programstandards2012.ashx

American Nurses Association. (2000). *Scope and standards of practice for nursing professional development.* Washington, DC: American Nurses Publishing.

American Nurses Association. (2010). *Nursing's social policy statement: The essence of the profession* (3rd ed.). Silver Spring, MD: Author.

American Nurses Association. (2015). *Nursing: Scope and standards of practice* (3rd ed.). Silver Spring, MD: Author.

American Nurses Association & National Nursing Staff Development Organization. (2010). *Nursing professional development: Scope and standards of practice.* Silver Spring, MD: American Nurses Association.

American Nurses Credentialing Center. (n.d.-a). ANCC Magnet Recognition Program®. Retrieved from http://www .nursecredentialing.org/magnet.aspx

American Nurses Credentialing Center. (n.d.-b). Nursing professional development certification eligibility criteria. Retrieved from http://www.nursecredentialing.org/NPD-Eligibility.aspx

Benedict, M.B., & Bradley, D. (2010). A peek at the revised nursing professional development: Scope and standards of practice. *Journal of Continuing Education in Nursing, 41,* 195–196. doi:10.3928/00220124-20100423-07

Clyne, M.E. (2011). Strategic planning, goal-setting, and marketing. In P.S. Yoder-Wise (Ed.), *Leading and managing in nursing* (5th ed., pp. 329–333). St. Louis, MO: Elsevier Mosby.

Fowler, M.D.M. (Ed.). (2015). *Guide to the code of ethics for nurses with interpretive statements: Development, interpretation, and application* (2nd ed.). Silver Spring, MD: American Nurses Association.

Jacobs, L.A., & Mayer, D.K. (2015). *Standards of oncology nursing education: Generalist and advanced practice levels* (4th ed.). Pittsburgh, PA: Oncology Nursing Society.

Joint Commission. (n.d.). What is accreditation? Retrieved from http://www.jointcommission.org/accreditation/ accreditation_main.aspx

Mancini, M.E. (2011). Understanding and designing organizational structures. In P.S. Yoder-Wise (Ed.), *Leading and managing in nursing* (5th ed., pp. 137–156). St. Louis, MO: Elsevier Mosby.

Manning, L., & Neville, S. (2009). Work-role transition: From staff nurse to clinical nurse educator. *Nursing Praxis in New Zealand, 25*(2), 41–53.

Oncology Nursing Society. (n.d.-a). Approver unit. Retrieved from https://www.ons.org/education/approver-unit

Oncology Nursing Society. (n.d.-b). Educator Resource Center. Retrieved from https://erc.ons.org

Oncology Nursing Society. (2015). Putting evidence into practice: Prevention of infection. Retrieved from https:// www.ons.org/practice-resources/pep/prevention-infection/prevention-infection-general

Polit, D.F., & Beck, C.T. (2012). *Nursing research: Generating and assessing evidence for nursing practice* (9th ed.). Philadelphia, PA: Wolters Kluwer/Lippincott Williams & Wilkins.

Professional Nurse Educators Group. (n.d.). About. Retrieved from http://pneg.org

Ravin, C.R. (2012). Implementation of a journal club on adult learning and nursing professional development. *Journal of Continuing Education in Nursing, 43,* 451–455. doi:10.3928/00220124-20120702-16

Shellenbarger, T. (2009). Time and project management tips for educators. *Journal of Continuing Education in Nursing, 40,* 292–293.

CHAPTER 4

Orienting Clinical Nurses to the Organization, Assessing Competence, and Promoting Lifelong Learning

C HAPTER 2 introduced the *Nursing Professional Development: Scope and Standards of Practice* document published by the American Nurses Association (ANA) and the National Nursing Staff Development Organization (NNSDO) in 2010. These standards included the Nursing Professional Development Specialist Practice Model that was also depicted in Figure 2-1. This system-based framework of inputs, throughputs, outputs, and a feedback loop guides NPDSs in their professional roles and responsibilities in various educational and clinical practice settings (ANA & NNSDO, 2010). This chapter will focus on two of the model's throughputs—orientation and competency programs.

Although orientation has existed as part of NPD for nearly two decades, it was often grouped with in-service educational and continuing education (CE) programs under the umbrella domain of "staff development" (ANA, 2000). Each of these focused on assessing, validating, and developing the competencies of professional nurses central to safe, quality patient care (ANA, 2000). Today, competency programs are identified as a separate throughput within the NPDS practice model (ANA & NNSDO, 2010).

It is important to understand the orientation and competency components of NPD and your specific roles and responsibilities related to these activities within your healthcare organization. Understanding this information will help you coordinate your unit-based efforts; determine what to include in your orientation and competency programs; and decide how to plan, organize, implement, evaluate, and sustain these programs in a cost-conscious manner.

Continuing Competence and Nursing Professional Development

Continuing competence and lifelong learning are the primary aims of professional development activities for nurses (ANA, 2000). The ultimate goal of these activities is to ensure that consumers receive safe, quality health care provided by competent nurses (ANA, 2000).

Understanding the Language of Competence

NPDSs and unit-based educators need to understand the language associated with the terms *competency*, *continuing competence*, and *core competencies*. NPDSs should also familiarize themselves with professional nursing standards and related competencies to appropriately guide clinical nurses within their organizations.

Oermann and Gaberson (2014) stated that the terms *competency* and *outcome* may be used interchangeably by some experts when describing what is evaluated in clinical practice. While both are used throughout this book, *competency* will predominantly be used in this chapter because of its congruence with verbiage referenced in various scopes and standards of practice, such as those published by ANA and specialty organizations like the Oncology Nursing Society (ONS) (ANA, 2015; ANA & NNSDO, 2010; Brant & Wickham, 2013).

According to ANA (2015), *competency* refers to the "expected level of performance that integrates knowledge, skills, abilities, and judgment" (p. 44). Therefore, nurses who are "performing at an expected level" (ANA, 2015, p. 44) are referred to as demonstrating competence in their roles. Similarly, the phrase *core competencies* refers to a "fundamental level of knowledge, ability, skill, or expertise that is essential to a particular job" (ANA & NNSDO, 2010, p. 43). The core competencies of NPDSs, addressed in *Nursing Professional Development: Scope and Standards of Practice*, are categorized under the headings of career development, education, leadership, and program and project management (ANA & NNSDO, 2010).

ANA (2000) defines *continuing competence* as the "ongoing professional nursing competence according to level of expertise, responsibility, and domains of practice as evidenced by behavior based on beliefs, attitudes, and knowledge matched to and in the context of a set of expected outcomes as defined by nursing scope of practice, policy, code of ethics, standards, guidelines, and benchmarks that ensure safe performance of professional activities" (p. 23).

Continuing competence is an important aspect of health care, as it enables nurses to continuously provide safe, quality nursing care to patients who expect a high standard of care (ANA, 2000). Continuing competence is a key feature of nursing professionalism and provides an accountability to society (ANA, 2000).

Given the importance of competent patient care, NPD departments sponsor ongoing competency programs to systematically evaluate the performance of nurses (ANA & NNSDO, 2010) and other healthcare professionals. NPDSs usually play a key role in developing, coordinating, administering, facilitating, conducting, and evaluating competency programs (ANA & NNSDO, 2010).

Ensuring the Continuing Competence of Nurses

Although nurses are primarily responsible for assuring the public of their continuing competence, others also participate in this important obligation (ANA, 2014). In its position statement on professional role competence, ANA claims that the competence of professional nurses is the "shared responsibility of the profession, individual nurses, professional organizations, credentialing and certification entities, regulatory agencies, employers, and other key stakeholders" (ANA, 2014, para. 1).

Professional Nurses

Professional nurses are expected to be self-directed learners (ANA, 2000). They are supposed to recognize their own learning needs and actively participate in educational experiences that will maintain their professional competence in current nursing practice (ANA, 2000, 2014). Nurses have a professional responsibility to keep abreast of the Nurse Practice Act in the state or states in which they practice. Nurses are expected to demonstrate continuing competency using a variety of methods and assessment options, which will be discussed later in this chapter.

Professional Nursing Associations and Organizations

Professional nursing associations and organizations assume a leadership role in creating strategies to verify nursing competence (ANA, 2014). ANA also assumes responsibility for the continuing competence of nurses through its involvement in the legislative and health policy arenas, CE and nursing certification efforts, and research (ANA, 2000). In *Nursing: Scope and Standards of Practice*, ANA identified six standards of practice (Standard 5 has two subsections) and 11 standards of professional performance that all RNs are expected to demonstrate depending on their work setting, role, patient population, and specialty (ANA, 2015).

The standards of practice describe a "competent level of nursing care as demonstrated by the critical-thinking model known as the nursing process" (ANA, 2015, p. 4), while the standards of professional performance delineate the "competent level of behavior in the professional role" (p. 5). Figure 4-1 illustrates the key concepts included in both sets of standards. Specific competencies listed within each of these 17 standards offer examples of how nurses can comply with each standard (ANA, 2015). Additionally, higher-level competencies are included for advanced practice nurses (APNs) and nurses prepared at the graduate level. Although not inclusive, these competencies can assist NPDSs and unit-based educators in determining sources of evidence regarding nursing performance. Standard 12: Education states that an RN "seeks knowledge and competence that reflects current nursing practice and promotes futuristic thinking" (ANA, 2015, p. 5). This standard includes 12 competencies that address the expectation that nurses should engage in ongoing educational offerings and commit to lifelong learning initiatives. APNs are also expected to strengthen their performance by integrating research and other evidence-based resources into their practice.

Many specialty nursing organizations, such as ONS (Brant & Wickham, 2013), have developed standards of practice for their generalist and advanced practice. ONS standards, similar to those of ANA, emphasize the individual nurse's responsibility in attaining and maintaining continuing competence, especially in light of the rapid changes in cancer care and technology. This commitment to lifelong learning also is emphasized in ONS's position statement Lifelong Learning for Professional Oncology Nurses, which offers oncology nurses 12 strategies to become engaged in lifelong learning throughout their careers (ONS, 2014). These strategies include precepting and mentoring novice nurses, sharing expertise via presentations at professional conferences, writing for publication, obtaining certification in oncology, and continually assessing personal learning needs (ONS, 2014). In addition, ONS sponsors CE activities

---

Figure 4-1. Standards of Professional Nursing Practice

Standards of Practice	Standards of Professional Performance

• Assessment
• Diagnosis
• Outcomes identification
• Planning
• Implementation
  – Coordination of care
  – Health teaching and health promotion
• Evaluation
	• Ethics
	• Culturally congruent practice
	• Communication
	• Collaboration
	• Leadership
	• Education
	• Evidence-based practice and research
	• Quality of practice
	• Professional practice evaluation
	• Resource utilization
	• Environmental health

Note. Based on information from American Nurses Association, 2015.

and provides various learning materials and opportunities to help oncology nurses maintain or develop the knowledge, skills, and values that are essential in cancer care. The Oncology Nursing Certification Corporation, the certifying corporation of ONS, provides opportunities for oncology nurses to demonstrate competency through its certification process.

Nursing Employers

Healthcare organizations that employ nurses are responsible for establishing a work environment that makes it possible for patients to receive safe, quality care from competent nursing staff (ANA, 2014). Hospitals can use various strategies to accomplish this goal, such as offering sufficient staffing on clinical units, sponsoring professional development and CE programs for nurses to maintain and develop their competencies, and providing a process to assess and validate nursing competencies (ANA, 2000).

Accreditation Agencies

Accreditation agencies, such as the Joint Commission, also take responsibility for ensuring the continuing competency of nurses (ANA, 2014). The mission of the Joint Commission (n.d.) is "to continuously improve health care for the public, in collaboration with other stakeholders, by evaluating healthcare organizations and inspiring them to excel in providing safe and effective care of the highest quality and value" (para. 2). The Joint Commission supports improved performance by establishing accreditation standards that address competence. Hospitals voluntarily seeking accreditation from the Joint Commission need to comply with these standards. Each standard is accompanied by an intent that explains the rationale and significance of the standard and ways that hospitals can demonstrate the standard. For example, one of the Joint Commission's Human Resources standards requires staff to engage in ongoing training and education to develop or maintain competencies related to the care needs of the patient population of their healthcare organization (Joint Commission, 2015). This standard details specific training topics associated with the safety priorities of the Joint Commission, such as team communication, collaboration, coordination of care, unanticipated adverse events, fall reduction, deteriorating patient condition, and change in staff responsibilities (Joint Commission, 2015).

Another standard states that "staff are competent to perform their responsibilities" (Joint Commission, 2015). Staff competency should be assessed upon hire, during orientation, and on an ongoing basis as determined by the hospital's policies and procedures, although the Joint Commission mandates competency assessment once every three years after hire (Joint Commission, 2015). This standard also addresses the qualifications of the person who conducts the assessment, possible assessment methods used in the process, and the hospital's obligation to manage staff who do not meet competency requirements (Joint Commission, 2015).

Regulatory Agencies

Regulatory agencies, such as the licensing establishments within the National Council of State Boards of Nursing (NCSBN) jurisdiction, aim to protect the public by determining the minimum competency of new graduate nurses (ANA, 2014; NCSBN, 2012). State boards of nursing ensure that "standards of nursing practice are met and nurses are competent in their practice" (ANA, 2012, p. 3). These boards issue licenses to graduate nurses who successfully pass the National Council Licensure Examination (NCLEX-RN), designed to measure the "competencies needed to perform safely and effectively as a newly licensed, entry-level registered nurse" (NCSBN, 2012, p. 3). The NCLEX-RN examination is based on an analysis of the current practice of entry-level nurses (NCSBN, 2012).

Boards also grant relicensure to RNs who meet respective state requirements for continuing competency, assuring the public that nurses remain current in their practice (American Nurses

Credentialing Center [ANCC], n.d.-c). These requirements often include a predetermined number of contact hours awarded through participation in CE programs (see Chapter 13). As of 2014, 36 states required mandatory CE for RNs to maintain their licenses (ANCC, n.d.-c).

In addition to NCSBN, the Occupational Safety and Health Administration (OSHA) within the U.S. Department of Labor also supports the need for staff competency with safety guidelines and resources for healthcare organizations (OSHA, n.d.). These guidelines protect nurses from injuring themselves while they provide patient care. Expectations exist that nurses will properly use equipment, such as a mechanical lift, and function safely and without injury in the work setting (OSHA, n.d.).

The Orientation Component of Nursing Professional Development

Chapter 2 provided an overview of the orientation component of the NPDS practice model (ANA & NNSDO, 2010). The orientation process provides newly employed nurses with information and experiences to function effectively in their assigned roles within an organization (ANA, 2000). Accreditation agencies, such as the Joint Commission, require hospitals to provide an orientation for their staff (Joint Commission, 2015).

Easing the transition of newly licensed nurses from the student role to that of a practicing professional nurse through transition-to-practice models has been an ongoing focus of experts at NCSBN (Spector & Echternacht, 2010) and with faculty in schools of nursing (Foster, Benavides-Vaello, Katz, & Eide, 2012). In 2010, Spector and Echternacht proposed a national, evidence-based model to be put into effect through regulation, citing similar international programs that existed in nursing and other healthcare professions. With similar intentions to ease the transition for newly hired nurses, Foster et al. (2012) designed the Generative Leadership Model, which guided curriculum changes at their school of nursing. These changes were intended to better prepare students to cope with work-related issues that often resulted in burnout and job turnover. Key elements of the model included "embracing paradox, seeking ambiguity, and reframing" (Foster et al., 2012, p. 253). The authors also offered recommendations for nurse educators framed within the model.

Newly graduated nurses often comprise a large portion of nurses who participate in nursing orientation activities; however, experienced nurses may attend an orientation program if they change jobs, alter their roles or responsibilities within the same organization, or are assigned to a new clinical unit or department. NPDSs and unit-based educators may be responsible for developing orientation programs for individuals at their organization or for members of the professional community (ANA, 2000). The specific learning needs of each of these groups of orientees will be discussed later in this chapter.

Jeffery and Jarvis (2014) offered a different perspective, using the terms *orientation* and *onboarding* when referring to new employees. For these authors, orientation designates an event that a newly hired nurse participates in upon being hired by an organization, whereas onboarding refers to a process that begins once the nurse first accepts the position.

Purposes of Orientation

Orientations focus on three main purposes: competency, socialization, and role transition (ANA, 2000). As stated earlier, the primary emphasis of an orientation is assessing, validating, and developing specific competencies needed for nurses to function effectively in their roles (ANA, 2000). Orientation socializes new employees to a work environment and helps orientees understand what is expected of them. These programs also help ease the transition from student to professional.

Orientations also play an important role in helping healthcare organizations recruit and retain nurses (Crimlisk, McNulty, & Francione, 2002; Krugman et al., 2006; Pine & Tart, 2007). Newly hired nurses who experience educational support, guidance, and a positive work environment may be more likely to stay at an organization than those who have a negative experience upon hire (Crimlisk et al., 2002). The availability of a well-developed orientation program guided by experienced preceptors also may encourage nurses to seek employment at a particular organization.

Competency-Based Orientation Programs

Given the national emphasis on delivering safe, quality care to consumers and cost-effective, outcome-focused education to providers, some healthcare organizations prefer a competency-based approach, rather a traditional time-based method, when orienting new employees. In a traditional time-based program, orientees progress through a preplanned orientation schedule with a start and end date that varies based on setting (Jeffery & Jarvis, 2014). At the conclusion of the program, orientees who have not demonstrated the expected behaviors may be provided an extended orientation period, with reevaluation at the end.

Conversely, a competency-based orientation (CBO) not only varies in length based on orientees and their learning needs (Jeffery & Jarvis, 2014) but also focuses on the outcomes expected of orientees rather than what knowledge they possess about performing their job (Alspach, 1996). The outcome of a CBO is the ability of orientees to carry out the specific responsibilities defined in their position descriptions (Abruzzese, 1996). Jeffery and Jarvis (2014) advocated for CBOs that provide a more individualized, effective learning experience during orientation, believing that this approach may result in more competent nurses.

In a CBO, the healthcare organization determines a set of competencies (knowledge, skills, or values) that all orientees must adequately demonstrate before they are considered qualified to provide safe, quality care to patients without the supervision of a preceptor (Alspach, 1996). Demonstration of these competencies indicates that the orientee has successfully completed orientation (Jeffery & Jarvis, 2014). It is important to realize that selected nurse competencies are assessed on an ongoing basis after the orientation period.

A variety of competency programs have been reported in the nursing literature. Whereas some programs have focused on strengthening nursing care received by age-specific groups of patients (e.g., adults, children) (Beauman, 2001), others have dealt with specialty units, such as emergency departments (Gurney, 2002; Proehl, 2002), critical care units (Leonard & Plotnikoff, 2000), and medical or oncology units (Johnson, Opfer, VanCura, & Williams, 2000). Some organizations have developed competencies in specific areas, such as genetics (Jenkins, 2002) and culturally congruent care (Leonard & Plotnikoff, 2000), that support the goals of the healthcare organization.

Culley et al. (2012) produced an innovative, learner-centered orientation setting that resembled an academic setting and focused on reducing patient errors and strengthening nurse retention. "Nursing U" combined two hours of classroom sessions (each focused on a single topic) with another two hours of hands-on experience in a simulation lab. Results revealed participant satisfaction, improved retention at 82% after six months (previously 69% for newly hired nurses who attended the traditional orientation), and reduced patient errors (Culley et al., 2012).

In some healthcare organizations orientees may progress through a CBO at different rates (Amerson, 2002; Jeffery & Jarvis, 2014). Once orientees attain specific competencies, they advance to the next phase of the orientation program, which includes a new list of competencies to demonstrate. Orientees are expected to attend additional educational activities for competencies they are unable to adequately demonstrate.

The benefits of using the Performance-Based Development System (PBDS), a commercially produced, customized competency assessment tool, were reported in the nursing literature during the 1980s and 1990s (Performance Management Services, 2012). The tool is still available for use today. Based on a model originally developed by del Bueno in 1985, PBDS focuses on management and clinical competencies using criterion-based performance standards. PBDS describes competency as having three overlapping dimensions applied within the context of a given situation: critical-thinking skills, interpersonal skills, and technical skills (Anthony & del Bueno, 1993).

In this system, both new and experienced nurses must demonstrate their competencies in assessment centers during orientation before they can provide direct patient care on the clinical units. Within a particular specialty (i.e., medical-surgical, neonatal intensive care, obstetrics, critical care), various methods are used to assess competency in critical thinking, interpersonal relations, and technical skills (Anthony & del Bueno, 1993). These computer-based assessment centers actively engage learners through the use of videotaped scenarios, simulations, self-learning packets, and other active learning exercises. Although initial startup may be costly, this system offers the benefit of decreased orientation time for hospitals (Abruzzese, 1996). Despite reports that address the psychometric properties of PBDS (del Bueno, 1990, 1994, 2001, 2005; Whelan, 2006) and its use by more than 500 hospitals over the past 25 years (Performance Management Services, 2012), critics have identified the need for stronger research evidence to support the system's psychometric value in assessing critical thinking (AllNurses, 2009).

CBOs offer several advantages to the orientee, preceptor, and healthcare organization. First, by focusing on the learning needs and abilities of individual learners, CBOs allow experienced RNs to demonstrate their fundamental nursing competencies within a short period of time. Newly graduated nurses with less experience have an opportunity to validate familiar competencies and develop new ones at their own pace. Orientees can identify their own strengths and weaknesses based on their performance related to competency evaluation criteria. Although most CBOs do not have specific time limitations, some experts suggest using target dates to help orientees complete the program within a reasonable time period (Abruzzese, 1996).

CBOs also provide preceptors with clearly defined expectations of orientees during their clinical experience on the unit (Abruzzese, 1996). This minimizes the chances of preceptors and other staff providing inconsistent information to orientees.

Finally, because CBOs may reduce the amount of time that experienced orientees spend in orientation, these programs can offer a cost savings to healthcare organizations (Abruzzese, 1996). The competency statements and critical behaviors recorded as part of the orientees' competency validation process provide organizations with a performance document, or evidence that orientees demonstrated safe, quality care at the time of assessment (Abruzzese, 1996). This recording system also complies with Joint Commission standards.

CBOs may also pose some challenges. For example, preceptors need to be familiar with the main concepts of CBOs and consistently hold orientees to the same performance outcomes (Alspach, 1996). Also, although each clinical unit within a healthcare organization may identify unique competencies based on their needs, all clinical units within that organization should use a similar format and approach to verify competencies. The majority of competencies should also focus on essential high-risk procedures, despite their volume.

Implementing Competencies in an Orientation Program

Demonstrating nursing competencies is a very familiar practice for newly graduated nurses. Prior to graduating from their prelicensure RN programs, nursing students must attain particular outcomes or competencies (knowledge, skills, and values) outlined in national curriculum standards published by professional nursing organizations (American Association of Colleges of Nursing, 2008; National League for Nursing [NLN], 2012) and in school program outcomes. Nurses enrolled in APN programs are also expected to attain specific program outcomes (American Association of Colleges of Nursing, 2011; NLN, 2012). Although newly graduated nurses must pass the NCLEX-RN as a means of demonstrating minimal competency as a beginning practitioner (NCSBN, 2012), passing does not ensure complete competency (Cooper, 2002).

Upon employment, newly graduated RNs continue a lifelong journey of professional development by participating in the various throughputs included in the NPDS model (ANA & NNSDO, 2010). Although these nurses demonstrated select competencies prior to being employed, their competencies need to be validated and further developed upon hire. Employers also require more experienced RNs to validate competencies during orientation to verify that they can function safely in their roles.

Before implementing a CBO program at your healthcare organization, you will need to identify core competencies that you expect all nurses to successfully demonstrate by the end of orientation or at various points during the orientation process. You will need to develop a process to evaluate or validate these competencies and provide nurses with various learning options they can use to develop or strengthen these competencies.

Identifying Core Competencies

Identifying core competencies is the first step in developing a CBO program (Alspach, 1996) and is a process similar to that used by faculty in schools of nursing when they design a new curriculum for an academic program or revise a current one. Ideas for competencies can come from a variety of sources, such as nursing staff, the healthcare organization, external experts, and professional nursing organizations. Use a variety of methods to retrieve this information, including literature reviews, interviews or focus groups with key stakeholders, surveys, and internal and external aggregated data that may be available. Wright (2005, 2015) suggested identifying competencies based on new, changing, high-risk, or problematic aspects of one's position within an organization.

Once identified, organize these competencies in order of their importance within the context of ensuring safe, quality patient care at your healthcare organization.

Nursing Staff

Nursing staff members are excellent resources for identifying competencies that should be included in an orientation program (Exstrom, 2001). Because nurse managers evaluate nursing staff and manage patient care issues on the unit, they are in a prime position to identify competencies that are vital to safe, quality patient care. Results of patient satisfaction surveys, quality assurance reports, policies and procedures, and incident reports often provide ideas for competencies.

Nurses in leadership roles can be instrumental in identifying competencies needed by staff nurses as well as future leaders. Strong, Kane, Petras, Johnson-Joy, and Weingarten (2014) surveyed nurse leaders and direct care nurses to gain their perspectives regarding competencies needed by clinical nurses to provide safe, quality patient care. The survey included 10 competencies adapted from the Massachusetts Department of Higher Education's (2010) *Nurse of the Future: Nursing Core Competencies*: leadership, informatics and technology, therapeutic communication, evidence-based practice, quality improvement, patient-centered care, professionalism, systems-based practice, teamwork and collaboration, and safety.

Data obtained from this gap analysis also were used for NPD purposes. Results obtained from more than 60 nurses revealed that the informatics and technology competency was perceived by clinical nurses as being more "appropriate, important, and incorporated into their practice" than nurse leaders perceived it (Strong et al., 2014, pp. 199–200). Also, participants with a baccalaureate degree or higher considered the patient-centered care and informatics and technology competencies as being "more appropriate and important" (p. 199) than did nurses with a degree lower than baccalaureate. Strong et al. emphasized the need to expand the focus from psychomotor skills of competencies to a more comprehensive perspective using application of evidence-based knowledge and skills and "managing patient-centered care" (p. 196).

NPDSs and unit-based educators also play an important role in determining baseline competencies that orientees must demonstrate before the conclusion of an orientation. Competencies should reflect expectations outlined in a nurse's job description and also can include those identified through past orientations and other sources of evidence.

As a unit-based educator, you should encourage nursing staff on your clinical unit to identify the specific competencies that orientees need to demonstrate before the conclusion of a unit-based orientation. Wright (2015) believed that a competency model should include competencies that matter to an organization and its employees; incorporate appropriate strategies for verification; define the roles and responsibilities of the nurse being assessed, the educator, and the manager; and foster a "culture of engagement and commitment" (p. 5) during "employee-centered competency verification" (p. 5). The Wright Competency Assessment Model advises educators to foster a work culture that supports success by addressing key components in competency assessment programs: ownership, empowerment, and accountability (Wright, 2015). For example, NPDSs should help nurses assume "ownership of the competency assessment process" (Wright, 2015, p. 6). They also can empower nurses by placing them at the "center of the verification process for competency assessment" (Wright, 2015, p. 8) and creating a supportive work environment in which nurses are held accountable for attaining their competencies in a timely, ongoing fashion.

Cooper (2002) described an approach in which all nursing staff had input in identifying the competencies required for their unit's orientation program. A group of staff nurses from diverse levels brainstormed possible competencies that they believed new nurses should possess at the completion of orientation. They ranked these competencies by importance and sought input from other unit staff before developing the details of these competencies and determining ways to evaluate them. Obtaining input from staff on all shifts may be helpful in capturing time-specific competencies related to patient care.

Accreditation and Regulatory Agencies

Many accreditation and regulatory agencies provide guidance related to staff competencies. Therefore, it is important for NPDSs and unit-based educators to familiarize themselves with current standards and guidelines and be alert for new or changing opportunities for their healthcare organizations. Speak with leaders at your healthcare organization to gain their perspectives regarding these sources.

Joint Commission: This agency shares in the responsibility of ensuring safe, quality nursing care through published accreditation standards (Joint Commission, 2015). The Joint Commission allows hospitals to identify their own competencies expected of staff based on job responsibilities (Joint Commission, 2015). However, it advises hospitals to take into account the "needs of its patient population, the types of procedures conducted, conditions or diseases treated, and the kinds of equipment it uses" (Joint Commission, 2015). Hospitals are required to assess, validate, and appraise the competencies of their nursing staff beginning at orientation and at least once every three years, unless hospital policy dictates assessment more often (Joint Commission, 2015). Hospitals are expected to determine their own patient safety content and ensure that staff are competent (Joint Commission, 2015). Content may include topics such as fire and life safety, security, hazardous materials and waste, infection control, restraints, medication errors, patient falls, and pain management. Hospitals are required to appropriately manage instances in which staff do not meet required competencies (Joint Commission, 2015). Documentation regarding all Joint Commission requirements is essential.

Because nursing care should be adapted to a patient's age, nurses need to demonstrate age-specific competencies (Joint Commission, 2015). For example, a nurse should consider the age of a cardiac arrest victim (i.e., infant, child, or adult) when providing cardiopulmonary resuscitation (CPR).

Hospitals have the flexibility to determine the age ranges and labels for each age-specific group they recognize (Cooper, 2002). For example, a pediatric hospital may choose to designate age ranges with categories such as neonate, infant, toddler, preschool, school age, adolescent, and adult.

Although the Joint Commission allows hospitals to determine their own safety competencies and validation frequencies for staff after orientation, it does mandate specific topics during orientation and ongoing CE offerings (Joint Commission, 2015).

Wright (2015) stated that it is an organization's responsibility to not only define what competency means within its environment but also to create a competency assessment plan that begins during orientation and continues on an ongoing basis. In addition, the organization must address employees who do not successfully meet expected competencies and document these cases.

Occupational Safety and Health Administration: OSHA supports a safe and healthy work environment through standards and education (OSHA, n.d.). OSHA's protective standards can be a valuable source of expected competencies for nurses and other healthcare workers. These topics may overlap with those of the Joint Commission and include job safety and health, protective equipment, blood-borne pathogens, emergency evacuation, ergonomics, and hazardous chemicals.

American Nurses Credentialing Center Nursing Skills Competency Program: ANCC offers accreditation for skills programs offered by various constituents, such as schools of nursing, hospitals, state nurses associations, companies that produce healthcare products, and simulation centers (ANCC, n.d.-b). This voluntary accreditation serves as an "independent national standard to measure the quality of courses designed to validate a nurse's skill or skill set in the clinical setting" (ANCC, n.d.-b, para.1).

Organizations that seek ANCC accreditation need to comply with specific criteria, including program design, curriculum, teaching-learning methods, reliability and validity of testing methods, outcomes criteria, and qualifications of faculty who evaluate learner performance (ANCC, 2015). The program can target anyone from nursing students to experienced RNs working in specialty practice areas (ANCC, n.d.-b). According to ANCC, current accredited skills programs focused on specialty topics include cardiovascular care, renal replacements, breast-feeding and lactation, chemotherapy, intrathecal care, and dysrhythmias (ANCC, n.d.-a).

ANCC's Nursing Skills Competency Program offers advantages to various stakeholders, including nurses who successfully pass this proficiency standard, healthcare employers, NPDSs, schools of nursing, faculty who can offer quality education and training based on a national performance benchmark, and patients who receive care (ANCC, n.d.-b). Nurses may transfer their competency validation among employers and obtain partial contact hours for completing the course (ANCC, n.d.-b). According to ANCC, this accreditation offers cost savings to organizations, decreases the chance of clinical errors, and strengthens patient outcomes (ANCC, n.d.-b). The process is fee-based and reviewed by a panel of experts.

Professional Nursing Organizations

Many professional nursing organizations, especially those with a clinical specialty focus, have developed field-related core competencies for beginning and advanced practice roles. For example, ONS has published several sets of role-based core competencies for oncology nurses (ONS, n.d.-b). These competencies range from oncology nursing core competencies to high-level practice roles, such as nurse navigators, clinical trial nurses, nurse practitioners, clinical nurse specialists, and general leadership.

Research and Other Sources of Evidence

Consider investigating other sources of evidence that may help you identify competencies for newly hired and currently employed nurses, such as published research studies, integrative reviews, and organization-specific quality improvement data. Evaluate each study's level of evidence, how its setting compares with that of your organization, and how its purpose aligns with your patient population and services (see Chapter 12). If appropriate, replicate some of the studies at your organization. Similarly, consult with experts in quality improvement and research departments at your organization or local school of nursing who can help you interpret the study results and data sources or collect additional data to capture needs specific to your healthcare organization. Theisen and Sandau (2013), for example, reviewed 26 studies published from 2000 to 2012 to identify essential psychomotor and cognitive competencies needed by newly graduated nurses for a nurse residency program. Although only five of the studies included quasi-experimental, experimental, or meta-analysis designs, the results revealed six key competencies: communication, leadership, organization (prioritization and time management), critical thinking and clinical reasoning, specific situations, and stress management. Theisen and Sandau (2013) also recommended evidence-based interventions, such as "nurse residency programs, simulation, debriefing, preceptorships, and the use of valid measurement tools" (p. 412) for healthcare organizations and schools of nursing.

Some healthcare organizations have adopted and tested models to guide identification of nurse competencies in clinical practice. Nearly two decades ago, the American Association of Critical-Care Nurses developed the Synergy Model for Patient Care to connect clinical nursing practice with patient outcomes (American Association of Critical-Care Nurses, 2014a). This model guides certification examination and the performance of nurses employed in acute and critical care clinical settings (American Association of Critical-Care Nurses, 2014a). It consists of eight patient characteristics (needs), such as vulnerability and complexity, and a separate set of eight nurse competencies, such as clinical judgment and response to diversity. Each component comprises several levels that increase in complexity. The basic premise of this model is that quality patient care outcomes result when patient and nurse elements are appropriately matched. According to the American Association of Critical-Care Nurses (2014a), patient needs determine the specific competencies of nurses and synergy results when the needs and characteristics of a patient, clinical unit, or system are matched with a nurse's competencies.

This model also has been used to guide various initiatives within healthcare organizations, such as preceptor programs, nursing rounds, performance evaluations, and clinical advancement programs (American Association of Critical-Care Nurses, 2014b). In addition, schools of nursing have adopted the model to formulate undergraduate program outcomes (competencies), curriculum, teaching-learning strategies, and evaluation processes (Zungolo & Leonardo, 2007).

Prioritizing and Organizing Competencies

After you identify a list of competencies that newly hired nurses need to demonstrate before completing their orientation period, prioritize this list in order of importance based on work setting and the populations served at your healthcare organization. Also, identify and prioritize key competencies that nurses must demonstrate thereafter on an annual basis. Consider risk, volume, and problem areas when ranking your competencies (Cooper, 2002).

Depending on your organization, duties included in a job description may be the starting point, as well as annual competencies mandated by accreditation and regulatory agencies. Because the clinical practice setting is a dynamic environment, it is important to systematically review these competencies and modify them based on new requirements or changes in practice. Many healthcare organizations focus on nurses' job expectations and include both high-risk, high-volume and high-risk, low-volume competencies congruent with the organization's standards, policies, and procedures (Krozek & Scoggins, 2000).

High-risk, high-volume competencies are those (knowledge, skills, and attitudes) that can cause serious damage to patients or nurses if performed incorrectly. If a nurse performs this high-risk competency every day (high-volume), then it should be included among the baseline competencies demonstrated during orientation, rather than in an annual competency review (Cooper, 2002). Some organizations refer to these as *essential competencies*. For example, nurses who work on a surgical head and neck unit perform tracheostomy care every day. If they do not perform it correctly, then the patient may experience difficulty breathing, a condition that may greatly worsen over time. Nurses on this unit should demonstrate this skill as part of their unit-based orientation program. Because these nurses perform tracheostomy care daily, this competency may not be included in their annual competency review.

High-risk, low-volume competencies are those (knowledge, skills, and attitudes) that could pose harm to a patient if a nurse performs them incorrectly but are not often conducted on the clinical unit (Cooper, 2002). These competencies may be reviewed during an annual competency assessment to ensure that nurses will be able to perform these skills when the situation arises. For example, some patients admitted to a surgical head and neck unit require chest tubes after surgery. This event does not occur often, but when it does, unit nurses need to know how to safely care for these patients. If a nurse does not perform this care appropriately, patients could suffer serious consequences, including death. You may decide to include this competency during orientation, but, at minimum, it should be included in an annual review.

Some competency ideas arise from internal sources, such as incident and quality assurance reports (Cooper, 2002) or other data sources. For example, a clinical unit may have had several medication errors related to incorrect dosage calculations or a high incidence of wound infections in postoperative patients. These incidents may require investigation into their causes and warrant further education of staff through in-service educational or CE programs.

Wright (2015) further classified high-risk, low volume skills into those that are time sensitive versus those that are not. A time-sensitive skill needs to be performed very quickly, as it needs to become an automatic behavior (e.g., performing CPR) (Wright, 2015). Conversely, in situations where skills are considered high-risk, low volume but not time sensitive, nurses often have the luxury of time to prepare for that skill; however, their correct performance is vital, as indicated in Wright's (2015) example of preparing a high-risk medication drip. The author advised incorporating these latter skills into the procedure itself, rather than annually assessing nursing performance.

Writing Competency Statements and Evaluation Criteria

After organizing your list of competencies, you will need to format them in a way that conveys a clear understanding to both learners and evaluators. Although there may be some differences, a competency generally consists of a competency statement with a set of evaluation criteria. These criteria may also be called *critical behaviors* (Cooper, 2002), *performance criteria* or *statements* (Alspach, 1996), or *measurement criteria* in some scope and standards documents (ANA, 2015; ANA & NNSDO, 2010; Brant & Wickham, 2013). After drafting the competency statements and evaluation criteria, consider what strategies would be most appropriate to use for the learner to demonstrate the competencies.

As you draft competencies for nurses within your organization, consider reviewing competency examples written by national organizations. For example, ANA's *Nursing: Scope and Standards of Practice* lists competencies that all professional nurses must be able to perform (ANA, 2015). Its first standard, Assessment, begins with this descriptive statement: "The registered nurse collects pertinent data and information relative to the healthcare consumer's health or the situation" (p. 53). The competency delineated under this standard is as follows: "Uses evidence-based assessment techniques, instruments, tools, available data, information, and knowledge relevant to the situation to identify patterns and variances" (ANA, 2015, p. 54). According to ANA, competencies linked to each standard provide evaluators with possible evidence of the nurse's compliance with that particular standard. ONS, ANA, and NNSDO used a similar format in their respective scope and standards of practice publications (ANA & NNSDO, 2010; Brant & Wickham, 2013). However, these sources use the label *measurement criteria* rather than *competencies* when listing examples of evidence for standards.

Competency Statements

A competency statement describes specific knowledge, skills, or attitudes (outcomes) that an orientee needs to attain or demonstrate (Cooper, 2002). For example, a competency statement targeted toward orientees assigned to a surgical head and neck unit may read, "Conducts an accurate respiratory assessment in a patient with a total laryngectomy."

Evaluation Criteria

The second part of a competency consists of a set of evaluation criteria that describe behaviors or actions that need to be demonstrated as "evidence of competency" (Alspach, 1996, p. 89). In an orientation program, preceptors are often responsible for observing these behaviors and determining if an orientee's performance is acceptable. In other organizations, unit-based educators or NPDSs may validate a set of core competencies in a skills laboratory or clinical setting for a group of orientees. Evaluation criteria for the head and neck competency statement mentioned earlier may include the following: "Develops a plan of care that includes assessing these potential complications of surgery: airway obstruction, bleeding from the surgical incision, wound infection, fistula formation, and fluid and electrolyte problems."

Rather than stating the particular aspects of the assessment, the criteria may instead refer the reader to a set of hospital-based standards of care or policies where the plan of care is specifically outlined, such as "Develops a plan of care that includes the critical assessments according to the General Hospital Standards of Nursing Care for Postoperative Head and Neck Oncology Patients."

Evaluation criteria often include several elements (Alspach, 1996). For example, each criterion must be learner centered and describe a single behavior in measurable and observable terms (Alspach, 1996). Critical behaviors should begin with an action verb. Each criterion should be described clearly enough so that the orientee and evaluator (preceptor) will understand the specific behavior that is being evaluated (Alspach, 1996). Criteria also need to include any conditions that may be placed on an orientee's performance as well as a performance standard that provides the preceptor a baseline against which the orientee's behavior can be deemed acceptable (Alspach, 1996). A standard may require the orientee to perform an expected behavior within the first 15 minutes of the patient's arrival to the clinical unit after surgery. Only the key aspects of the behavior should be included in performance criteria (Alspach, 1996).

Assessing and Evaluating the Competencies of Nurses

After identifying specific core competencies essential for delivering safe, quality patient care, explore available methods that will allow nurses to accurately convey their ability to integrate knowledge, skills, abilities, and judgment (ANA, 2015). Remember that the purpose of competency assessment is to determine if nurses are able to demonstrate specific skills and apply knowledge to their assigned patient care responsibilities as expected (Joint Commission, 2015). While the Joint Commission (2015) indicated that assessment methods "may include test taking, return demonstration, or the use of simulation" (p. 7), Wright (2005) advocated providing nurses with more than one assessment method to accommodate preferred learning styles. Because competencies are considered to be "situational and dynamic" (ANA, 2015, p. 44), it is important that their inclusion is reevaluated over time based on available evidence. ANA (2015) noted that one single evaluation approach cannot ensure competence.

Wright (2015) recommended careful consideration when choosing validators to verify an employee's competence and suggested limiting their use for assessing technical skills that require return demonstrations. Rather than using educators or managers as validators, the author proposed actively engaging the nurses themselves in the verification process by allowing them to present evidence to support their competence.

Consider accessing commercially produced evidence-based educational resources, such as those available from ONS's Educator Resource Center (ERC) (ONS, n.d.-a). This subscription-based website contains many resources that NPDSs can incorporate into their competency-based orientation program for an oncology setting or an ongoing competency assessment series for new and experienced oncology RNs. Teaching-learning resources include slideshows, learner handouts and assessments, case studies, educator guides, journal articles, and skill development tools. Commercial products are available that contain policies and procedures with customizable clinical templates, forms, checklists, and other documents that can be used for accreditation, such as the one published by ONS (Esparza, 2014).

Cardiopulmonary Resuscitation as an Example

As you explore methods to assess clinical competencies, it may be helpful to reflect upon the current competency process required by the American Heart Association (AHA) regarding CPR (Field et al., 2010). Because learning CPR, according to AHA standards, is a common mandatory competency for all healthcare workers, it is easily accessible to learners.

Ongoing research regarding resuscitation efforts that result in the best patient outcomes provides AHA with a high level of evidence to establish their CPR curriculum standards, policies and procedures, and specific competencies. These are outlined in the *American Heart*

Association Guidelines for Cardiopulmonary Resuscitation and Emergency Cardiovascular Care Sciences (Field et al., 2010).

The process required to become certified is clearly stated for designated CPR instructors and interested learners. For example, learners must participate in an approved educational program offered either face-to-face or online. Following the program, the learners must use their cognitive skills to successfully pass a written, valid, and reliable examination created by AHA and based on course objectives. After passing the examination, learners must demonstrate their psychomotor skills by performing CPR on a mannequin resembling an adult, child, or infant, depending on the type of course. This activity often occurs in a laboratory or classroom setting.

This model may vary in fidelity depending on available resources. During the demonstration process, learners need to respond appropriately to questions based on various emergency scenarios.

Evaluators are required to be competent in CPR and formally trained as AHA CPR instructors. These evaluators use several checklists developed by AHA to rate the observed performance of learners. These checklists include specific skills and steps, critical performance criteria, and descriptors. The evaluator records whether each step was correctly demonstrated by the learner and signs and dates the form. If the learner did not perform the steps according to expectations, the evaluator recommends and documents specific remediation. The learner must successfully complete the performance according to the checklist. Learners and instructors have an opportunity to evaluate their overall experience after completing the session.

In the CPR example provided, it is important to note that an AHA standardized educational program with scenarios, a written test, and return demonstrations using a simulated scenario were all used to evaluate competency. Specific evaluation criteria outlined in AHA checklists were used to evaluate performance. Careful documentation was recorded, filed, and tracked by the evaluators over time. Participants received a wallet card indicating that they successfully completed the cognitive and skills evaluation according to AHA standards. The card includes an issue date and a date of recommended renewal.

Think about the process of evaluation that was used during CPR training as you plan your competencies for nurses during and after orientation. The following section will provide a brief review of some possible assessment methods to consider.

Written Tests

Written examinations may be used by some educators to assess competencies that are cognitive (knowledge-based) in nature (Exstrom, 2001). If written tests are needed to assess particular competencies, some educators suggest using them for only a portion of the orientees' assessment. Oermann and Gaberson (2014) recommended using context-dependent test items to evaluate the cognitive skills of learners. Rather than requiring the nurse to memorize certain terms, these items include some form of introductory information that test-takers must analyze and problem solve related to clinical practice.

Return Demonstrations (Checklists)

Because most competencies focus on specific behaviors that orientees must demonstrate, performance checklists can be used to evaluate the attainment of these competencies (Alspach, 1996). Preceptors may use checklists as a standard guide to assess orientees' behaviors as they care for patients on the clinical unit or in a setting that simulates a clinical unit.

However, Wright (2015) emphasized that checklists can be used in two different ways. First, a checklist can be used as a "competency verification method" (p. 23), as when observing a nurse's return demonstration in performing a technical skill. The author noted that these types of checklists tend to be used too often and advised educators to use them appropriately. Second, a checklist can be used as a step-like list to follow each time a nurse performs a procedure that requires high-risk, low volume skills that are not time-sensitive (Wright, 2015). The use of the latter checklist is not intended for verification of competencies.

For example, a preceptor can observe an orientee performing a dressing change on a real patient on the clinical unit or on a mannequin in a nursing skills laboratory. The clinical unit is the preferred setting for assessing competencies because it best reflects an orientee's ability to function appropriately in the clinical setting (Alspach, 1996).

Performance checklists may vary among healthcare organizations and usually include a table or grid format (Alspach, 1996). Similar to the CPR checklist, most checklists contain a competency statement and associated evaluation criteria with space for the preceptor to document the method used and the orientee's performance. Although the assessment should indicate whether the behavior was observed, it should not reflect a rating or a grade (Alspach, 1996). The preceptor should sign and date each observed criterion, indicating he or she observed the orientee demonstrating the behavior appropriately on that specific date. This does not guarantee continuing competency.

Rather than checklists, Frentsos (2013) recommended rubrics to assess competency, acknowledging their value and popularity with faculty in academic courses. Suskie (2009) described a rubric as a "scoring guide" that educators can use to evaluate or assign a grade to a learner's performance. Some rubrics include a "list or chart that describes the criteria" (Suskie, 2009, p. 137) used during the evaluation process (Suskie, 2009). Rubrics are also preferred because of their degree of clarity, accuracy, and alignment with adult learning principles—all appropriate elements for evaluating a nurse's performance. Frentsos (2013) recommended that educators pilot test their rubrics to establish validity and reliability prior to official use.

Simulation

Clinical simulation, an effective means of evaluating student performance in academic courses (Shellenbarger & Hagler, 2015), has become an increasingly popular method of demonstrating competencies of nurses in hospital settings. Simulation can offer a safe, realistic environment that resembles an actual clinical setting. It also provides learners with an opportunity to strengthen not only their simple psychomotor skills (like starting an IV) but also their "clinical reasoning, clinical judgment, problem-solving, and critical-thinking" skills (Shellenbarger & Hagler, 2015, p. 210). Various levels of simulation are available, ranging from traditional low levels that rely on static anatomic models to human high-fidelity mannequins that allow dynamic interaction. Educators need to be trained on how to appropriately use simulation as a teaching strategy and assessment method. They also will need to integrate learner preparation, clear objectives and outcomes, appropriate scenarios, guided reflection, and debriefing into these simulations (Shellenbarger & Hagler, 2015).

Disher et al. (2014) reported positive outcomes in their pilot study that examined the influence of using a unit-based, high-fidelity simulation to help 26 cardiovascular nurses identify and manage deteriorating patients encountered in the clinical setting. This intervention resulted in statistically significant increases in the nurses' knowledge and self-confidence scores measured from baseline to post-program.

Similarly, Hooper (2014) reported that case studies and videotaped vignettes were effective in strengthening the critical-thinking skills of 18 newly hired nurses engaged in a nurse residency program. Statistically significant increases were noted using the Health Sciences Reasoning Test on the first day of the program and after program completion.

In addition to simulations conducted in a skills laboratory setting, some organizations may use commercially prepared, computer-based programs such as PBDS, which focuses on critical-thinking and interpersonal and technical skills (Anthony & del Bueno, 1993).

Documenting Competencies, Credentials, and Qualifications

Documenting the results of competency assessments during and after orientation, per hospital policy, is an essential element included in Joint Commission (2015) standards. Any actions taken with individuals who do not successfully complete their competency validation, such as remediation and reassessment, also need to be recorded and tracked. Hospitals are responsible for ensuring that nursing staff competence is evaluated, maintained, demonstrated, followed, and continually strengthened (Joint Commission, 2015). The nurse manager, NPDSs, unit-based educators, and preceptors experienced in assessing competencies may be involved in this major and ongoing responsibility. However, managers assume the ultimate responsibility for ensuring that employees are competent (Jeffery & Jarvis, 2014; Wright, 2015).

Because documenting and tracking validation of competencies for all healthcare workers can be a monumental and continuous task, organizations have relied on technology to document, update, and track these data on a continuous basis. Wright (2015) referred to these available tracking systems as talent management systems and recommended that users determine not only what they want a system to produce but also who will use the system to enter assessment data. Competency and training needs also may be discussed during the employee's performance review (Joint Commission, 2015).

To help manage their hospital's nurse competency assessment process, Dumpe, Kanyok, and Hill (2007) transitioned from a traditional classroom approach to using an online learning management system (LMS) that allowed them to sponsor competency training programs, validate staff performance, and record results. This hospitalwide LMS allowed the authors to modify 24 annual competencies, including many mandatory programs about patient safety, record confidentiality, environment of care, and fire safety. This LMS approach reduced costs associated with educator and staff time, promoted the standardization and timely completion of competencies, and improved stakeholder satisfaction.

In addition to competencies, hospitals need to verify the credentials and qualifications of nurses and other healthcare workers (Joint Commission, 2015; Joint Commission International, 2013). This task may be assumed by the human resources department at a nurse's pre-employment interview or prior to orientation. These credentials and qualifications include evidence of a nurse's education and training, licensure, competence, and experience (Joint Commission, 2015; Joint Commission International, 2013). Credentials and qualifications are based on prerequisites identified in job descriptions. Health screenings and criminal background checks may also be required (Joint Commission, 2015).

Baseline Competencies During Orientation

Depending on the healthcare organization, new nurse employees may attend various orientation sessions such as organizational, departmental, specialty, and unit-based programs. During this orientation period, the organization assesses the nurses' competencies based on specific job duties. Some organizations ask orientees to complete a checklist indicating their familiarity with select skills. Because this checklist represents the perceptions of orientees, these skills need to be validated before assuming competency.

In the event that an orientee does not successfully attain a competency, the preceptor should discuss the situation with the orientee, identify specific learning needs, develop an action plan to remedy deficiencies, and continue to support and guide the orientee. The orientee may need to review the competency through a learning activity or may need the preceptor's support to reduce anxiety experienced while demonstrating the competency. If the orientee does not successfully attain the expected competencies after repeated support, he or she may face dismissal.

A competency-based approach to orientation was studied by Bashford, Shaffer, and Young (2012) to assess knowledge and clinical judgment skills of RNs. While some newly hired nurses may find participating in a competency-based assessment during their orientation period stressful, the study discovered that the perceived value of the competency-based assessment during the first phase of orientation was rated positively by the majority of nurses. This study aligns with suggestions offered by Wright (2005), who recommended making the assessment process an enjoyable experience in which staff have input into the identified competencies within a supportive environment.

In addition to demonstrating competencies during the initial orientation period, new nurse orientees will be required to demonstrate the same or additional competencies on an ongoing, time-specific basis (Joint Commission, 2015). These reviews are frequently scheduled and associated with an employee's annual performance appraisal. If a nurse does not perform satisfactorily during this annual review, an action plan needs to be developed to assist the nurse in strengthening any deficiencies. Although these annual competencies are based on the nurse's job description, they may change each year based on unit priorities such as the introduction of new equipment or findings from incident and quality assurance reports. Wright (2015) recommended including competencies as part of an employee's job description but conducting these reviews in two separately spaced sessions.

After orientation, NPDSs and unit-based educators continually help nurses to acquire, maintain, and increase their competencies through various activities such as in-service educational and CE programs (ANA, 2015). Nurses also can strengthen their competencies through outside CE programs and academic education such as formal programs sponsored by schools of nursing. In addition, nurses can obtain certification in their clinical area through a professional organization that validates qualifications, knowledge, and practice in a specific area of nursing (ANA, 2000).

Aggregate Competence Data, Patterns, and Trends

To obtain the outcomes of competency efforts, it is important to collect and review aggregated data related to patterns and trends so that appropriate interventions can be implemented for quality improvement. The review of aggregated data sources also can identify new competencies and help educators tailor educational programs for targeted nursing groups. For example, hospital-based aggregated data about patient race, ethnicity, and language may call for competencies related to the Joint Commission's focus on cultural competence, communication, and patient- and family-centered care (Joint Commission, 2010). Data can be used to "develop or modify services, programs, or initiatives to meet service population needs" (Joint Commission, 2010, p. 36).

Access to data sources related to competencies may be collected by various departments within the hospital. Selected data might also be collected by the nurse manager or the NPDS with the help of unit-based educators using performance evaluations, performance improvement reports, staff surveys, needs assessments, and outcomes of professional development programs. These data should be analyzed, and patterns and trends should be noted. Remedies for correcting problem areas should be followed by reassessment of competencies to determine the influence of the interventions. More specifically, Wright (2015) suggested using education as a possible remedy only if the problem was the result of a lack of knowledge or skills. The author advised educators to consider other sources that may have contributed to the problem, such as system issues, lack of tools, communication issues, departmental obstacles, and attitude problems. Competency assessment programs can provide evidence that supports cost savings, quality outcomes, and employee performances for healthcare organizations (Wright, 2015).

Establishing a Practical Record-Keeping System

Competency documents, regardless of type, should be considered confidential and treated accordingly in the clinical setting. Such documents should be easily accessible by appropriate individuals, such as nurses, preceptors, unit-based educators, and nurse managers. Information about an orientee's qualifications may be kept in a confidential employee file in the human resources department. A nurse manager also may maintain competency assessments, allowing the manager to access these records for performance evaluations.

As a unit-based educator, you should consider offering a variety of appropriate learning activities that orientees and other nursing staff can use to develop and demonstrate the behaviors included in competencies. These activities should be creative, cost-effective, encouraging of self-directed learning, and appropriate for the competency being assessed. For example, if the competency focuses on a psychomotor skill such as IV insertion, the assessment method should include a return demonstration on a mannequin or actual patient.

Some examples of learning activities include videos, print materials, self-learning packets, games, puzzles, posters, computer-assisted instruction, skill demonstrations, bedside clinical teaching rounds (Guin, Counsell, & Briggs, 2002), and online modules. It is important to understand that self-assessment alone is not an acceptable approach in validating a nurse's competency (Joint Commission, 2015).

Fostering Adult Learning in Orientation and Competency Programs

Adults view and comprehend learning experiences in different ways than children and adolescents (Knowles, 1990). These differences require NPDSs and unit-based educators to develop learning activities that will appeal to newly hired adult nurses and use strategies that will encourage successful learning.

Information about adult learning will help you assess the learning needs of orientees, clarify your role and the role of learners, and develop creative strategies to help learners attain their orientation and professional goals. Applying adult learning principles will encourage orientees to be self-directed learners, supporting their professional responsibility for continuing competence and lifelong learning.

You are responsible for ensuring that nursing staff on the unit, particularly preceptors, understand how adults learn and how they can develop their own clinical teaching skills. The skills that preceptors develop can be used in various NPD throughputs involving adult learners such as orientation, in-service education, competency programs, and CE offerings.

Hohler (2003) described a preceptor program in perioperative nursing that incorporated key principles of adult learning. Overall, this program created an atmosphere that enabled new nurses to develop their competencies within an environment of "mutual trust and respect" (p. 833). While learning about perioperative nursing, the educators built upon the nurses' prior knowledge and life experiences and actively engaged them throughout the learning experience with the use of repetition, small tasks, choices, and available resources. The use of frequent and ongoing feedback regarding their performance was instrumental in the nurses' attainment of goals (Hohler, 2003).

Andragogy and Adult Learning Principles

Andragogy is a term used by educators to describe the "art and science of helping adults learn" (Knowles, 1980, p. 43). Andragogy is based on a philosophy and set of learning assumptions that can help guide unit-based educators, preceptors, and others involved in teaching adult learners in the work setting. These principles should be applied when planning and implementing orientation programs and other NPD activities. With adult learners, NPDSs and unit-based educators should focus on being facilitators of learning, rather than experts on a topic providing information to learners.

Knowing the Reasons for Learning

Adults need to know why they are expected to learn something before they learn it (Knowles, 1990). They also need to realize the benefits of learning and the negative consequences that may result from not learning.

You should clarify the purposes of an orientation program to newly employed nurses and share evidence that supports the benefits of their participation. Conversely, orientees also need to understand the negative consequences of not participating in orientation. For example, you may explain how the orientation program is designed to help orientees develop key competencies that will enable them to provide safe, quality care to patients. Discuss how orientation will help them become socialized to the work environment and provide them with a sense of belonging. Give orientees frequent and continuous feedback on their progress through written and verbal evaluation and counseling (Hohler, 2003).

Self-Concept and Self-Directedness

Adults have a general need to be self-directed in their learning (Knowles, 1990). They know what they want to learn and when they need to learn it. You need to work collaboratively with orientees when assessing their learning needs and in developing a plan that includes experiences that build upon their career goals. Provide orientees with a variety of learning options. Encourage their responsibility for and active participation in these learning experiences. If possible, allow orientees to make choices and provide them with information about various learning options (Hohler, 2003). Avoid telling orientees what to do or imposing your own beliefs on them. This principle of adult learning is congruent with ANA's emphasis on self-directed, lifelong learning and continuing competence in nurses (ANA, 2000).

Experience

Adults are products of their life experiences (Knowles, 1990). These experiences are diverse and can influence learning in positive or negative ways. Adults recall their life experiences when learning; therefore, past experiences are good resources for learning (Knowles, 1990).

Encourage orientees to share their experiences with others during the orientation program. You need to consider these life experiences when assessing learning needs and build upon these experiences through experiential learning activities such as clinical practice or reality-based simulations (Hohler, 2003). Promote peer learning and group discussions of clinical issues.

You should assist orientees in conducting a self-evaluation of their learning needs in light of their past experiences, helping them realize biases and fostering new ideas and alternative ways of thinking (Knowles, 1990).

Readiness to Learn

Adults are ready to learn when a need exists for them to know information, such as in assuming a new role (Knowles, 1990). Adults also may be ready to learn if they realize they lack knowledge in a specific area or need to perform something more effectively (Knowles, 1990).

You should time learning experiences for orientees based on their readiness to learn (Knowles, 1990). Conducting a self-assessment at the beginning of the orientation period will help orientees identify any gaps in what they are expected to demonstrate. Review job expectations to help them understand what competencies they need in their new roles. Promote the orientees' readiness to learn by having them spend time working with experienced nurses who are good role models. Develop a trusting relationship with orientees by providing them with learning information and experiences when they need them (Hohler, 2003). Allow orientees an opportunity to apply and demonstrate their skills as soon as they learn them.

Orientation to Learning

Adult orientation to learning is task centered, problem centered, or life centered, rather than subject centered (Knowles, 1990). Adults are motivated to learn something if they believe it will help them perform a task or deal with potential problems.

You need to provide orientees with experiential learning activities that they can readily apply and use to solve problems in clinical practice. This approach to learning is congruent with CBOs that focus on learner performance. Use realistic scenarios, such as high-fidelity human simulation, when assessing and developing their competencies. Allow orientees to advance at their own pace.

Motivation to Learn

Adults are motivated to learn something largely by internal factors such as their desire for self-esteem, recognition, job satisfaction, improved quality of life, and increased self-confidence (Knowles, 1990). However, sometimes adults are motivated by external factors including obtaining a better job, getting promoted, or gaining a higher salary.

You can use these internal sources to motivate orientees to learn during the orientation period and other NPD activities. Demonstrate respect toward orientees and their expertise, knowledge, and accomplishments. Create an atmosphere on the clinical unit that is conducive to learning and fosters mutual trust and respect (Hohler, 2003). Encourage staff to extend their hospitality to orientees through simple gestures that will give them a feeling of belonging to the unit, such as inviting them out to lunch (Hohler, 2003).

Understanding Learners' Needs in Orientation Programs

As mentioned in Chapter 1, recent changes in healthcare organizations have affected the nature of the work performed by nurses and other healthcare professionals. These changes, in turn, have influenced what nurses need to learn in order to deliver competent nursing care to patients and assume leadership roles among a team of diverse healthcare workers. Educators in NPD departments need to utilize innovative strategies that will help nursing staff meet their learning needs.

Unit-based educators frequently assume responsibility for orienting nursing staff. As a unit-based educator, you may be involved in certain phases of the orientation process or be entirely responsible for conducting the orientation.

The unit-based educator role may include responsibility for meeting the learning needs of various healthcare professionals, not just RNs. Therefore, it is important to understand the background and learning needs of the workers you may encounter during the unit-based orientation process. Understanding how these orientees learn may help you in supporting their success in their new roles. Jeffery and Jarvis (2014) advised educators to explore currently available formal learning tools and models to better understand how each orientee processes and learns.

Figure 4-2 lists the types of healthcare workers you may encounter during orientation. The learning needs of each group and suggestions are provided in the following section. Regardless of the orientees' educational background or experience, the focus should be on helping them provide safe, quality care to their patients.

Figure 4-2. Possible Employees Encountered in a Nursing Orientation

- Newly hired nurses (novice and experienced nurses)
- Newly hired nurses (nurse residents)
- Nurses from other units (cross-trained or retrained)
- Nurses assuming a new role on a familiar unit (charge nurse or unit-based educator)
- Foreign-educated nurses
- Nursing faculty
- Nursing students
- Student externs/interns
- Licensed practical and licensed vocational nurses
- Assistive personnel and nursing assistants
- Healthcare workers from disciplines other than nursing (e.g., physical therapists, occupational therapists, nutritionists, social workers)
- Volunteers on clinical units
- Forensic personnel on clinical units (e.g., security guards, law enforcement officers)

Professional Nurses

Most healthcare organizations hire both inexperienced, newly graduated nurses and experienced RNs. These nurses possess varied work histories, clinical competencies, educational preparations, and specialty interests. Regardless of their background, newly hired nurses need information to help them understand the healthcare organization and contribute to its goals (ANA, 2000). These new employees need to learn how to function safely and effectively in their assigned roles on the clinical unit (ANA, 2000). These roles may vary and can include direct patient care provider, educator, researcher, or manager.

Intergenerational differences that exist among new and existing nursing staff are also important for NPDSs to understand, recognize, and manage (Lipscomb, 2010). Generation-based groups identified by birth years (i.e., traditionalists, baby boomers, generation X, millennials) are credited as having their own unique characteristics and perspectives (Lipscomb, 2010). Challenges related to interpersonal communication, role expectations, and priorities may surface in the work setting when nursing staff fail to understand generational perspectives and recognize the value of these diverse views. Intergenerational differences need to be considered by NPDSs when pairing more experienced nurses with newer, younger nurses in mentoring or preceptor roles.

Nurses with diverse backgrounds have unique learning needs that often pose challenges for the unit-based educator. Although these nurses have similar learning needs as new employees within the same healthcare organization, each individual nurse has unique learning needs that should be addressed during the orientation program.

Newly Hired, Inexperienced Nurses

Inexperienced nurses, such as graduates who recently passed their NCLEX-RN examination, have learning needs that differ from those of more experienced RNs. New RNs need your guidance in making the transition to a professional role. Being a professional nurse may be the first time these RNs have provided patient care without the supervision of a nursing instructor or preceptor. This process takes time and support from preceptors and other colleagues on the clinical unit.

The orientation experience may elicit mixed feelings among new RNs. Although new graduates may find excitement in finally meeting their goal of being a professional nurse, they also may feel anxious, afraid of failing, and overwhelmed by the reality of the work environment. Unit-based educators and preceptors can help RNs manage these emotions by mentoring them during orientation.

The challenges and stress encountered by newly graduated nurses in professional roles were described in a study by Casey, Fink, Krugman, and Propst (2004). Repeated assessments of 270 nurses in six hospitals were conducted throughout the nurses' first year of employment. Feelings of unpreparedness, lack of confidence, discomfort, and lack of support from preceptors were among perceptions that often lingered.

Related work challenges were reported in a survey by Naholi, Nosek, and Somayaji (2015). In this study, 42 oncology nurses with less than three years of experience identified seven major sources of workplace stress: workload, death and dying, inadequate preparation, conflict with physicians, uncertainty concerning treatment, conflict with other nurses, and lack of support. They used various strategies to cope with this stress such as sleeping, eating, drinking coffee, developing a personal perspective about the value of their work, and participating in entertaining activities (Naholi et al., 2015). Study results and the respondents' recommendation for a nurse educator coach may offer guidance for NPDSs who prepare orientation programs for new nurses, especially in cancer care settings.

Similar experiences have been reported in studies with newly hired nurses in other countries. Kumaran and Carney (2014) obtained the personal perspectives of 10 newly hired nurses in Ireland regarding their role transition. The participants felt overwhelmed with the responsibility and accountability in their new role. However, this transition was made less stressful with staff support, teamwork, and assistance from experienced preceptors.

New graduates also may differ from more experienced nurses regarding their mastery of clinical skills. For example, some nurse managers and staff educators may claim that new RNs need assistance organizing care for multiple patient assignments, setting priorities, and delegation. Others may need help perfecting their fundamental nursing skills and gaining self-confidence in performing procedures (e.g., inserting an indwelling urinary catheter, providing discharge instructions, administering injections) or mastering specialty skills (e.g., suctioning a tracheostomy tube, interpreting a patient's heart rhythm on an electrocardiogram [ECG] tracing).

Some new RNs may have worked as nursing assistants (NAs) or externs while enrolled in their nursing programs. These opportunities may have helped them master fundamental nursing skills and understand unit routines.

Experienced Nurses

Experienced nurses also present challenges to unit-based educators. These seasoned nurses are most likely proficient in basic nursing skills, unlike new RNs, and may have no issues progressing rapidly through the orientation process. Instead, these experienced nurses may need help adjusting to their new work environment, transferring previous competencies, or developing new competencies required on a specialty unit.

It is also important to focus your attention on experienced nurses transitioning to new roles within the same healthcare organization (see Chapter 1). Some nurses may be reassigned to units similar to their previous clinical specialty, whereas others may be expected to care for patients within an entirely different specialty. To function safely and effectively on these units, nurses may need to develop additional clinical competencies. Although they are experienced clinical practitioners, experienced RNs may need assistance in developing new leadership roles, such as that of a nurse manager or an NPDS.

In addition to hiring experienced full-time nurses, most organizations also hire a pool of part-time or full-time nurses, often referred to as *per diem*, *casual*, or *float pool staff*, who are assigned daily to various units throughout the healthcare organization based on staffing needs. Some organizations contract with private agencies that provide nurses to supplement staffing pools as needed. These nurses also need to be oriented to their roles and responsibilities on their assigned units to function effectively. Wright (2015) recommended tailoring a competency assessment program for permanent float nurses around "understanding crisis management options" (p. 21), rather than a myriad of diverse competencies.

Nurses who are retrained or cross-trained need time to adjust to their new role, work setting, and coworkers. They also need time to gain the knowledge and clinical skills vital to a new specialty unit. For example, suppose a nurse experienced in caring for patients with ear, nose, and throat (ENT) conditions is asked to cross-train and function on a head and neck surgical unit. Although proficient in caring for ENT patients, the nurse is unfamiliar with the core knowledge and competencies related to the head and neck specialty. To function effectively in this new specialty, this nurse needs an orientation to the head and neck unit that focuses on these competencies.

In another example, an experienced intensive care unit (ICU) nurse is reassigned to a medical-surgical unit. Although this nurse may be proficient in organizing and performing multiple tasks for one or two critically ill patients, this nurse may need assistance and time to adapt to providing nursing care to five or more patients who have a lower level of acuity than patients in the ICU.

Nurses who change their roles and responsibilities within the same organization also require an orientation to function effectively (ANA, 2000). For example, think about a clinical staff nurse who accepts a nurse manager position within an organization. Even if this nurse is familiar with the organization or the clinical unit, the nurse may need to learn about the organization and unit from the perspective of this new position. Because the work of a staff nurse is quite different from that of a nurse manager, so is the focus of the learning need. A nurse with several years of clinical experience may need assistance in mastering the management skills required of a nurse manager, whereas a staff nurse must focus on perfecting direct patient care skills.

It is important to understand the emotions that experienced RNs who are being cross-trained or retrained may feel. These nurses may fear losing their jobs, developing competencies in a new specialty, or meeting new coworkers. You can help these nurses in becoming socialized to their new work environment and feeling valued for their contributions within the organization.

English-as-a-Second-Language and Foreign-Educated Nurses

The nursing shortage in the United States has led some healthcare organizations to recruit and hire foreign-educated nurses (Pittman, Folsom, & Bass, 2010). This hiring practice may pose unique workforce challenges for nurse managers, NPDSs, and unit-based educators regarding language and interpersonal communication; psychological stress; problem-solving approaches; physical assessment skills; CPR and emergency code procedures; pharmacology; accountability, collaboration, and assertiveness; time management and priority setting; and perspectives in healthcare practices (Robinson, 2009).

Schools of nursing, in an effort to create a more diverse nursing workforce that mirrors the population, have aligned with national efforts to recruit and retain students from racial and ethnic groups who have been underrepresented in nursing (Robert Wood Johnson Foundation, 2013). However, Olson (2012) reported that a portion of minority, or English-as-a-second-language (ESL), students, often encounter challenges throughout their studies and on their licensure examination. Language barriers were identified as the top obstacle for ESL students, followed by cultural, academic, and personal barriers. Language barriers included issues related to medical terminology and communicating with patients and colleagues (Olson, 2012).

Consider these potential barriers during orientation and help newly hired ESL and foreign-educated nurses to understand not only the healthcare organization but also American culture, its healthcare system, and its expectations of nurses (Amerson, 2002). Attention to recognizing and supporting language development is essential (Olson, 2012). Educators also need to help nursing staff strengthen their cultural competence within this diverse work environment and assist ESL and foreign-educated nurses in their transition into nursing practice in the United States.

Licensed Practical and Vocational Nurses, Assistive Personnel, and Nursing Assistants

Recent changes in healthcare reimbursement have led many administrators to reexamine both the number and mix of healthcare workers providing patient care. Some organizations changed staffing patterns by increasing their pool of licensed practical and licensed vocational nurses (LPNs and LVNs), assistive personnel (AP), and NAs to assist with patient care.

Troubles arise in evaluating the capabilities of these various roles. AP are often responsible for drawing blood, inserting urinary catheters, and performing ECGs. These procedures are often more than what is expected of NAs. As such, educators need to understand potential issues they may face with NAs during the orientation program and provide them with proper assistance and guidance. Although individuals who are hired for NA positions are expected to have a high school diploma or equivalent, they may have unique learning needs related to their role. Therefore, it is important that you explore the availability of appropriate resources in your organization to help these individuals develop their skills.

As a clinical educator, you may be expected to develop a unit-based orientation program for LPNs and LVNs, AP, or NAs who are newly hired or need to be cross-trained to your clinical unit. Some newly hired employees also may be certified nursing assistants (CNAs), which means they successfully completed a state-approved NA training course, passed a competency examination (written and skills performance), and completed supervised clinical hours (Han et al., 2014). This may add an additional element to consider when devising your plan. You should take into account several key points in planning your program.

First, understand the role expectations and responsibilities of LPNs, AP, and NAs by reviewing their job descriptions and related policies and procedures in your organization. Be aware of ongoing proposed changes in their roles and responsibilities and make sure they are practicing within their regulated scope of practice at your workplace. It is important to remember that AP and NAs need to perform the various tasks assigned to them and understand why and when these tasks need to be performed.

Second, when planning their orientation, realize the strength of the life experiences that these healthcare workers bring with them. Build upon these experiences in their classes and clinical experiences.

Third, create a work environment in which LPNs, AP, and NAs feel valued for the services they perform and the role they play on the healthcare team. They should feel comfortable discussing ways to meet their learning needs.

Finally, develop an orientation program that is an appropriate educational level for specific learners. This will help them successfully develop the competencies they need to function effectively in their roles. Provide them with explanations of medical terms or the rationale behind why particular clinical decisions are made by nurses when a patient's condition changes. They need to be able to function effectively as team members on the clinical unit.

Province (2008) developed a successful orientation program for CNAs who were transitioning from working in a long-term care setting to an acute care hospital. Key elements of the program included immediately applying classroom learning to the clinical setting, being flexible, and tailoring learning based on individual needs. These changes resulted in a shortened orientation time, stronger performance, and increased retention rates.

Similarly, Ward, Stewart, Ford, Mullen, and Makic (2014) implemented a CE program that included "just-in-time" teaching for CNAs employed at their healthcare organization. In this method, learners are provided with educational resources in an efficient and time-effective manner when they need it the most (Lengetti, Monachino, & Scholtz, 2011). Just-in-time strategies have been successfully reported with nursing students in preparing for their patient care assignments (White, 2006) and with clinical nurses engaged in a central venous catheter simulation program (Lengetti et al., 2011). The CNA program designed by Ward et al. (2014) included weekly educational fliers, in-service programs, and a simulation-based skills laboratory. The cost-effective educational fliers were referred to as the "Educational Offerings on the Run" or the "eDOOR" program because they were posted on the linen closet doors where CNAs could view the bulleted information and apply it while on the job. The fliers focused on various topics of interest to the CNA role and healthcare organization, such as fall prevention, skin care, stroke, and pain. Program outcomes demonstrated increased levels of knowledge and role satisfaction.

In addition to orienting staff nurses and other ancillary personnel, unit-based educators often have an opportunity to support other healthcare professionals from disciplines other than nursing. These individuals may include physicians, physical therapists, dentists, social workers, respiratory therapists, and nutritionists. You may be responsible for orienting these individuals to nursing practice after they are hired or if they are reassigned to your clinical unit.

It is important to develop a mutual understanding of the contributions that each discipline makes to patient outcomes. This experience is a unique opportunity to develop a collaborative relationship and understand each other's role in patient care from an interdisciplinary perspective. This approach also can help identify immediate learning needs that can be addressed during orientation or later through in-service education. Increases in patient acuity combined with shortened lengths of stay make this partnership essential in order to have a coordinated, effective, and efficient healthcare team.

National guidelines that support collaborative team-based education for health professionals prepared within the United States have been developed in an effort to benefit patient outcomes in clinical practice (Interprofessional Education Collaborative, 2011). Given the importance of interprofessional education, representatives from nursing, pharmacy, medicine, dentistry, and public health industries prepared guidelines, called *Core Competencies for Interprofessional Collaborative Practice: Report of an Expert Panel*. This document identified core interprofessional competencies in four domains: values and ethics for interprofessional practice, role and responsibilities, interprofessional communication, and teams and teamwork (Interprofessional Education Collaborative, 2011). These domains may offer NPDSs direction for hospital-based educational activities.

Nursing Faculty and Students

Prior to allowing a school of nursing's faculty and students to practice within a healthcare organization, a legal affiliation (contract) is developed and signed by both parties. Some agencies partner with multiple schools of nursing with each school assigned to a clinical unit on designated days and times (ANA & NNSDO, 2010).

Although faculty and students from schools of nursing are not employees when working within the context of an academic course, they still need to be oriented to the organization and their assigned clinical units. Because their time at a clinical setting often lasts less than a semester, orientation programs targeted to these groups need to be provided in a concise, creative, and timely manner. In some organizations, faculty members attend the orientation and are responsible for sharing this information with students.

NPDSs are responsible for orienting these faculty members and nursing students to the healthcare organization prior to the start of their clinical practicum. Figure 4-3 provides possible topics that may be included in an orientation for academic partners. The faculty orientation should include meeting with the unit's nurse manager and staff and shadowing a nurse on the clinical unit to become familiar with unit protocol. Faculty orientations may consist of prescheduled face-to-face sessions and printed or online self-study learning modules. Faculty are often responsible for verifying student completion of learning modules and other requirements.

Figure 4-3. Content That May Be Included in Faculty and Student Orientation

- Blood-borne pathogens
- Cultural competence
- Emergency preparedness
- Environment of care
- Prevention of infection
- Patient safety
- Privacy, security, compliance, and ethics review
- Health Insurance Portability and Accountability Act training
- Team effectiveness
- Improving line safety
- Use of restraints
- Rapid response teams (numbers to call)
- Change-of-shift reports
- Unit-based patient processes
- Orientation to the electronic patient record
- Environmental logistics (e.g., parking, food, lockers, conference room, communication policies, dress code)
- Orientation to hospital environment, directions
- Access codes needed for records and administration

A staff member (e.g., clinical coordinator, assistant dean) at the school of nursing usually begins this process by making a request to the NPDS (who is the liaison) to access a particular type of clinical unit based on course objectives. The school's clinical coordinator oversees the contract process with the NPDS liaison and also confirms clinical requirements that are communicated to students and faculty. These requirements must be completed and validated prior to the start of clinical. Orientation plans for faculty and students are also scheduled and communicated. Copies of the course syllabus, schedule, student and faculty names, and other required documentation are shared. For example, students enrolled in an adult medical-surgical course will be assigned to a patient care unit that admits patients with such conditions. Students receive classroom instruction on the nursing care of these patients and clinical skills training in a laboratory at the school of nursing. Students are supervised by faculty members who evaluate each student based on the clinical objectives. Each course has a required number of clinical hours determined by academic credits. Clinical courses and credit hours often vary among schools of nursing.

Administrators determine which course faculty members will teach based on their educational preparation and clinical expertise. Faculty members who teach the clinical component of a nursing course may be employed on either a full-time or part-time basis. Full-time faculty, such as clinical staff in healthcare organizations, assume multiple roles, including teaching in the classroom setting, publishing, conducting research, presenting at conferences, and serving on various school, university, and professional committees. Full-time faculty often participate in more than one clinical course during an academic year. Part-time faculty members usually are hired on a semester basis to supervise students in the clinical setting. Both full-time and part-time faculty often work per diem in a clinical setting to maintain their clinical competencies.

Although faculty members on the clinical unit often supervise nursing students, students enrolled in senior-level courses are frequently paired with experienced nurses in a special learning partnership called a *preceptorship*. In this arrangement, a staff nurse (preceptor) directly supervises the clinical learning of a student nurse (preceptee). Preceptor arrangements also are used with newly hired nurses during orientation (see Chapter 5).

Healthcare agencies usually identify a contact person who acts as a liaison between faculty at schools of nursing and the healthcare organization. This person, who may or may not be the unit-based educator, is responsible for communicating with faculty and arranging the clinical placements for students. The liaison, in conjunction with the unit-based educator and nurse manager, may schedule unit-based orientations and select qualified preceptors for these nursing students. As part of the school's program evaluation process, unit-based educators may be asked to provide formal and informal feedback concerning the performance of graduates.

As an NPDS or unit-based educator working with faculty and students from various schools of nursing, you need to be familiar with each school's scheduled dates and times on the clinical units, faculty and students assigned to the units, clinical course objectives, and students' level of performance.

Confusion can result on the clinical unit when staff members assume that nursing students from various schools possess similar skills, clinical interests, and learning needs. Ask faculty to share course profiles and clinical expectations with nursing staff on the unit. Meet with faculty prior to the scheduled clinical rotation to clarify role expectations and to discuss learning needs of students. Ask faculty to post students' weekly clinical objectives on the unit's assignment board so that staff can help them meet their learning needs. Meet with faculty before the start of the clinical experience and communicate regularly. Help faculty and students feel welcome on the clinical unit and offer your services as a resource for them. As appropriate, refer faculty to available specialty-specific educational resources, such as ONS's ERC (ONS, n.d.-a), as many aids are designed for prelicensure RN students.

Volunteers and Community Liaisons or Laypeople

National efforts to reduce racial and ethnic health disparities and "advance the health, safety, and well-being of the American people" (U.S. Department of Health and Human Services, 2011, p. 25) are increasing in community-based programs and policies. Therefore, volunteers may require orientation to function effectively in their role within a healthcare organization (Joint Commission, 2015) and its programs. These volunteer groups needs to be able to demonstrate competence in patient care skills, including safety and infection control procedures and patient confidentiality.

Recommendations for such community-based programs include implementing "culturally and linguistically evidence-based initiatives" (p. 26) that address health issues including obesity, tobacco use, maternal-child health, flu vaccination rates, and asthma (U.S. Department of Health and Human Services, 2011). Given these priorities and existing community-based collaborations, it is important for NPDSs to identify and address the learning needs of community liaisons or laypeople and community health workers.

Law Enforcement and Security Guards

Forensic personnel without clinical backgrounds (e.g., security guards, correctional officers) also need to be oriented to their responsibilities in patient care settings (Joint Commission, 2015). These individuals need to understand appropriate ways to interact with patients, respond to unexpected clinical events, and follow appropriate communication lines with hospital staff, administrative staff, and security. Forensic officers also need to understand the differences between "administrative and clinical seclusion and restraint" (Joint Commission, 2015). Unit-based educators need to develop creative strategies that can help forensic personnel develop the knowledge and skills they need to function effectively in the healthcare setting. For example, one healthcare organization developed a brochure to orient forensic personnel (Grove & Bush, 2002).

Gathering Information About Orientation at the Organization

Now that you have an idea about the possible learners you may interface with in your orientation program, gather additional information about the orientation program offered at both organizational and departmental levels. Clarify the process that new employees experience once they are hired and before they arrive on your unit. Contact appropriate representatives in your organization and arrange to attend these programs, or meet with them to discuss the purpose and specific content of these orientation programs.

Learning about the organization's orientation programs can benefit both you and new nursing employees. Although this task may seem time consuming, it can help you clarify and coordinate your own unit-based orientation with organizational and departmental orientations. Knowing the competencies that new employees have already attained before they arrive on your clinical unit will help you in focusing on unit-specific competencies.

A careful review of the entire orientation process will enable you to reduce duplication among these orientations, saving the organization both time and money. It is important for new employees to successfully complete the orientation in the designated time so that they can be prepared to assume their responsibilities in providing patient care.

Being familiar with other orientations also can assist you in identifying learning needs of nursing staff that can be addressed through other staff development activities, including in-service educational and CE programs. Conversely, you may realize that some topics delivered through these programs need to be moved to the orientation phase. This is especially helpful given the limited resources (nursing staff and time) that may be available to you on the clinical unit.

Gaining an organizational perspective of orientation programs can make you aware of resources that may be available to you at the unit-based level. These resources may include guest speakers, audiovisual equipment, supplies, and assessment and evaluation documents.

Reviewing the orientation process at your organization can help you develop professionally as a unit-based educator. This process gives you an opportunity to observe and model the teaching skills and behaviors of various experts within your organization. It also provides the opportunity to network with other educators and offer your own expertise.

Orientation Pathways for Newly Hired Nurses

Bumgarner and Biggerstaff (2000) and Johnston and Ferraro (2001) applied the concept of critical pathways used in patient care to the orientation experience of newly hired nurses. These pathways can benefit orientees, newly hired experienced RNs, preceptors, and the organization in many ways.

First, pathways provide a framework that promotes individualized orientation based on a nurse's past clinical experience while simultaneously focusing on specific job expectations related to patient care (Johnston & Ferraro, 2001). Second, pathways help educators identify target dates and competencies that need to be strengthened (Johnston & Ferraro, 2001). Third, an orientation pathway serves as a guide or road map for preceptors and orientees in providing direct patient care, promoting critical-thinking skills, and applying the nursing process (Bumgarner & Biggerstaff, 2000). Finally, pathways can positively influence nurses' job satisfaction and retention (Bumgarner & Biggerstaff, 2000).

Organizationwide (Hospital) Orientation Programs

The orientation process may vary among healthcare organizations. Most organizations require all new employees to attend an organizationwide (institutionwide or hospitalwide) orientation program.

The primary purpose of an organizationwide orientation program is to introduce all new employees to the organization's mission, philosophy, goals, and objectives. This orientation also includes a review of key hospitalwide policies, procedures, and rules and regulations that affect all employees (Joint Commission, 2015). Topics mandated by the healthcare organization's accreditation and regulatory agencies also may be included in this orientation phase (O'Shea & Smith, 2002). Figure 4-4 lists possible topics that may be addressed during an organizationwide orientation program.

The organizationwide orientation may be when employers verify the credentials and job requirements of new employees. For nurses, this may include providing the display portion of their current RN license and other documents needed to complete their employee file such as

---

Figure 4-4. Content That May Be Included in an Organizationwide Orientation Program

- Welcome and introduction to organization-level personnel
- Mission, values, and vision statements of the organization
- Philosophy of the organization
- Goals and objectives
- Policies and procedures
- Rules and regulations
- Strategic plan of the organization
- Payroll compensation and benefits
- Tour of physical layout of organization
- Communication systems (e.g., email, telephone, fax, newsletter, paging system, intranet)
- Fire and safety procedures (e.g., drug-free workplace, smoking policy, hazardous substances)
- Emergency disaster plan, emergency numbers, and procedures
- Employee accident and illness procedures
- Infection control
- Health promotion services
- Systemwide expected behaviors (e.g., customer relations, communication skills, quality services)
- Diversity in the workplace

---

evidence of current immunizations and drug testing. This also may be when new employees obtain their photo identification badges and complete paperwork related to parking, payroll, and benefits.

The length of this organizationwide orientation program varies among agencies and may last a day or longer. Representatives from the organization's human resources or training and development departments often coordinate this program. NPDSs may participate in some aspect of the program.

For nurses, a department orientation program designed by NPDSs usually follows this organizationwide orientation program. The department orientation might be followed by an additional orientation that often focuses on a specialty area such as critical care, oncology, or transplantation. The orientation process then concludes at the unit-based level. Figure 4-5 illustrates a process that a newly hired nurse may experience in an organization.

Nursing Department Orientation

Following the hospitalwide orientation, new employees hired within the nursing department usually proceed to a general nursing orientation program sponsored by the centralized NPDD. Other new employees, such as social workers, housekeepers, and physical therapists, proceed to their respective departments or units for further orientation.

The nursing department orientation may be provided to all nursing personnel (i.e., RNs, LPNs,

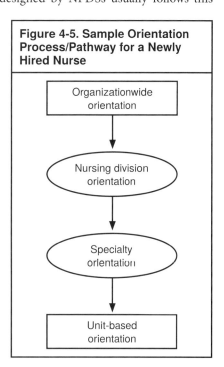

Figure 4-5. Sample Orientation Process/Pathway for a Newly Hired Nurse

Organizationwide orientation → Nursing division orientation → Specialty orientation → Unit-based orientation

LVNs, AP) at once or in different programs entirely. In some organizations, these groups are temporarily combined for portions of the orientation in which they have common needs (Amerson, 2002). Combining these groups may save staff costs and time.

The nursing department orientation focuses on patient care activities and prepares nurses for their specific roles and responsibilities within the organization. It centers on the information needed by all nurses, regardless of their specialty, and reviews relevant departmentwide policies and procedures related to patient care (Joint Commission, 2015). Mandatory requirements that affect patient care are explained during this orientation, if not already covered in the organizationwide program. Figure 4-6 provides examples of content that may be included in a nursing department orientation, including specific elements required by the Joint Commission (2015). Some organizations may choose to introduce this content earlier, during the hospitalwide orientation, or later, as part of the unit-based period of orientation.

The purpose of a nursing orientation program is to familiarize new nurses with the nursing department's philosophy, goals, and objectives and illustrate how these are congruent with those presented in the hospitalwide orientation. Orientees are introduced to the structure and communication pathway of the nursing department and often have an opportunity to meet key leaders in the department.

Figure 4-6. Content That May Be Included in a Nursing Department Orientation Program

- Welcome and introductions to key nursing department personnel
- Mission statement of the nursing department
- Philosophy of the nursing department
- Department goals and objectives
- Departmental structure and communication lines
- Tour of department and other areas of interest
- Policies and procedures; rules and regulations*
- Strategic plan of the department (and fit with organization's plan)
- Collaborative relationship with other departments and professionals
- Review of job descriptions and performance standards*
- Performance appraisal system (evaluation process)
- Nursing role in fire, safety, emergency, and disaster plans
- Cardiopulmonary resuscitation training and verification and crash cart review
- Medication administration
- Blood administration
- Charting and documentation
- Introduction to evidence-based practice
- Pain assessment and management*
- Patient rights: addressing ethics of care, treatment, and service
- Fall reduction*
- Environment of care*
- How to report unanticipated events*
- Sensitivity related to cultural diversity*
- Needs of the population served at the healthcare organization*
- Team collaboration, coordination, and communication*
- Early identification of changes in patient condition*
- Response to a deteriorating patient*
- Patient handoff
- Situation, Background, Assessment, and Recommendation (SBAR) communication

* These elements are required by Joint Commission standards (Joint Commission, 2015).

This orientation program is often when general competencies, such as CPR, medication administration, and documentation, are assessed and validated. These competencies should be evaluated before orientees begin the clinical portion of the orientation program. Competencies specific to a nurse's clinical unit may be reviewed later during the specialty and unit-based orientation programs.

The nursing department orientation also provides nurse orientees with an opportunity to socialize with nurses on other clinical units and introduces them to how professional nursing is viewed by the organization. The length of the nursing orientation may vary among organizations, but it often lasts a day or longer.

Specialty Orientations

Some healthcare organizations may require nurse orientees to attend a specialty orientation following the nursing department orientation, as various specialty units require different knowledge and skills to function safely and effectively. The purpose of specialty orientation programs is to prepare nurses for the competencies unique to their assigned clinical areas (e.g., oncology, critical care, dialysis, cardiac care, burn unit). For example, suppose a nurse was hired to work in a surgical ICU at your organization. That nurse would attend the scheduled hospitalwide orientation program, proceed to the nursing department orientation, and then complete a critical care orientation and an arrhythmia course. The critical care orientation would include all nurses who were hired to work in any of the organization's six critical care units. The specific unit would be used to provide the nurse with clinical experience in this area.

Although specialty orientation programs differ in content and learning experiences, they often include classroom presentations and clinical experiences. Clinical experiences may be integrated with classes or scheduled after the orientee successfully completes required course work. Consider incorporating commercially prepared evidence-based educational resources, such as the ONS ERC, for use in your specialty orientation (ONS, n.d.-a).

As a unit-based educator for a surgical ICU, you may be involved in planning and implementing a critical care orientation program or coordinating a clinical portion of the orientation on your ICU unit. Consider an interdepartmental team approach when designing a specialty orientation, such as the program described by Kuhrik, Laub, Kuhrik, and Atwater (2011), who saw a need for newly hired and experienced nurses to gain a better understanding of the many cancer care services offered to patients at their center. They also wanted their nurses to perceive themselves as part of a hospitalwide cancer care team and to realize the multiple job opportunities available to them within the center's oncology departments. They constructed an orientation program that was scheduled at monthly and bimonthly intervals and limited to five orientees per session. It included specialty-focused topics, speaker-guided clinical tours, and an outpatient shadowing experience with an oncology nursing team. Evaluation data captured from more than 200 participants reflected successful attainment of program goals (Kuhrik et al., 2011).

Student Internships and Externships

Many healthcare organizations offer special clinical opportunities for internships and externships to nursing students or recent graduates. These programs have been reported in various hospital settings (Lott, Willis, & Lyttle, 2011), including specialty units such as oncology (Childress & Gorder, 2012), critical care (Duvall, 2009; Letourneau, 2010), and emergency care (Glynn & Silva, 2013). Internships and externships may have different meanings, participants, outcomes, requirements, and compensations based on the sponsoring healthcare organization. It is important to understand the details and participants of these experiences.

In some organizations, internships may refer to part-time paid positions similar to that of an NA or nurse technician (Johns Hopkins University School of Nursing Career Center, n.d.). However, many published accounts have referred to newly hired graduate nurses as being in internships during their orientation to the facility (Childress & Gorder, 2012; Glynn & Silva, 2013; Letourneau, 2010; Phillips & Hall, 2014).

Externships might be full-time paid positions scheduled over summer months, varied in duration, and targeted to nursing students entering their senior year. Conversely, other organizations call this kind of position an internship, with various options regarding scheduling, time commitment, and compensation (Indiana University Health, 2014). Some commitments also involve postgraduation employment for a predetermined amount of time.

Healthcare organizations also reap the benefits of these arrangements. The externship program is viewed as a recruitment strategy. Students who return to the organization as employees following graduation already are familiar with the organization and may require less orientation time. It is important to weigh the costs of these programs against their benefits of easing the shortage of specialty nurses.

A summer experience, in this case referred to as an externship, often provides students with clinical time under the direction of a preceptor (Lott et al., 2011). Both externships and internships may include an orientation to the healthcare facility as well as didactic and laboratory instruction using various active teaching-learning strategies such as role play, reflective journaling, case studies, and simulation. These programs help learners strengthen their evidence-based nursing skills through direct patient care activities and ease their transition to a professional nursing role (Lott et al., 2011). Many programs strive to increase learners' level of confidence and focus on strengthening skills in critical thinking, time management, organization, and priority setting. Externs may engage in various professional development activities over the summer and network with other externs. While extern programs are often used as a recruitment strategy for organizations, externs can personally use this experience to assess the organization as a potential employer and direct patient care as a specialty of choice after graduation. Externs can also use this opportunity to demonstrate their professional behaviors and clinical expertise to nurse managers and clinical staff.

Whether called an internship or externship, both professional development opportunities provide students and new nurses with focused clinical experience under the guidance of an experienced RN.

A 10-week summer externship program for nursing students described by Lott et al. (2011) focused on developing select competencies of student externs with the intention of later recruiting them after graduation. This program was a revised version of their prior externship program with more attention paid to organizational collaboration, program structure and formality, standardization across units, and the recruitment process. It was anticipated that the program would decrease orientation time and associated costs for soon-to-be-hired participants. Externs were paired with experienced RNs who mentored them and shared patient assignments. Outcomes revealed strong extern satisfaction scores, increased confidence and competence, and a 73% retention rate (Lott et al., 2011). Upon hire, the externs' baseline assessment rate was 12% higher than that of RNs who were nonparticipants. According to Lott et al. (2011), this difference in scores reflected higher critical-thinking skills among externs.

Similarly, Childress and Gorder (2012) reported positive outcomes from their four-month oncology internship that focused on recruiting graduating students and hiring them as they developed their competencies. The interns completed a curriculum based on national oncology standards that included formal classes, readings, quizzes, and weekly feedback and discussions. Clinical experience under the direction of a preceptor focused on bone marrow transplant and medical-surgical oncology units and was enhanced with visits to related sites such as radiation and outpatient settings. Reported outcomes over a five-year period reflected an 80% retention rate, positive performance evaluations, increased confidence, and positive relationships. Many graduates assumed leadership roles after program completion and offered to mentor future interns as preceptors. While the recruitment of graduating students initially posed a challenge, by the program's third year, new graduates were applying from across the country (Childress & Gorder, 2012).

Outcomes consistent with other internships were reported by Glynn and Silva (2013), who obtained the personal perspectives of eight new nurses in an emergency department internship. Themes of this qualitative study included the "acquisition of new knowledge and skills in a specialty area, becoming more proficient, and assistance with role transition" (Glynn & Silva, 2013, p. 173). Key factors of this intern program included structured classroom and clinical learning and the guidance of preceptors and unit-based clinical specialists.

Nurse Residency Programs

Although nurse residency programs have been discussed in the nursing literature for nearly two decades, the Institute of Medicine (IOM) recently appealed to healthcare organizations and other constituents, such as state boards of nursing, the federal government, and accrediting bodies, to support these programs (IOM, 2010). IOM included this request among five other recommendations in their landmark report *The Future of Nursing: Leading Change, Advancing Health* (IOM, 2010). IOM also suggested that these "transition-to-practice programs" target not only nurses who have successfully completed their prelicensure RN but also those who either completed their academic program as an APN or are transitioning into new practice specialties (IOM, 2010). This recommendation was accompanied by the expectation for healthcare organizations to assess residency program outcomes regarding nurses' retention, competencies, and influence on patient outcomes (IOM, 2010).

In 2000, the American Association of Colleges of Nursing (AACN) assumed an early leadership role in nurse residency programs by collaborating with the University Health-System Consortium (UHC) to form the UHC/AACN Residency Program (AACN, 2014). This national program aims to help newly graduated nurses transition to their professional RN role and provide care to patients in hospital-based acute care settings. Residents complete the one-year program consisting of structured classroom and clinical experiences. To date, 92 practice sites in 30 states offer the UHC/AACN Residency Program (AACN, 2014). Reports of program outcomes indicate a first-year retention rate of greater than 95%, as well as positive changes in residents' "perceptions of their competence, ability to communicate, and satisfaction with their work" (American Association of Colleges of Nursing, 2014, para. 2).

In addition to programs for new graduates, Longo et al. (2014) described a successful one-year residency program designed to help experienced RNs transition from being competent to proficient in pediatrics. The Transitioning the Experienced Registered Nurse (TERN) Residency Program revealed positive outcomes related to decision-making and point-of-care principles. TERN also engaged RNs in reflective journaling.

Many healthcare organizations have developed their own successful residency programs for new hires. Programs may vary in depth, length, curriculum, teaching-learning strategies, and resident expectations. Some programs are offered at scheduled times during the year and require an application process, while others provide automatic entry into the program for new nurses. Residents are usually assigned to preceptors to develop core competencies.

Favorable outcomes have been reported related to various types of residency programs for both the individuals involved in the programs and their organizations (Harrison & Ledbetter, 2014). A decade-long study conducted in UHC/AACN postbaccalaureate nurse residency programs revealed statistically significant increases in residents' retention rates; organization, priority-setting, and communication skills; and participation in leadership efforts in the clinical setting (Goode, Lynn, McElroy, Bednash, & Murray, 2013).

Dedicated Education Units

Some healthcare organizations have partnered with their affiliated schools of nursing to create dedicated education units (DEUs) for nursing students contracted within their facilities. DEUs were first reported in the nursing literature in 2009 (Burke, Moscato, & Warner, 2009; Warner & Burton, 2009). The global shortage of nurses, nurse faculty, and clinical sites has recently fueled the development of this new clinical practice model in various settings such as acute care hospitals (Freundl et al., 2012; Jeffries et al., 2013; Krampe, L'Ecuyer, & Palmer, 2013; Rhodes, Meyers, & Underhill, 2012), long-term care (Melillo et al., 2014; O'Lynn, 2013), rural (Harmon, 2013), community (Betany & Yarwood, 2010), oncology (Dean et al., 2013), and interprofessional education (McVey, Vessey, Kenner, & Pressler, 2014). Some partners have used models to guide their DEU development (Melillo et al., 2014; Murray & James, 2012), including the Quality and Safety Education for Nurses (QSEN) Initiative (McKown, McKeon, & Webb, 2011; QSEN Institute, n.d.). The intended impact of DEUs aligns with many national initiatives that support patient safety, nurse competency, and collaboration for nursing excellence and quality patient outcomes.

A DEU provides a controlled and designated clinical learning environment for nursing students and other healthcare professionals as they engage in direct patient care during a clinical course or program. Unlike the traditional clinical teaching model where a faculty member oversees the clinical performance of a group of nursing students assigned to different clinical units for each course by semester, a DEU model uses experienced clinical staff nurses employed by the healthcare organization as clinical teachers on one designated clinical unit. The role of faculty members changes to that of mentors or coaches on the DEU (Hannon et al., 2012). The clinical staff may be referred to as preceptors (Krampe et al., 2013) or clinical instructors (Hannon et al., 2012).

Creating a successful DEU experience requires a great deal of collaboration and planning between an academic program and healthcare organization, with some teams reporting their first efforts as pilot projects (Hannon et al., 2012; Harmon, 2013; Melillo et al., 2014). Careful selection of a DEU-appropriate unit is among the first steps in this process. To help facilitate unit selection, Parker and Smith (2012) relied on a tool called the Revised Professional Practice Environment Scale to identify inpatient acute care units at their workplace that could be used as DEUs. It is important that all stakeholders (i.e., nurse managers, staff educators, nursing staff, faculty, and students) engaged in a DEU understand the process, role expectations, workloads, and intended outcomes. Burke et al. (2009) also emphasized building trust and relationships, communicating, and setting mutual goals when developing a DEU program.

Research and quality improvement efforts exploring the influence of DEUs on students, clinical unit nurses, faculty, and organizations have generally revealed positive outcomes in quality student learning (Mulready-Shick, Flanagan, Banister, Mylott, & Curtin, 2013; O'Lynn, 2013); satisfaction (O'Lynn, 2013); nurse-to-nurse collaboration (Moore & Nahigian, 2013) and mentoring (Nishioka, Coe, Hanita, & Moscato, 2014b); QSEN competencies (McKown et al., 2011); and critical thinking, clinical judgment, and self-confidence (Hannon et al., 2012). Positive perspectives also exist at the organizational level including observations of increased professionalism among staff (O'Lynn, 2013), a welcoming clinical environment for students (Nishioka, Coe, Hanita, & Moscato, 2014a), stronger and sustained relationships and communication between academic-service partners (Mulready-Shick & Flanagan, 2014; Rhodes et al., 2012), a win-win situation for all participants of the DEU (Hannon et al., 2012), and cost-effectiveness (Springer et al., 2012).

Developing a Competency-Based Orientation for Your Clinical Unit

Now that you have a general understanding of the orientation programs that a nurse orientee needs to complete, focus on developing your unit's CBO program. Clarify whether your unit-based orientation program is considered part of the nursing department, a specialty orientation, or a separate clinical experience that builds upon prior orientations.

Start this process by gathering information about the learners and resources available on your clinical unit. Your assessment also should evaluate the readiness of unit staff and preceptors tasked with educating orientees. This will help you develop a detailed plan for your program.

Begin your assessment by meeting with the nurse manager of the clinical unit and developing a good working relationship. The nurse manager, as administrator of the clinical unit, is responsible for ensuring that staff provide safe, quality nursing care to patients on the unit. The nurse manager also has the authority to implement unit-based strategies and resources to make this happen.

Be sure that you have the understanding and support of the unit's nurse manager as it relates to your role as a unit-based educator. Develop a regular meeting schedule and communication system. Express your specific needs related to your role in the unit-based orientation program. Keep the manager informed of the orientees' progress toward program outcomes.

Talk with the NPDS or nurse manager to obtain information about the number of orientees assigned to your unit. Obtain their names and credentials, including information about their past experiences. If available, discover their particular strengths and areas that need improvement. Review any documentation describing the orientees' performances to date.

Although you may have a general idea of their learning needs based on your past experiences, gaining additional information about these particular learners can help you match them with preceptors and develop individual orientation plans. Jeffery and Jarvis (2014) emphasized the importance of engaging orientees not only before they begin orientation but also daily after the onboarding process begins. For example, the authors suggested contacting new employees at your organization even before they arrive for orientation to share some positive comments about their upcoming experience. Once orientation formally begins, continue to involve them in meaningful activities.

If you are not familiar with the nursing and specialty orientations offered by your organization, investigate these programs and the outcomes expected of orientees. If the specialty orientation includes unit-based clinical experience, review clinical competencies. If it does not, then you will need to develop these outcomes. Consider including the unit's preceptors in this process. Regardless of your approach, this information will help you build upon the orientees' prior experiences at your organization and plan appropriate clinical learning experiences.

Clarifying Unit-Based Competencies

Clarify the unit-based competencies that you, the unit manager, clinical staff, and NPDSs have developed for the unit's CBO and make any needed changes. Make sure that everyone on the unit is familiar with these competencies, which will be further defined as more information is gathered about orientees, preceptors, available resources, and the learning environment.

Selecting Qualified Preceptors

After you have information about the number of orientees and their skill levels, identify qualified unit staff who can serve as preceptors. Be sure that they have successfully completed a preceptor preparation program and are familiar with the CBO process. Discuss your selections with the unit's nurse manager, and clarify any staffing or scheduling changes that need to be made for these preceptors while they are working with their orientees.

Consider matching less-experienced preceptors with orientees who are newly hired, inexperienced nurses and teaming seasoned preceptors with experienced RNs (see Chapter 5). Include these preceptors in planning a unit-based orientation and keep them abreast of information regarding their orientees.

Confirming Resources Available on the Clinical Unit

In addition to qualified preceptors, determine other resources that are available to you for the unit-based orientation program. For example, check with the nurse manager or NPDS to determine if the program is included in their budget and if expenses are incurred for duplication, supplies, equipment, services, or refreshments. Secure a private room that can be used by preceptors and orientees for clinical conferences and evaluation sessions. Assess the patient census on the unit to determine if it will be sufficient for the appropriate type and number of clinical assignments. Inquire about access to a clinical skills and simulation laboratory to assist with competency testing, if needed. In addition to these resources, consider inviting a team of staff nurses, such as experienced preceptors, to work with you in developing the unit-based orientation program.

Assessing the Learning Environment

Assess the environment on the unit and determine if it is conducive to orientee learning. Discuss the orientation needs with staff and assess their willingness to participate in the overall program. Ensure that nursing staff possess knowledge about the orientation process and are able to provide orientees with proper guidance and direction. Interactions that occur between new orientees and nurses on the clinical unit during the orientation period can have a significant influence on the orientees' professional development and socialization.

Defining the Outcomes

After analyzing the results of your assessment data, determine the specific learning needs of the orientees assigned to your clinical unit. Clarify these learning needs with appropriate individuals at your organization, including the unit's nurse manager and the NPDS.

If you have an opportunity to meet with orientees beforehand, assist preceptors in reviewing learning needs and obtain their feedback. If you do not have access to orientees at this point, include this step when orientees begin the unit-based program.

Establishing the Purpose of the Unit-Based Orientation

After defining the orientees' learning needs, clarify the general purpose of the unit-based orientation program. Orientation programs introduce orientees to the healthcare organization and assist with their socialization (ANA, 2000). The focus is on assessing the orientees' competencies and developing them to support safe, quality patient care.

Developing Unit-Based Competencies

After identifying the purpose of your unit-based program, clarify that the unit-specific competencies are congruent with the purpose and principles of adult learning (ANA, 2000). Make sure that orientees will be able to attain these outcomes within a reasonable time frame. Discuss these competencies with the nurse manager, staff development educator, and preceptors of your unit.

Unit-based competencies also should be congruent and build upon those included in the specialty and nursing department orientations. Because clinical competencies may be integrated within the competencies of the specialty orientation, check with appropriate individuals within your organization to determine this. Your unit-based orientation efforts may be considered an integral part of the specialty orientation rather than as a separate entity.

Planning the Unit-Based Orientation

After you have determined the purpose and competencies for your unit-based orientation, develop a detailed plan to implement the program. Although planning takes time and energy, it will help you determine the work and who is responsible for the work that needs to be completed before orientees arrive on your clinical unit. Planning also helps you determine the relative time frame for the orientation, clarify outcomes, identify appropriate clinical assignments, and determine the evaluation plan. Your plan also can help orientees successfully attain program outcomes and, ultimately, become productive members of the unit.

Recognizing the Importance of Planning and Team Building

To further understand the importance of developing a plan for your unit-based orientation program, take into consideration this analogy of a football team.

When planning to face an opponent, a coach's ultimate goal is for his team to win the game. At the beginning of the week, the coach and his assistants start planning and discussing various plays or strategies that they believe will help in this goal. Players are then tasked to learn a final game plan based on these strategy discussions. Veteran players may help rookies (the new players) in understanding the playbook, expectations of the coaches and organization, or any other unclear information. Once the game begins, coaches and players work together to implement their game plan in the midst of chaos, unexpected confusion, and time constraints. Players feel a responsibility toward their teammates to perform their best during every play.

After the game, the coach and team debrief. They discuss what they did well during the game and how they could have been better. The process then starts all over again, as the next week's opponent is just days away. Without this careful planning, the team would not be successful.

The planning process for developing a unit-based orientation program is quite similar to this analogy. The goals of the program are to develop the clinical competencies of orientees, help them become socialized, and facilitate their role transition. The ultimate goal of the unit or organization is for clinical nurses to deliver safe, quality care to patients. This is a "victory" in football terms. The nursing staff on your unit, with you as the coach, comprise the veteran players responsible for helping orientees, or the rookies, attain the outcomes of the orientation. The orientation team develops a plan to accomplish these goals, with each team member made aware of his or her roles and responsibilities. This is similar to the coaching staff developing a game plan and the players learning it throughout the week.

When orientees arrive on the clinical unit, team members work to help the orientees reach their goals. This occurs in the midst of an often busy and chaotic clinical unit. The team uses its resources wisely, recruiting experienced nurses to serve as preceptors and making good use of the time allotted for orientation. Like orientees, football rookies are coached on the job and often put in unfamiliar situations to assess their capabilities.

After orientees successfully complete the unit-based orientation program, they are able to provide competent nursing care to patients on the unit. This is similar to when a rookie finally learns the playbook and is able to execute the game plan with success. These new employees feel that they are valued members of the clinical unit and are more at ease in their roles.

Much like the end of a football game, the unit staff eventually debriefs, reviewing all aspects of the unit-based orientation program. The staff feel that they have made a significant contribution to the orientees' learning and to patient care. They discuss ways to improve the orientation and start planning for the next one.

Developing a Plan Based on Orientee Learning Needs and Goals

Use unit-specific competencies to help you develop a plan for the nurses attending the unit-based orientation. Start with a teaching plan. Figure 4-7 lists examples of content that may be included in the program. Next, outline any content and teaching strategies that will help the orientee attain the expected outcomes. After determining whether your unit-based orientation stands alone from the specialty orientation, determine a need for including didactic content in addition to clinical assignments.

Be sure to include various active learning exercises that are congruent with each competency (see Chapter 6). Provide the orientees with a variety of learning options that they

---

Figure 4-7. Content That May Be Included in a Unit-Based Orientation Program

- Philosophy
- Goals and objectives
- Policies and procedures
- Rules and regulations
- Strategic plan (and fit with nursing department plan)
- Organizational structure of the unit personnel
- Tour of physical plan of the unit
- Patient documentation system
- Documentation of work schedule, requests for vacations, call-off procedures, etc.
- Breaks and meals, designated eating areas
- Patient assignments
- Use of communication systems
- Location of emergency numbers and equipment
- Ordering equipment and supplies
- Unit educational plan
- Committee structure and assignments

- Review of job description and performance appraisal process at unit level
- Confidentiality of patient and health information
- Nutritional support
- Promotions (clinical ladder) and transfers
- Portfolio preparation
- Infection control and isolation procedures
- Patient's Bill of Rights
- Advance directives
- Body mechanics and patient transfers
- Ethical dilemmas
- Restraint use
- IV fluids and central lines
- Blood product administration
- Organ procurement
- Oxygen therapy
- Computer training

---

can complete at their own pace. Use learning activities that resemble the actual clinical environment. Preceptors need to observe the orientees as they demonstrate these competencies.

Familiarizing Unit Staff With Adult Learning Principles

Before the orientees arrive on the clinical unit, help the nursing staff develop an understanding of how adults learn, and provide them with practical strategies to use when interacting with the orientees. Although preceptors should already have an understanding of these principles as part of their preceptor preparation program, it is important that all staff who will be interacting with the orientees understand how adults learn. Consider conducting a unit-based in-service for staff on adult learning principles, or develop a packet of information that they can review at their own pace or at a journal club session.

When preparing staff for the orientation program, ask them to reflect on the emotions they experienced when they were new to the clinical unit. Explore staff behaviors that were most effective in making them feel welcome. Ask nursing staff to recall specific teaching strategies and learning activities that were most effective in helping them develop their clinical competencies.

Creating a Unit-Based Schedule With Target Dates

After developing your plan, create a schedule for the unit-based orientation and assign target dates when orientees are expected to complete particular competencies. Although no pre-established end dates usually exist for CBOs, target dates may keep orientees on their timeline. In some healthcare organizations, orientees progress through a unit-based orientation at their own rate. It is likely that some orientees, such as experienced RNs, may complete the unit-based orientation in less time than newly hired, inexperienced nurses.

When developing a schedule for your unit-based program, include the day of the week, date, times, the learning activity, its location, and the guest speaker or person responsible for overseeing each activity. Also include the names of the orientees and their respective preceptors.

Distribute the schedule to appropriate individuals in your organization, such as the nurse manager, staff development educator, orientees, and preceptors. Post the schedule on the unit's bulletin board or your hospital's intranet so it is available to all staff. Save a copy of the schedule for your education files along with your plan.

Consider inviting staff from the clinical unit to serve as guest speakers for the orientation program. Invite members of the interprofessional team to participate, including the unit's social worker, physical therapist, and nutritionist.

It is important to develop an evaluation plan for the CBO program before orientees arrive on the unit. Kirkpatrick's Four-Level Evaluation Model (Kirkpatrick, 1998; Kirkpatrick & Kirkpatrick, 2006) may be a helpful framework to use. The model includes four levels of outcomes: reaction, learning, behavior/transfer, and results. Regardless of the model you use in evaluating the CBO program, your plan should include key individuals involved in the unit-based program such as the orientees, preceptors, and the nurse manager. This plan should consider both formative and summative evaluations.

Formative Evaluation

Formative evaluation occurs on an ongoing basis during the unit-based orientation and provides learners with timely feedback regarding their progress toward program outcomes (Gaberson, Oermann, & Shellenbarger, 2015). It also enables orientees to seek learning experiences that will strengthen their competencies. Formative evaluation helps to determine the orientees' learning needs and does not determine whether the orientee successfully completed the orientation program.

Because preceptors observe orientees as they provide direct patient care and understand the behaviors expected of orientees during their clinical experience, they are in a prime position to evaluate the orientees' performance. Preceptors should provide orientees with timely verbal and written feedback about their clinical performance and work closely with orientees to develop strategies to improve.

A variety of methods can be used to evaluate the orientee's performance during the unit-based orientation program. First, preceptors can document the orientee's performance through daily, written anecdotes. Anecdotes are narrative descriptions of an orientee's performance based on the preceptor's observations (Gaberson et al., 2015). Anecdotes may or may not include the preceptor's interpretation of the observation. These observations should be discussed privately with the orientees, providing them with immediate feedback about their behavior and an opportunity to clarify misconceptions. Together, the preceptor and orientee can develop a personal plan to strengthen any deficiencies.

Second, preceptors should assess and validate the orientee's performance related to unit-specific competencies. Clinical competencies often are evaluated using performance checklists. These checklists include key competency statements and evaluation criteria. Appendix 4-1 is an example of a competency validation tool that was developed for nurses employed on a bone marrow and cellular transplant unit. The tool lists the competency, along with criteria that indicate successful completion of the competency. The method of validation used (documentation, observation, or testing) and selection criteria (high-risk, problem prone, or essential) are recorded. The preceptor indicates gender- and age-specific information (neonate, pediatric, adolescent, adult, and geriatric) and provides an opportunity for the preceptor to comment on an orientee's performance. Both the orientee and preceptor, as the validator, sign and date each competency. The nurse manager and orientee sign and date the checklist after it is completed.

Preceptors also may summarize an orientee's overall progress during the orientation program on a weekly basis by using a tool that may include a summary of the orientee's experiences, strengths, and areas for improvement. Daily anecdotes and the competency validation tool can be used to develop this evaluation. Specific goals for the orientee are developed based on these data. Both the orientee and the preceptor have an opportunity to provide comments. The orientee, preceptor, nurse manager, and educator sign this weekly evaluation.

Third, some organizations may include additional forms to document the progress of the orientee during orientation. Appendix 4-2 is an example of a competency validation tool that was developed for nurses employed on a bone marrow and cellular transplant unit at three months to one year after hire. The preceptor and orientee identify specific goals based on these accomplishments and provide comments, as needed. This evaluation may be used near the end of the orientation period, once the orientee has successfully completed the program, or at specific intervals in the event that an orientee is not performing as expected. The nurse manager and educator may be present during this evaluation.

Depending on the clinical unit, validation of specific competencies may be determined to be necessary by the healthcare organization. Appendix 4-3 provides an example of a skills checklist for chemotherapy/targeted therapy spill management. Similar checklists exist for nurses and include chemotherapy/targeted therapy administration, extravasation, and hypersensitivity/anaphylactic management.

Summative Evaluation

In addition to formative evaluation, conduct a summative evaluation at the conclusion of the unit-based orientation to determine if the orientees have attained expected competencies and if program outcomes have been achieved (Oermann & Gaberson, 2014). The summative evaluation should include input from anyone who actively participated in the orientation program. In addition to using a traditional survey to collect evaluation data, Jeffery and Jarvis (2014) suggested other approaches as well, such as individual interviews and focus group sessions.

Table 4-1 illustrates the possible perspectives that you can obtain for this evaluation. The grid lists the individuals mentioned previously across the top axis. The vertical axis indicates the various perspectives you may obtain. For example, you may wish to obtain the orientees' self-evaluation and feedback on the effectiveness of program teachers. Repeat this process with the remaining individuals. The completed competency valida-

Table 4-1. Grid for Determining Unit-Based Orientation Program Evaluation

	Orientee	Preceptor	Unit-Based Educator	Nurse Manager
Orientee	Self-evaluation	x	x	x
Preceptor	x	Self-evaluation	x	x
Unit-based educator	x	x	Self-evaluation	x
Nurse manager	x	x	x	Self-evaluation

tion form can serve as evidence of an orientee's performance related to unit-specific competencies.

In addition, obtain feedback from all individuals on the orientation program. This evaluation should include the orientees' feedback on the degree in which the program enabled them to attain their competencies and their overall satisfaction with the program. Ask participants for their ideas for future orientations.

Establishing a Documentation and Record-Keeping System

Determine the documents that you will need to maintain as part of the unit-based orientation program, along with a system to maintain these records. Start by meeting with the staff development educator responsible for the specialty orientation and the nurse manager to help you identify these items. Regardless of the system you choose, be sure that it offers privacy and allows records to be easily retrieved and accessed. Consider how you will organize your records, such as an alphabetical order or by hiring date (Jeffery & Jarvis, 2014).

You will need to maintain certain documents related to the unit-based program. For example, each orientee's competency validation form should be maintained. Some organizations prefer to keep these forms in the nurse manager's office on the clinical unit, whereas others prefer they be kept in the orientee's personnel file in the human resources department. Copies of the unit-based plan, schedules, and completed evaluations also should be maintained, most often in secure professional development education files. Be sure that the competency documents are signed by the orientee, educator, and manager (Jeffery & Jarvis, 2014).

Determining Expenses

With careful planning, you should be able to determine the anticipated costs for the unit-based orientation program. Talk with the nurse manager and the staff development educator to clarify this procedure. It is important to plan a program that is cost-effective.

Implementing the Unit-Based Orientation Program

Careful planning of your unit-based orientation program will help you get organized and keep you on track once the orientees arrive on the clinical unit. Spend this time welcoming the orientees to the clinical unit, orienting them to the CBO and their expectations, and pairing them with their preceptors. Preceptors can work with their respective orientees in developing individualized plans for meeting their learning needs.

Creating an Environment Conducive to Learning on the Clinical Unit

Clinical units often can be very stressful, chaotic, and busy places for patients and unit staff. Attempt to transform the clinical unit into a place that is conducive to learning and makes orientees feel comfortable and welcome. This is especially important given the nursing shortage and the personal and financial investment an organization makes during orientation. Although there are some elements in the work environment you may not be able to change, focus your energy on the things that you can positively influence.

Start by coordinating a welcoming reception on the unit when the orientees arrive. This will give them an opportunity to meet their preceptor, nurse manager, and other staff in the organization. Consider taking photographs of this event, with permission, and post them on the unit's intranet, social media page, or bulletin board.

Provide orientees with an opportunity to share their past experiences and professional goals. Have preceptors build upon these experiences in developing individualized learning options for each of their orientees.

Introducing Orientees to the Unit-Based Orientation Program and Preceptors

Introduce the orientees to the goals of the unit-based CBO program, review the competencies they are expected to demonstrate, and educate them on how they can successfully progress through the program. Clarify their specific roles and responsibilities and those of the preceptors, unit-based educators, and nurse managers. Inform orientees of the various learning opportunities available to them. Explain the program's evaluation plan and how it will provide them with ongoing feedback about their progress. Orient the new nurses to the physical layout of the unit and the locations of the supplies and equipment needed to provide patient care.

Selecting Meaningful and Appropriate Clinical Assignments

Assist preceptors in designing learning experiences that will allow orientees to demonstrate or develop expected unit-specific competencies. These competencies may be completed while providing patient care under preceptor supervision or through other available learning options. Support preceptors in selecting appropriate patient care assignments, if needed. If the orientees require additional information and practice to attain these competencies, provide them with additional learning opportunities. Ensure that the preceptors' evaluation of the orientees' performance is objective and consistent among all learners.

Providing Support and Guidance

Although it is vital that the orientees receive ongoing support and guidance from their preceptors during the orientation program, it is also important that preceptors receive support. Consider scheduling private meetings with preceptors on a regular basis to determine their learning needs and provide them with support and direction in their role. Be available to preceptors on a daily basis in the event that problems arise. Provide preceptors with feedback about their performance and ways to strengthen their behaviors.

Encourage preceptors to allow their orientees to progress through the orientation program at their own pace while keeping them on target. Remind preceptors that newly graduated nurses may require more support than more experienced nurses. Alert them to nonverbal cues that may indicate that an orientee may be experiencing difficulties.

Lepianka (2014) recommended introducing newly hired graduate nurses to weekly reflective journaling during their orientation to decrease their anxiety while strengthening their competencies. Orientees are asked to identify a "memorable and significant practice experience" for their reflection and share personal feelings (Lepianka, 2014, p. 342). Staff nurses who are paired with the orientees review these journals.

Documenting the Progress of the Orientees

Assist the preceptors as they document the orientees' progress. Help them in developing individualized action plans to strengthen the competencies of the orientees or in dealing with unique issues such as attitude problems, lack of motivation, or an inability to meet performance expectations (Joint Commission, 2015).

Evaluating Outcomes of the Unit-Based Orientation

Rely on the comprehensive plan you previously developed to evaluate key aspects of the orientation program, focusing on orientee performance related to unit-specific competencies and job duties. Consider scheduling a focus group with nursing staff and preceptors to gain their input regarding the orientation program's process and outcomes. Determine the cost of the program and consider ways to streamline it while ensuring strong outcomes. Consider calculating the return on investment or cost–benefit ratio for your orientation program (Jeffery & Jarvis, 2014). This evidence will allow you to determine if the benefits of an orientation are greater than its costs.

Wright (2005) suggested asking key stakeholders questions to gain their perspectives on the competency program. Questions may ask what portions of the program worked well and what could have been stronger, what competencies posed the greatest challenges for orientees, and whether sufficient support was provided to evaluators.

Use evaluation data to revise future unit-based orientation programs. Finally, monitor the unit-based outcomes that may have been influenced by the orientation program, including staff satisfaction, recruitment, and retention rates.

Summary

The orientation component of NPD focuses on assessing and developing the competencies of both new and experienced nurses in healthcare organizations. The ultimate goal of ensuring competency is for nurses to effectively provide safe, quality care to patients. Although the primary responsibility for continuing competence belongs to individual nurses, others, including unit-based educators and managers, play an important role in contributing to this goal. Educators need to understand the orientation process at their organization and develop quality, cost-effective unit-based programs that will ensure the competency of orientees and meet their educational needs as adult learners. These programs need to include a comprehensive evaluation program that can determine the outcome of these interventions on orientees, nursing staff, patient care, and the healthcare organization.

Helpful Websites

• Joint Commission—About The Joint Commission: www.jointcommission.org/about_us/about_the_joint_commission_main.aspx

- National Council of State Boards of Nursing: www.ncsbn.org/index.htm
- Occupational Safety and Health Administration—Education and Training: www.osha.gov/dsg/hospitals/education_training.html

References

Abruzzese, R.S. (1996). *Nursing staff development: Strategies for success* (2nd ed.). St. Louis, MO: Mosby.

AllNurses. (2009). Performance Based Management System (PBMS). Retrieved from http://allnurses.com/nursing-educators-faculty/performance-based-development-393490.html

Alspach, J.G. (1996). *Designing competency assessment programs: A handbook for nursing and health-related professions.* Pensacola, FL: National Nursing Staff Development Organization.

American Association of Colleges of Nursing. (2008). *The essentials of baccalaureate education for professional nursing practice.* Washington, DC: Author.

American Association of Colleges of Nursing. (2011). *The essentials of master's education in nursing.* Retrieved from http://www.aacn.nche.edu/education-resources/MastersEssentials11.pdf

American Association of Colleges of Nursing. (2014). Nurse residency program. Retrieved from http://www.aacn.nche.edu/education-resources/nurse-residency-program

American Association of Critical-Care Nurses. (2014a). The AACN Synergy Model for Patient Care. Retrieved from http://www.aacn.org/wd/certifications/content/synmodel.pcms?menu=\\

American Association of Critical-Care Nurses. (2014b). The Synergy Model in practice. Retrieved from http://www.aacn.org/wd/certifications/content/syninpract.pcms?menu=certification

American Nurses Association. (2000). *Scope and standards of practice for nursing professional development.* Washington, DC: Author.

American Nurses Association. (2012). Frequently asked questions. Roles of state boards of nursing: Licensure, regulation and complaint investigation. Retrieved from http://www.nursingworld.org/MainMenuCategories/Tools/State-Boards-of-Nursing-FAQ.pdf

American Nurses Association. (2014). Professional role competence. Retrieved from http://www.nursingworld.org/MainMenuCategories/ThePracticeofProfessionalNursing/NursingStandards/Professional-Role-Competence.html

American Nurses Association. (2015). *Nursing: Scope and standards of practice* (3rd ed.). Silver Spring, MD: Author.

American Nurses Association & National Nursing Staff Development Organization. (2010). *Nursing professional development: Scope and standards of practice.* Silver Spring, MD: American Nurses Association.

American Nurses Credentialing Center. (n.d.-a). Accredited competency programs. Retrieved from http://www.nursecredentialing.org/AccreditedCompetencyCourses

American Nurses Credentialing Center. (n.d.-b). Nursing Skills Competency Program. Retrieved from http://www.nursecredentialing.org/NursingSkillsCompetencyProgram.aspx

American Nurses Credentialing Center. (n.d.-c). State boards of nursing CE renewal requirements. Retrieved from http://www.nursecredentialing.org/StateCERequirements

American Nurses Credentialing Center. (2015). American Nurses Credentialing Center's Nursing Skills Competency Program Criteria. Retrieved from http://www.nursecredentialing.org/NSCP-CriteriaList.aspx

Amerson, R. (2002). Orientation. In K.L. O'Shea (Ed.), *Staff development nursing secrets* (pp. 161–174). Philadelphia, PA: Hanley and Belfus.

Anthony, C.E., & del Bueno, D.J. (1993). A performance-based development system. *Nursing Management, 24*(6), 32.

Bashford, C.W., Shaffer, B.J., & Young, C.M. (2012). Assessment of clinical judgment in nursing orientation: Time well invested. *Journal for Nurses in Staff Development, 28,* 62–65. doi:10.1097/NND.0b013e31824b4155

Beauman, S.S. (2001). Didactic components of a comprehensive pediatric competency program. *Journal of Infusion Nursing, 24,* 367–374. doi:10.1097/00129804-200111000-00003

Betany, K., Yarwood, J. (2010). Adapting the dedicated education unit model for student learning in the community. *Kai Tiaki: Nursing New Zealand, 16*(5), 22–23.

Brant, J.M., & Wickham, R. (Eds.). (2013). *Statement on the scope and standards of oncology nursing practice: Generalist and advanced practice.* Pittsburgh, PA: Oncology Nursing Society.

Bumgarner, S.D., & Biggerstaff, G.H. (2000). A patient-centered approach to nurse orientation. *Journal for Nurses in Staff Development, 16,* 249–256. doi:10.1097/00124645-200011000-00003

Burke, K., Moscato, S., & Warner, J.R. (2009). A primer on the politics of partnership between education and regulation. *Journal of Professional Nursing, 25,* 349–351. doi:10.1016/j.profnurs.2009.10.002

Casey, K., Fink, R., Krugman, M., & Propst, J. (2004). The graduate nurse experience. *Journal of Nursing Administration, 34,* 303–311. doi:10.1097/00005110-200406000-00010

Childress, S.B., & Gorder, D. (2012). Oncology nurse internships: A foundation and future for oncology nursing practice? *Oncology Nursing Forum, 39,* 341–344. doi:10.1188/12.ONF.341-344

Cooper, D.C. (2002). The "c" word: Competency. In K.L. O'Shea (Ed.), *Staff development nursing secrets* (pp. 175–184). Philadelphia, PA: Hanley and Belfus.

Crimlisk, J.T., McNulty, M.J., & Francione, D.A. (2002). New graduate RNs in a float pool: An inner-city hospital experience. *Journal of Nursing Administration, 32*(4), 211–217.

Culley, T., Babbie, A., Clancey, J., Clouse, K., Hines, R., Kraynek, M., … Wittmann, S. (2012). Nursing U: A concept for nursing orientation. *Nursing Management, 43*(3), 45–47. doi:10.1097/01.NUMA.0000412950.80510.95

Dean, G.E., Reishtein, J.L., McVey, J., Ambrose, M., Burke, S.M., Haskins, M., & Jones, J. (2013). Implementing a dedicated education unit: A practice partnership with oncology nurses. *Clinical Journal of Oncology Nursing, 17,* 208–210. doi:10.1188/13.CJON.208-210

del Bueno, D.J. (1990). Experience, education, and nurses' ability to make clinical judgments. *Nursing and Health Care, 11,* 290–294.

del Bueno, D.J. (1994). Why can't new grads think like nurses? *Nurse Educator, 19*(4), 9–11. doi:10.1097/00006223-199407000-00008

del Bueno, D.J. (2001). Buyer beware: The cost of competence. *Nursing Economics, 19,* 250–257.

del Bueno, D.J. (2005). A crisis in critical thinking. *Nursing Education Perspectives, 26,* 278–282. doi:10.1043/1536-5026(2005)026[0278:ACICT]2.0.CO;2

Disher, J., Burgum, A., Desai, A., Fallon, C., Hart, P.L., & Aduddell, K. (2014). The effect of a unit-based simulation on nurses' identification of deteriorating patients. *Journal for Nurses in Professional Development, 30,* 21–28. doi:10.1097/NND.0b013e31829e6c83

Dumpe, M.L., Kanyok, N., & Hill, K. (2007). Use of an automated learning management system to validate nursing competencies. *Journal for Nurses in Staff Development, 23,* 183–185. doi:10.1097/01.NND.0000281418.50472.2e

Duvall, J.J. (2009). From novice to advanced beginner: The critical care internship. *Journal for Nurses in Staff Development, 25,* 25–27. doi:10.1097/NND.0b013e318194b4fc

Esparza, D. (Ed.). (2014). *Oncology policies and procedures.* Pittsburgh, PA: Oncology Nursing Society.

Exstrom, S.M. (2001). The state board of nursing and its role in continued competency. *Journal of Continuing Education in Nursing, 32,* 118–125.

Field, J.M., Hazinski, M.F., Sayre, M.R., Chameides, L., Schexnayder, S.M., Hemphill, R., … Vanden Hoek, T.L. (2010). 2010 American Heart Association guidelines for cardiopulmonary resuscitation and emergency cardiovascular care: Part 1: Executive summary. *Circulation, 122,* S640–S656. doi:10.1161/CIRCULATIONAHA.110.970889

Foster, K.I., Benavides-Vaello, S., Katz, J.R., & Eide, P. (2012). Using the Generative Nursing Model to reframe nursing student transition to practice. *Nurse Educator, 37,* 252–257. doi:10.1097/NNE.0b013e31826f27c1

Frentsos, J.M. (2013). Rubrics role in measuring nursing staff competencies. *Journal for Nurses in Professional Development, 29,* 19–23. doi:10.1097/NND.0b013e31827d0a9c

Freundl, M., Anthony, M., Johnson, B., Harmer, B.M., Carter, J.M., Boudiab, L.D., & Nelson, V. (2012). A dedicated education unit VA Medical Centers and baccalaureate nursing programs partnership model. *Journal of Professional Nursing, 28,* 344–350. doi:10.1016/j.profnurs.2012.05.008

Gaberson, K.B., Oermann, M.H., & Shellenbarger, T. (2015). *Clinical teaching strategies in nursing* (4th ed.). New York, NY: Springer.

Glynn, P., & Silva, S. (2013). Meeting the needs of new graduates in the emergency department: A qualitative study evaluating a new graduate internship program. *Journal of Emergency Nursing, 39,* 173–178. doi:10.1016/j.jen.2011.10.007

Goode, C.J., Lynn, M.R., McElroy, D., Bednash, G.D., & Murray, B. (2013). Lesson learned from 10 years of research on a post-baccalaureate nurse residency program. *Journal of Nursing Administration, 43,* 73–79. doi:10.1097/NNA.0b013e31827f205c

Grove, J., & Bush, B. (2002). First hand: Developing an orientation brochure to make sure forensic staff get the information they need. *Joint Commission Benchmark, 4,* 6–7.

Guin, P., Counsell, C.M., & Briggs, S. (2002). Round out your department. *Nursing Management, 33*(5), 24. doi:10.1097/00006247-200205000-00010

Gurney, D. (2002). Developing a successful 16-week "transition ED nursing" program: One busy community hospital's experience. *Journal of Emergency Nursing, 28,* 505–514. doi:10.1067/men.2002.129707

Han, K., Trinkoff, A.M., Storr, C.L., Lerner, N., Johantgen, M., & Gartrell, K. (2014). Associations between state regulations, training length, perceived quality and job satisfaction among certified nursing assistants: Cross-sectional secondary data analysis. *International Journal of Nursing Studies, 51,* 1135–1141. doi:10.1016/j.ijnurstu.2013.12.008

Hannon, P.O., Hunt, C.A., Haleem, D., King, L., Day, L., & Casals, P. (2012). Implementation of a dedicated education unit for baccalaureate students: Process and evaluation. *International Journal of Nursing Education, 4,* 155–159.

Harmon, L.M. (2013). Rural model dedicated education unit: Partnership between college and hospital. *Journal of Continuing Education in Nursing, 44,* 89–96. doi:10.3928/00220124-20121217-62

Harrison, D., & Ledbetter, C. (2014). Nurse residency programs: Outcome comparisons to best practices. *Journal for Nurses in Professional Development, 30,* 76–82. doi:10.1097/NND.0000000000000001

Hohler, S.E. (2003). Creating an environment conducive to adult learning. *AORN Online, 77,* 833–835. doi:10.1016/S0001-2092(06)60802-8

Hooper, B.L. (2014). Using case studies and videotaped vignettes to facilitate the development of critical thinking skills in new graduate nurses. *Journal for Nurses in Professional Development, 30,* 87–91. doi:10.1097/NND.0000000000000009

Indiana University Health. (2014). Patient care internships (formerly known as student nurse externships). Retrieved from http://iuhealth.org/education/nursing-and-patient-care/student-nurse-extern-program

Institute of Medicine. (2010). *The future of nursing: Leading change, advancing health.* Washington, DC: National Academies Press.

Interprofessional Education Collaborative. (2011). *Core competencies for interprofessional collaborative practice: Report of an expert panel.* Retrieved from http://www.aacn.nche.edu/education-resources/ipecreport.pdf

Jeffery, A.D., & Jarvis, R.L. (2014). *Staff educator's guide to clinical orientation: Onboarding solutions for nurses.* Indianapolis, IN: Sigma Theta Tau International.

Jeffries, P.R., Rose, L., Belcher, A.E., Dang, D., Hochuli, J.F., Fleischmann, D., … Walrath, J.M. (2013). A clinical academic practice partnership: A clinical education redesign. *Journal of Professional Nursing, 29,* 128–136. doi:10.1016/j.profnurs.2012.04.013

Jenkins, J. (2002). Genetics competency: New directions for nursing. *AACN Clinical Issues: Advanced Practice in Acute and Critical Care, 13*(4), 486–491.

Johns Hopkins University School of Nursing Career Center. (n.d.). Clinical nurse intern/extern programs: An opportunity to develop nursing skills. Retrieved from http://nursing.jhu.edu/life-at-hopkins/center/documents/nursing_intern.pdf

Johnson, T., Opfer, K., VanCura, B.J., & Williams, L. (2000). A comprehensive interactive competency program: Part II: Implementation, outcomes, and follow-up. *MEDSURG Nursing, 9,* 308–310.

Johnston, P.A., & Ferraro, C.A. (2001). Application of critical pathways in the maternity nursing orientation process. *Journal for Nurses in Staff Development, 17,* 61–66. doi:10.1097/00124645-200103000-00001

Joint Commission. (n.d.). About the Joint Commission. Retrieved from http://www.jointcommission.org/about_us/about_the_joint_commission_main.aspx

Joint Commission. (2010). Advancing effective communication, cultural competence, and patient- and family-centered care: A roadmap for hospitals. Retrieved from http://www.jointcommission.org/assets/1/6/ARoadmapforHospitalsfinalversion727.pdf

Joint Commission. (2015). The Joint Commission E-dition: Human resources. Retrieved from http://www.jointcommission.org/standards_information/edition.aspx

Joint Commission International. (2013). *Joint Commission International accreditation standards for hospitals* (5th ed.). Retrieved from http://www.jointcommissioninternational.org/jci-accreditation-standards-for-hospitals-5th-edition

Kirkpatrick, D.L. (1998). *Evaluating training programs: The four levels* (2nd ed.). San Francisco, CA: Berrett-Koehler.

Kirkpatrick, D.L., & Kirkpatrick, J.D. (2006). *Evaluating training programs: The four levels* (3rd ed.). San Francisco, CA: Berrett-Koehler.

Knowles, M.S. (1980). *The modern practice of adult education: From pedagogy to andragogy.* Chicago, IL: Follett.

Knowles, M.S. (1990). *The adult learner: A neglected species* (4th ed.). Houston, TX: Gulf Publishing.

Krampe, J., L'Ecuyer, K., & Palmer, J.L. (2013). Development of an online orientation course for preceptors in a dedicated education unit program. *Journal of Continuing Education in Nursing, 44,* 352–356. doi:10.3928/00220124-20130617-44

Krozek, C., & Scoggins, A. (2000). *Ambulatory medicine department competencies: Registered nurse.* Glendale, CA: CINAHL Information Systems.

Krugman, M., Bretschneider, J., Horn, P.B., Krsek, C.A., Moutafis, R.A., & Smith, M.O. (2006). The national postbaccalaureate graduate nurse residency program: A model for excellence in transition to practice. *Journal for Nurses in Staff Development, 22*(4), 196–205.

Kuhrik, N., Laub, L., Kuhrik, M., & Atwater, K. (2011). An interdepartmental team approach to develop, implement, and sustain an oncology nursing orientation program. *Oncology Nursing Forum, 38,* 115–118. doi:10.1188/11.ONF.115-118

Kumaran, S., & Carney, M. (2014). Role transition from student nurse to staff nurse: Facilitating the transition period. *Nurse Education in Practice, 14,* 605–611. doi:10.1016/j.nepr.2014.06.002

Lengetti, E., Monachino, A.M., & Scholtz, A. (2011). A simulation-based "just in time" and "just-in-place" central venous catheter education program. *Journal for Nurses in Staff Development, 27,* 290–293.

Leonard, B.J., & Plotnikoff, G.A. (2000). Awareness: The heart of cultural competence. *AACN Clinical Issues: Advanced Practice in Acute and Critical Care, 11,* 51–59. doi:10.1097/00044067-200002000-00007

Lepianka, J.E. (2014). Using reflective journaling to improve the orientation of graduate nurses. *Journal of Continuing Education in Nursing, 45,* 342–343. doi:10.3928/00220124-20140724-14

Letourneau, R.M. (2010). Attract the best and brightest with comprehensive internships. *Nursing Management, 41*(4), 12–16. doi:10.1097/01.NUMA.0000370872.17725.20

Lipscomb, V.G. (2010). Intergenerational issues in nursing: Learning from each generation. *Clinical Journal of Oncology Nursing, 14,* 267–269. doi:10.1188/10.CJON.267-269

Longo, M.A., Young, D., Jones, C., Shaw, C.A., Werner, R., Minor, D., & Hoying, C. (2014). TERN residency program: Transitioning the experienced registered nurse. *Journal for Nurses in Professional Development, 30,* 181–184. doi:10.1097/NND.0000000000000063

Lott, T., Willis, L., & Lyttle, E. (2011). The successful redesign of a student nurse extern program. *Journal for Nurses in Staff Development, 27,* 236–239. doi:10.1097/NND.0b013e31822d6f14

Massachusetts Department of Higher Education. (2010). *Nurse of the future: Nursing core competencies.* Retrieved from http://www.mass.edu/currentinit/documents/NursingCoreCompetencies.pdf

McKown, T., McKeon, L., & Webb, S. (2011). Using quality and safety education for nurses to guide clinical teaching on a new dedicated education unit. *Journal of Nursing Education, 50,* 706–710. doi:10.3928/01484834-20111017-03

McVey, C., Vessey, J.A., Kenner, C.A., & Pressler, J.L. (2014). Interprofessional dedicated education unit. *Nurse Educator, 39,* 153–154. doi:10.1097/NNE.0000000000000051

Melillo, K.D., Abdallah, L., Dodge, L., Dowling, J.S., Prendergast, N., Rathbone, A., … Thornton, C. (2014). Developing a dedicated education unit in long-term care: A pilot project. *Geriatric Nursing, 35,* 264–271. doi:10.1016/j.gerinurse.2014.02.022

Moore, J., & Nahigian, E. (2013). Nursing student perceptions of nurse-to-nurse collaboration in dedicated education units and in traditional clinical instruction units. *Journal of Nursing Education, 52,* 346–350.

Mulready-Shick, J., & Flanagan, K.M. (2014). Building the evidence for dedicated education unit sustainability and partnership success. *Nursing Education Perspectives, 35,* 287–293. doi:10.5480/14-1379

Mulready-Shick, J., Flanagan, K.M., Banister, G.E., Mylott, L., & Curtin, L.J. (2013). Evaluating dedicated education units for clinical education quality. *Journal of Nursing Education, 52,* 606–614. doi:10.3928/01484834-20131014-07

Murray, T.A., & James, D.C. (2012). Evaluation of an academic service partnership using a strategic alliance framework. *Nursing Outlook, 60,* e17–e22. doi:10.1016/j.outlook.2011.10.004

Naholi, R.M., Nosek, C.L., & Somayaji, D. (2015). Stress among new oncology nurses. *Clinical Journal of Oncology Nursing, 19,* 115–117. doi:10.1188/15.CJON.115-117

National Council of State Boards of Nursing. (2012). *2013 NCLEX-RN detailed test plan: Item writer/item reviewer/nurse educator version.* Retrieved from https://www.ncsbn.org/2013_NCLEX_RN_Detailed_Test_Plan_Educator.pdf

National League for Nursing. (2012). *Outcomes and competencies for graduates of practical/vocational, diploma, baccalaureate, master's practice doctorate, and research doctorate programs in nursing.* Washington, DC: Author.

Nishioka, V.M., Coe, M.T., Hanita, M., & Moscato, S.R. (2014a). Dedicated education unit: Nurse perspectives on their clinical teaching role. *Nursing Education Perspectives, 35,* 294–300. doi:10.5480/14-1381

Nishioka, V.M., Coe, M.T., Hanita, M., & Moscato, S.R. (2014b). Dedicated education unit: Student perspectives. *Nursing Education Perspectives, 35,* 301–307. doi:10.5480/14-1380

Occupational Safety and Health Administration. (n.d.). Worker safety in hospitals: Education and training. Retrieved from https://www.osha.gov/dsg/hospitals/education_training.html

Oermann, M.H., & Gaberson, K.B. (2014). *Evaluation and testing in nursing education* (4th ed.). New York, NY: Springer.

Olson, M.A. (2012). English-as-a-Second-Language (ESL) nursing student success: A critical review of the literature. *Journal of Cultural Diversity, 19,* 26–32.

O'Lynn, C. (2013). Comparison between the Portland Model dedicated education unit in acute care and long-term care settings in meeting medical-surgical nursing course outcomes: A pilot study. *Geriatric Nursing, 34,* 187–193. doi:10.1016/j.gerinurse.2013.01.001

Oncology Nursing Society. (n.d.-a). Educator Resource Center. Retrieved from https://erc.ons.org

Oncology Nursing Society. (n.d.-b). Practice resources: Oncology nursing core competencies. Retrieved from https://www.ons.org/practice-resources/competencies

Oncology Nursing Society. (2014). Lifelong learning for professional oncology nurses [Position statement]. Retrieved from https://www.ons.org/advocacy-policy/positions/education/lifelong

O'Shea, K.L., & Smith, L.S. (2002). The mandatories. In K.L. O'Shea (Ed.), *Staff development nursing secrets* (pp. 185–195). Philadelphia, PA: Hanley and Belfus.

Parker, K.M., & Smith, C.M. (2012). Assessment and planning for a dedicated education unit. *Journal for Nurses in Staff Development, 28,* E1–E6. doi:10.1097/NND.0b013e31825515da

Performance Management Services. (2012). Home. Retrieved from http://www.pmsi-pbds.com/Default.aspx

Phillips, T., & Hall, M. (2014). Graduate nurse internship program: A formalized orientation program. *Journal for Nurses in Professional Development, 30,* 190–195. doi:10.1097/NND.0000000000000069

Pine, R., & Tart, K. (2007). Return on investment: Benefits and challenges of a baccalaureate nurse residency program. *Nursing Economics, 25*(1), 13–18, 39.

Pittman, P.M., Folsom, A.J., & Bass, E. (2010). U.S.-based recruitment of foreign-educated nurses: Implications of an emerging industry. *American Journal of Nursing, 110*(6), 38–48. doi:10.1097/01.NAJ.0000377689.49232.06

Proehl, J.A. (2002). Developing emergency nursing competence. *Nursing Clinics of North America, 37,* 89–96. doi:10.1016/S0029-6465(03)00085-9

Province, J.L. (2008). Bridging the gap from long-term care nursing assistants to acute care nursing assistants. *Journal for Nurses in Staff Development, 24,* 290–294. doi:10.1097/01.NND.0000342236.20495.69

Quality and Safety Education for Nurses Institute. (n.d.). The evolution of the Quality and Safety Education for Nurses (QSEN) initiative. Retrieved from http://qsen.org/about-qsen/project-overview

Rhodes, M.L., Meyers, C.C., & Underhill, M.L. (2012). Evaluation outcomes of a dedicated education unit in a baccalaureate nursing program. *Journal of Professional Nursing, 28,* 223–230. doi:10.1016/j.profnurs.2011.11.019

Robert Wood Johnson Foundation. (2013). About NCIN. Retrieved from http://www.newcareersinnursing.org/about-ncin

Robinson, J.E. (2009). 10 suggestions for orienting foreign-educated nurses: An integrative review. *Journal for Nurses in Staff Development, 25,* 77–83. doi:10.1097/NND.0b013e31819d84b6

Shellenbarger, T., & Hagler, D. (2015). Clinical simulation. In K.B. Gaberson, M.H. Oermann, & T. Shellenbarger (Eds.), *Clinical teaching strategies in nursing* (4th ed., pp. 187–216). New York, NY: Springer.

Spector, N., & Echternacht, M.S. (2010). A regulatory model for transitioning newly licensed nurses to practice. *Journal of Nursing Regulation, 1*(2), 18–25.

Springer, P.J., Johnson, P., Lind, B., Walker, E., Clavelle, J., & Jensen, N. (2012). The Idaho dedicated education unit model: Cost-effective, high-quality education. *Nurse Educator, 37,* 262–267.

Strong, M., Kane, I., Petras, D., Johnson-Joy, C., & Weingarten, J. (2014). Direct care registered nurses' and nursing leaders' review of the clinical competencies needed for the successful nurse of the future: A gap analysis. *Journal for Nurses in Professional Development, 30,* 196–203. doi:10.1097/NND.0000000000000076

Suskie, L. (2009). *Assessing student learning: A common sense guide* (2nd ed.). San Francisco, CA: Jossey-Bass.

Theisen, J.L., & Sandau, K.E. (2013). Competency of new graduate nurses: A review of their weaknesses and strategies for success. *Journal of Continuing Education in Nursing, 44,* 406–414. doi:10.3928/00220124-20130617-38

U.S. Department of Health and Human Services. (2011). *HHS action plan to reduce racial and ethnic health disparities: A nation free of disparities in health and health care.* Washington, DC: Author.

Ward, S., Stewart, D., Ford, D., Mullen, A.M., & Makic, M.B. (2014). Educating certified nursing assistants educational offerings on the run and more. *Journal for Nurses in Professional Development, 30,* 296–302. doi:10.1097/NND.0000000000000102

Warner, J.R., & Burton, D.A. (2009). The policy and politics of emerging academic–service partnerships. *Journal of Professional Nursing, 25,* 329–334. doi:10.1016/j.profnurs.2009.10.006

Whelan, L. (2006). Competency assessment of nursing staff. *Orthopaedic Nursing, 25,* 198–202. doi:10.1097/00006416-200605000-00008

White, L.L. (2006). Preparing for clinical: Just-in-time. *Nurse Educator, 31,* 57–60.

Wright, D. (2005). *The ultimate guide to competency assessment in health care* (3rd ed.). Minneapolis, MN: Creative Health Care Management.

Wright, D. (2015). *Competency assessment field guide: A real world guide for implementation and application.* Minneapolis, MN: Creative Health Care Management.

Zungolo, E., & Leonardo, M. (2007). The synergy model as a framework for nursing curriculum. In M.A.Q. Curley (Ed.), *Synergy: The unique relationship between nurses and patients* (pp. 141–156). Indianapolis, IN: Sigma Theta Tau International.

Appendix 4-1. Sample Nurse Competency Verification Document (Upon Hire)

ALLEGHENY HEALTH NETWORK
ONCOLOGY COMPETENCY-BASED ORIENTATION (CBO) CHECKLIST

BONE MARROW AND CELLULAR TRANSPLANT - RN

PLEASE PRINT

NAME:	EMPLOYEE NUMBER:
DEPARTMENT:	MANAGER:
PRECEPTOR:	
HIRE / TRANSFER DATE:	

INSTRUCTIONS
- Completed form must be signed by employee, preceptor(s), and unit manager within six weeks of hire.
- Use the key below to document the orientation progress.
- Preceptor shall validate the orientee's level of competence by dating, initialing, and indicating the method of validation.
- If orientee is not competent in any area, preceptor and orientee shall discuss with manager and education specialist.
- An action plan should be developed and documented in collaboration with Human Resources.

KEY TO METHOD OF VALIDATION
D = Documentation O = Observation T = Test S = Simulation
R&D = Reviewed and discussed, no opportunity to perform
Signature Key:

Initials	Name	Title

Reviews at completion of orientation:

Employee Signature:_____Date: _____

Manager Signature:_____Date:_____

(Continued on next page)

Appendix 4-1. Sample Nurse Competency Verification Document (Upon Hire) *(Continued)*

KEY TO METHOD OF VALIDATION
D = Documentation O = Observation T = Test S = Simulation
R&D = Reviewed and discussed, no opportunity to perform

BY THE END OF ORIENTATION THE EMPLOYEE WILL BE ABLE TO:	Date	Initials	Competency Validation Method: D, O, T, S, R&D
PART 1 – Hospital Orientation Requirements			
Environment and Safety			
Identifies emergency codes (code blue, rapid response team, etc.)			
Locates key areas of the hospital List here:			
Utilizes doctor lift			
Initiates occurrence/errors/near miss reporting for adverse drug reactions, complications of procedures, equipment malfunction, medication errors, procedure errors, etc.			
Policies and Procedures			
Reviews the following policies/procedures and/or locates the following:			
☐ Assignment board: Unit assessment guideline policy			
☐ Chain of command			
☐ Beeper/nurse call system policy			
☐ Walking rounds/shift report guidelines policy			
☐ Schedule/time/attendance			
☐ Paging system			
☐ Guidelines for contacting a physician			
☐ Physician coverage/resident/fellow on-call schedule			
☐ Off-shift coverage for patient problems			
☐ Bed management			
☐ Daily code cart checklist			
☐ Infection control policy			
☐ Critical laboratory value policy			
Uses intranet effectively: ☐ Circular education			
☐ SharePoint			
☐ Access Policy Tech on the intranet			

(Continued on next page)

Appendix 4-1. Sample Nurse Competency Verification Document (Upon Hire) *(Continued)*

Equipment			
Demonstrates use of equipment: ☐ PCA pump			
☐ Fax machine			
☐ PYXIS machine			
☐ Telephones			
☐ Pneumatic tube			
☐ Lateral transfer equipment (SLIPP Sheet/Hover Mat)			
☐ Specialty beds			
☐ Feeding pumps			
☐ Continuous pulse oximetry			
☐ Suction			
☐ Blood glucose monitoring			
☐ Oxygen setup			
☐ IV pump setup			
Communication and Collaboration			
Describes the roles of the Care Model healthcare team members: ☐ RN			
☐ PCA/NA			
☐ Resource/Charge nurse			
☐ Manager			
☐ Resident			
☐ Fellow			
☐ Attending physician			
☐ Oncology clinical pharmacist			
☐ NPs/PA			
☐ Coordinator			
☐ Protocol nurse and staff			
☐ Case management			
☐ Social worker			
☐ Dietician			
☐ Enterostomal therapist			
☐ Respiratory therapist			
☐ Blood bank			
☐ EKG			
Communicates pertinent patient information to appropriate health team members effectively			

(Continued on next page)

Appendix 4-1. Sample Nurse Competency Verification Document (Upon Hire) *(Continued)*

Completes verbal/bedside report and handoff			
Delegates tasks to appropriate disciplines			
Demonstrates principles of service excellence when inter-acting with patients, visitors, and fellow employees			
Complies with current guidelines for case management utilization			
Patient Care and Assessment			
Performs nursing interventions consistent with the plan of care according to policy, procedures, and SOPs			
Performs assessment, including physical parameters, learning needs, age-specific/developmental needs, and discharge needs			
Completes oncology admission independently			
Provides care for 1–2 patients independently in timely fashion (organizing, prioritizing, and adapting to crisis/changes)			
Provides care for 2–3 patients independently in timely fashion (organizing, prioritizing, and adapting to crisis/changes)			
Provides care for 3–4 patients independently in timely fashion (organizing, prioritizing, and adapting to crisis/changes)			
Provides care for 4–5 patients independently (night shift) in timely fashion (organizing, prioritizing, and adapting to crisis/changes)			
Performs reassessments according to policy and proce-dure			
Notifies appropriate discipline for changes in patient status			
Patient education: ☐ Locates patient education materials			
☐ Documents using correct forms			
☐ Utilizes TEACH back methodology			
Completes patient discharge independently			
Develops Interdisciplinary Plan of Care			
Utilizes the EMR independently and with accuracy			
Maintains isolation protocols and proper use of PPE ☐ Contact			

(Continued on next page)

Appendix 4-1. Sample Nurse Competency Verification Document (Upon Hire) *(Continued)*

☐ Strict			
☐ Reviews postmortem care policy			
Documents accurately and independently: ☐ Enters preadmission orders independently			
☐ Patient/family teaching record			
☐ Pre-op checklist			
☐ Medication administration			
☐ Discharge instructions			
☐ Restraint/seclusion flow sheet			
☐ Fall risk assessment			
☐ Advance directive			
☐ Admission assessment			
☐ Blood glucose			
☐ Allergies			
☐ Height and weight using double check signature policy			
☐ I&O			
☐ Vital signs			
☐ Oncology daily physical assessment			
☐ Pain assessment			
Procedures/Skills			
Obtains cultures: ☐ Urine			
☐ Blood			
☐ Nasal			
☐ Wound			
Obtains specimens: ☐ Urine			
☐ Sputum			
☐ Stool			
Maintains drains: ☐ Foley			
☐ JP/hemovac			
☐ NGT			
Administers tube feedings			
Performs medication administration safely and accurately per policy and procedure: ☐ Intravenous			
☐ Subcutaneous			

(Continued on next page)

Appendix 4-1. Sample Nurse Competency Verification Document (Upon Hire) *(Continued)*

☐ Oral			
☐ All other routes (R&D)			
Assesses for OTC and herbal supplements			
Administers blood products safely to policy and procedure: ☐ Verifies written consent			
☐ Orders products			
☐ Completes accurate type and cross			
☐ Administers premedications			
☐ Packed RBCs			
☐ Single donor platelets			
☐ Random donor platelets			
☐ HLA platelets			
☐ Discusses CMV status			
☐ Verifies irradiation status			
☐ Ensures leukocyte-depleted products			
☐ Administers IVIG			
Central venous access devices: ☐ Identifies various lines (tunnel/nontunnel) • PICC • Ports • Temporary large central line • Neostar			
☐ Accesses ports			
☐ Flushes to protocol			
☐ Vanco lock when indicated			
☐ Blood cultures			
☐ Blood sampling			
☐ Dressing changes			
☐ Administers Cathflo			
Phlebotomy: ☐ Performs lab draws			
☐ Labels tubes correctly			
☐ Utilizes proper order of blood draws			
☐ FK506 levels (5–10)			
☐ MTX levels (protect in foil) – (less than 0.05)			
Tests/Procedures			
Describes diagnostic testing and results: ☐ Pulmonary function tests			

(Continued on next page)

Appendix 4-1. Sample Nurse Competency Verification Document (Upon Hire) (Continued)

☐ CT scan/PET scan			
☐ MRI			
☐ Lumbar puncture			
☐ Bone marrow biopsy and aspirate			
☐ Bronchoscopy			
☐ Bone scan			
☐ MUGA scan			
☐ Skin biopsy (Infiltrates/GVHD)			
PART 2 – Oncology Orientation Requirements by 6 Weeks			
Integrates key aspects of oncology nursing care: ☐ Absolute neutrophil count calculation			
☐ Dietary restrictions (neutropenia)			
☐ Induction treatment			
☐ Consolidation treatment			
☐ Mobilization therapy			
☐ Neutropenia/febrile illness			
☐ Anemia			
☐ Thrombocytopenia			
☐ Pain management			
☐ Reviews bone marrow and HSCT policies			
Describes supportive therapies including ESA and growth factors			
Provides care for specific oncology disease processes: ☐ Leukemia			
☐ Myelodysplastic syndrome			
☐ Lymphoma			
☐ Multiple myeloma			
Provides care for patients receiving: ☐ Autologous transplant			
☐ Allogeneic transplant			
☐ Tandem transplant			
☐ DLI			
☐ Cord transplants			
Care for immunocompromised patients (B6.6.4.1): ☐ Identifies an immunocompromised patient based on ANC ☐ Institutes neutropenic precautions ☐ Demonstrates proper use of PPE ☐ Implements antibiotic therapy when indicated ☐ Completes a thorough head-to-toe assessment			

(Continued on next page)

Appendix 4-1. Sample Nurse Competency Verification Document (Upon Hire) *(Continued)*			
Care for radiation patients: ☐ Reviews radiation safety			
a. Discusses TBI			
b. Care for patient receiving radiation therapy			
Documents on transplant infusion flow sheet and reaction form			
Completes oncology physical assessment: ☐ Toxicity grading			
Correlates lab findings with medical history, assessment, normal parameters, and standing orders: ☐ Administers electrolyte replacements as needed			
☐ Cyclosporine levels			
☐ FK506 levels			
☐ Methotrexate levels			
Note. Figure courtesy of A. Vioral, PhD, MEd, RN, OCN®, BMTCN™, Director, Oncology Education and Research, Allegheny Health Network, Pittsburgh, PA. Used with permission.			

Appendix 4-2. Sample Nurse Competency Verification Document (3 months – 1 year)

ALLEGHENY HEALTH NETWORK
ONCOLOGY COMPETENCY BASED ORIENTATION (CBO) CHECKLIST
BONE MARROW AND CELLULAR TRANSPLANT – RN
3 Months – 1 Year

PLEASE PRINT

NAME:	EMPLOYEE NUMBER:
DEPARTMENT:	MANAGER:
PRECEPTOR:	
HIRE / TRANSFER DATE:	

INSTRUCTIONS

- Completed form must be signed by employee, preceptor(s), and unit manager within six weeks of hire.
- Use the key below to document the orientation progress.
- Preceptor shall validate the orientee's level of competence by dating, initialing, and indicating the method of validation.
- If orientee is not competent in any area, preceptor and orientee shall discuss with manager and education specialist.
- An action plan should be developed and documented in collaboration with Human Resources.

KEY TO METHOD OF VALIDATION
D = Documentation O = Observation T = Test S = Simulation
R&D = Reviewed and discussed, no opportunity to perform

Signature Key:

Initials	Name	Title

Reviews at completion of orientation:

Employee Signature:_____Date: _____

Manager Signature:_____Date: _____

(Continued on next page)

Appendix 4-2. Sample Nurse Competency Verification Document (3 months – 1 year) *(Continued)*

KEY TO METHOD OF VALIDATION
D = Documentation O = Observation T = Test S = Simulation
R&D = Reviewed and discussed, no opportunity to perform

	Time Frame (months) 3-6-9-12	Date	Initials	Competency Validation Method: D,O,T, S, R&D
PART 1 – FACT Orientation Standards (out-patient oncology)				
Cellular therapy process (B3.6.3.1) ☐ Identifies key concepts of hematology/oncology patient care and cellular therapy process				
Blood products (B6.6.4.5), growth factors, cellular therapy products, and supportive therapy (B3.6.3.3) and (B6.6.4.5) ☐ Identifies key concepts of hematology/oncology patient care and cellular therapy process				
Transplant complications (neutropenia, fever, mucositis, nausea, vomiting, pain management, infectious, and noninfectious, etc.) – (B3.6.3.4) ☐ Identifies interventions to manage transplant complications, including neutropenia, fever, mucositis, nausea, vomiting, pain management, infectious, and noninfectious complications				
Cellular therapy complications and emergencies requiring rapid notification of the clinical transplant team (B3.6.3.5) ☐ Identifies complications and emergencies requiring rapid response				
Care for immunocompromised patients (B6.6.4.1) ☐ Identifies an immunocompromised patient based on ANC ☐ Demonstrates proper use of PPE ☐ Implements antibiotic therapy when indicated ☐ Completes a thorough head-to-toe assessment				
PART 2 – FACT Orientation Standards (in-patient oncology)				
Describes hematology/oncology patient care, including an overview of the cellular therapy process (B3.6.3.1)				
Discusses preparative regimens (B3.6.3.2)				
Administers preparative regimens (B.6.6.4.2) ☐ Discusses key side effects of the most commonly administered preparative regimens				

(Continued on next page)

Appendix 4-2. Sample Nurse Competency Verification Document (3 months – 1 year) *(Continued)*				
Administers: ☐ Blood products (B6.6.4.5)				
☐ Growth factors (B3.6.3.3)				
☐ Cellular therapy products (B6.6.4.3)				
☐ Other supportive therapies				
Administers cellular therapy products (B.3.6.4.3): ☐ Demonstrates the administration of thawed HPC and MNC products ☐ Demonstrates safe handling procedures during the administration process ☐ Discusses all documentation forms that apply to the cellular administration process *See attached skills checklist				
Care for immunocompromised patients (B6.6.4.1): ☐ Identifies an immunocompromised patient based on ANC ☐ Institutes neutropenic precautions ☐ Demonstrates proper use of PPE ☐ Implements antibiotic therapy when indicated. ☐ Completes a thorough head-to-toe assessment				
Provides care interventions to manage transplant complications including, but not limited to: (B3.6.3.4) ☐ Neutropenic fever				
☐ Infectious and noninfectious processes				
☐ Mucositis				
☐ Nausea and vomiting				
☐ GVHD				
☐ Pain management				
Recognizes cellular therapy complications and emergencies requiring rapid notification of the clinical transplant team (B3.6.3.5)				
Manages patients requiring palliative and end-of-life care (B3.6.3.6)				
PART 3 – Inpatient and Outpatient Oncology				
Procedures and Labs				
Describes the following specialty labs and requisitions: ☐ HLA typing				
☐ FISH				
☐ Flow cytometry				

(Continued on next page)

Appendix 4-2. Sample Nurse Competency Verification Document (3 months – 1 year) *(Continued)*

☐ Chimerism				
☐ Blood donor panel				
☐ Platelet refractory assay				
☐ EBV by PCR				
☐ HSV1, IgG and IgM				
☐ Toxoplasmosis IgG and IgM				
☐ BK virus by PCR				
Discusses nursing management and indications of granulocyte transfusions				
Describes blood transfusion reactions and treatment of specific conditions: ☐ Rigors				
☐ Hives				
☐ Abdominal pain				
☐ Increased fever				
☐ Hiccups				
☐ Nausea				
☐ Extrapyramidal symptoms				
☐ TRIALI				
Discusses clinical trials and protocols				
Manages oncology-specific symptom management: ☐ Weakness/Fatigue				
☐ Alopecia				
☐ Mucositis				
☐ Nausea/vomiting				
☐ Diarrhea				
☐ Constipation				
☐ Neurological effects				
☐ Cardiovascular effects/PE/VTE				
☐ Pulmonary effects				
Manages metabolic oncologic emergencies ☐ Hypercalcemia				
☐ Tumor lysis syndrome				
☐ Sepsis				
☐ Syndrome of inappropriate antidiuretic syndrome				
☐ Disseminated intravascular clotting				

(Continued on next page)

Appendix 4-2. Sample Nurse Competency Verification Document (3 months – 1 year) *(Continued)*

Manages structural oncologic emergencies: ☐ Spinal cord compression				
☐ Superior vena cava syndrome				
☐ Pleural effusion				
☐ Cardiac tamponade				
☐ Increased intracranial pressure				
Manages patients receiving radiation therapy: ☐ TBI				
☐ Reviews radiation safety				
☐ Completes RITN review				
Reviews NMDP confidentiality training				
Manages 3-way Foley: ☐ Insertion				
☐ Irrigation				
☐ I&O				
Completes the apheresis competency simulation (see checklist)				
Completes the circulars on GVHD and VOD				
Attends a transplant intake				
Oncology Courses and Chemotherapy SOPs				
Completes *Fundamentals of Oncology* course within six months of hire				
Completes *Fundamentals of Transplant* course within six months of hire				
Completes *Fundamentals of Chemotherapy and Targeted Therapy* course within six months of hire				
Discusses the Chemotherapy Standards of Practice:				
a. Overview				
b. Training and staffing				
c. Planning and documentation				
d. Consent and patient education				
e. Ordering				
f. Mixing				
g. Administration				
h. Extravasation				
i. Hypersensitivity and anaphylaxis				

(Continued on next page)

Appendix 4-2. Sample Nurse Competency Verification Document (3 months – 1 year) *(Continued)*

j. Monitoring and assessment				
k. Spills				
l. Safe handling				
m. Oral chemotherapy				
n. Special routes of administration (where applicable) • Intrathecal • Intravesicular • Intrahepatic • Intraperitoneal • Intrapleural • Hemodialysis				

Note. Figure courtesy of A. Vioral, PhD, MEd, RN, OCN®, BMTCN™, Director, Oncology Education and Research, Allegheny Health Network, Pittsburgh, PA. Used with permission.

Appendix 4-3. Sample Chemotherapy/Targeted Therapy Spills Management Competency Skills Checklist

ALLEGHENY HEALTH NETWORK
CHEMOTHERAPY/TARGETED THERAPY SPILLS MANAGEMENT COMPETENCY
SKILLS CHECKLIST 2014

Employee_____ Employee ID_____ Date_____

Evaluator Signature_____Initials___1st attempt___2nd Attempt___3rd Attempt___

Specific Facility (Check one):
□ AVH   □ AGH   □ AGH-Somerset   □ CGH   □ FRH   □ WPH   □ WPAON   □ SVH   □ RH
_____Office

1. Specially trained chemotherapy competent staff must demonstrate the proper procedure for managing a small and large chemotherapy/targeted therapy spill.
2. Evaluator is responsible to verbally review all aspects of this skills checklist prior to signature and initialing.

*** **The staff completing the competency will have the opportunity to review the procedure and competency expectations prior to demonstrating the standards for managing a small and large chemotherapy/targeted therapy spill.**

Objectives:
1. Initiate the steps to take in the event of a large chemotherapy/targeted therapy spill on a hard surface.
2. Demonstrate policy and procedure for cleaning up small hard surface chemotherapy/targeted therapy spill.
3. Discuss the documentation that occurs after a spill.

Criteria Elements References:	Initials
Oncology Nursing Society, *Chemotherapy and Biotherapy Guidelines and Recommendations for Practice*, 4th Edition (2014), and Allegheny Health Network Chemotherapy and Targeted Therapy Standards of Practice, Policy Name: Safe Handling; Spills, Exposure, Medical Surveillance	
Initiate the steps to take in the event of a large chemotherapy/targeted therapy spill on a hard surface.	
1. Verbalize what defines a large spill (> 5 ml).	
2. Alert others in the area of a large spill/call facility emergency number to report a spill/ gather a spill kit. • AVH x 66 • AGH x 1111 • AGH-Somerset x contact manager • CGH x 99 • FRH x 121 • WPH x 1111 • WPAON x Margie Leslie • SVH x • JRH x	
3. Ensure all patients and staff are removed from area.	
4. Immediately post a sign to warn others that there is a spill.	

(Continued on next page)

Appendix 4-3. Sample Chemotherapy/Targeted Therapy Spills Management Competency Skills Checklist *(Continued)*	
5. Don 2 pairs of gloves, disposable gown, face shield and NIOSH-approved respirator (all should be included in the spill kit).	
6. Contain the spill using the absorbent pads or pillows to keep the spill contained.	
Demonstrate policy and procedure for cleaning up small, hard surface chemotherapy/targeted therapy spill.	
1. Verbalize what defines a small spill (< 5 ml).	
2. Alert others in the area that there is a small spill/obtain a spill kit.	
3. Ensure all patients and staff are removed from area.	
4. Open spill kit and immediately post a sign.	
5. Wipe up liquids with absorbent pads or control pillows that are provided in the kit.	
6. Wipe up solids by using wet absorbent pads provided in spill kits.	
7. Pick up any glass fragments by using a small scoop that is supplied in spill kit.	
8. Place glass in puncture proof container.	
9. Place puncture proof container and contaminated materials into a leak proof waste bag. Seal the bag. Place sealed bag inside another bag appropriately labeled as hazardous waste.	
10. Clean spill area thoroughly from least contaminated to most contaminated areas using standard detergent solution (or as directed from the SDS sheets— located on intranet site), followed by rinsing with clean water.	
11. The area must be cleaned three times with a detergent followed by a water rinse. Notify environmental services to complete.	
12. Remove PPE and place disposable items in the unsealed waste disposable bag.	
13. Seal bag and place in puncture proof container.	
Discuss the documentation that occurs after a spill.	
1. Nurses notes need to contain: • Objective information • Interventions taken • MD notified and any additional orders • Supervisor notified • Patient assessment	
2. Complete an occurrence report.	
3. Complete an employee safety form.	

Note. Figure courtesy of A. Vioral, PhD, MEd, RN, OCN®, BMTCN™, Director, Oncology Education and Research, Allegheny Health Network, Pittsburgh, PA. Used with permission.

CHAPTER 5

Developing a Unit-Based Clinical Preceptorship Program

NURSES who work in clinical settings frequently are asked to share their expertise with less experienced nurses, other healthcare professionals, and nursing students and faculty from academic partnerships. One method of accomplishing this goal is through a preceptor program, a model of teaching used in clinical settings. In a preceptor program, an experienced nurse, referred to as a *preceptor*, is partnered with a less experienced nurse, or *preceptee*. The preceptor guides the learning experience of the preceptee through supervision and clinical instruction.

As an NPDS or unit-based educator, you may become involved with preceptor programs in a multitude of ways. You may be asked to develop a preceptor program for a clinical unit or manage an existing one. You also might be responsible for supervising nursing staff who currently serve as preceptors, selecting experienced nurses to become preceptors, developing these nurses for the preceptor role, and evaluating their performances. Additionally, you may be tasked with developing the curriculum for a preceptor program, serving as course faculty, coordinating clinical experiences, or acting as the liaison between your healthcare agency and faculty at affiliated academic programs.

From a different perspective, you may serve as a preceptor yourself, working on the clinical unit in a one-on-one arrangement with a new staff nurse. You may partner with a nurse who recently assumed the role of NPDS or unit-based educator for another clinical unit within your organization, a nursing student enrolled in a leadership course, or a graduate student completing a nursing education practicum in NPD.

On the contrary, you might be a preceptee working with an experienced NPDS. This arrangement can help you learn more about your role as an educator and help you develop required NPDS competencies.

Regardless of the nature of your involvement in preceptor programs, you will need to understand the key components of a successful preceptor program, how to develop and manage this program for your clinical units, ways to coordinate your efforts within your own organization, and how to evaluate the outcomes of the program. Each of these roles will be discussed throughout the chapter.

Understanding Preceptor Programs

The idea of partnering an inexperienced nurse with a more experienced one in a learning partnership has existed throughout the history of nursing. Using preceptors in clinical teaching has been evident in the nursing education literature for decades in the United States and has been documented globally, for example, in Australia, Canada, Ireland, Jordan, Oman, and Sweden (Al-Hussami, Saleh, Darawad, & Alramly, 2011; Bassendowski, Layne, Lee, & Hupaelo, 2010; Carlson,

2013; Duteau, 2012; Finn & Chesser-Smyth, 2013; Heffernan, Heffernan, Brosnan, & Brown, 2009; Kalischuk, Vandenberg, & Awosoga, 2013; Madhavanpraphakaran, Shukri, & Balachandran, 2014; McCarthy & Murphy, 2010; Myrick, Caplan, Smitten, & Rusk, 2010; Smedley & Penney, 2009).

Despite their current popularity, preceptorship programs may assume different meanings in various healthcare settings. In some organizations, the role of a preceptor is used interchangeably with that of a mentor or coach and associated with less formal teaching models than those used during an orientation. Regardless of the term used at your workplace, it is important to understand what a preceptor relationship entails as well as the roles and responsibilities of preceptors and preceptees.

Gaberson, Oermann, and Shellenbarger (2014) defined *preceptorship* as a "time-limited, one-to-one relationship between a learner and an experienced nurse who is employed by the healthcare agency in which the learning activities take place" (p. 273). This arrangement lasts for a predetermined length of time and focuses on a specific period of learning.

A variety of individuals can serve as preceptees, such as newly hired staff nurses, student nurses, faculty members, or experienced nurses who are unfamiliar with the specialty work of a clinical unit.

Before you become involved in any aspect of a preceptor program, take time to thoroughly prepare yourself for this role. One way to learn more about preceptor programs is to reflect upon your own experiences as both a student nurse and newly hired nurse. You were probably paired with an experienced nurse; this arrangement may or may not have been formally referred to as a preceptorship. The learning process you experienced during this partnership was probably very different than most of your experiences as a student, when a faculty member directly supervised your nursing care.

Think about the positives of this preceptorship. Although all of your experiences may not have been ideal, hopefully you learned from them. If you had a negative experience with your preceptor, think about what made it unsatisfactory. Try to relive your experience and determine what could have improved it. Reflect upon the relationship you had with your preceptor, focusing specifically on the professional goals that you were able to attain because of the preceptor's guidance. Figure 5-1 offers some questions to ask yourself when reflecting on these past experiences. Consider these questions when developing yourself and other nurses for a preceptor role.

Reasons for Preceptor Programs

Preceptor programs are used in clinical settings within a healthcare organization and between a healthcare organization and a partnered school of nursing. Figure 5-2 illustrates some common learners of preceptors.

Figure 5-1. Sample Questions to Ask Yourself About Previous Preceptors

- What did my preceptor do best to help me learn in the clinical setting?
- What could my preceptor have done differently that would have increased my learning?
- How did I best learn new clinical skills and concepts?
- How did I feel about learning with a preceptor versus an instructor or independently?
- What did I like best about my relationship with my preceptor?
- What did I like least about my preceptor?
- How did my preceptor provide me with feedback about my performance?
- What kind of learning environment did my preceptor create on the clinical unit?
- How did my preceptor's attitude (mood) influence my mood?
- Was my time with the preceptor sufficient? If not, how much more time did I need?

Figure 5-2. Types of Learners Taught by Preceptors

- Experienced and inexperienced nurses
- Nurses in residency programs
- Nurses being cross-trained, PRN/agency nurses
- Assistive personnel (nursing assistants)
- Unit secretaries
- Non-nursing staff (e.g., social workers, nutritionists, pharmacists, physical and occupational therapists)
- Nurses assuming a new role (e.g., leadership, educator)
- Students participating in special programs (e.g., internships, externships)
- Faculty employed by affiliating schools of nursing
- Student nurses enrolled in academic courses

Orientation of Nurses in a Healthcare Organization

When used within a healthcare organization, a preceptor program is often an integral part of orientation. For example, individuals who require an orientation may include not only novice, newly hired nurses, but also experienced RNs who either were relocated to a new unit or assumed a new position within the organization (American Nurses Association [ANA], 2000, 2015). Other individuals who may participate include faculty and students from affiliated schools of nursing, assistive personnel, and healthcare workers from other professions (e.g., pharmacists, social workers, physical and occupational therapists, nutritionists).

When used during orientation or residency programs, preceptors help new employees meet orientation goals. Through their expertise, preceptors introduce new nurses to information they need to function safely in their assigned roles on a clinical unit (ANA, 2000, 2010). Preceptors also help new staff in socializing into an organization or clinical unit, gaining an understanding of the work environment, and developing their clinical competencies (ANA, 2000; ANA & NNSDO, 2010).

Some preceptorships help students and nurses develop their competencies in specific areas: perioperative nursing (Wilson, 2012), critical care (Elmers, 2010), emergency departments (Glynn & Silva, 2013), long-term care (Aaron, 2011), public health and community nursing (Reilly et al., 2012), pediatric nursing (Chang, Douglas, Breen-Reid, Gueorguieva, & Fleming-Carroll, 2013), and leadership (Conley, Branowicki, & Hanley, 2007).

While most preceptorship literature focuses on its use within hospital-based contexts, Aaron (2011) described the pilot testing of a preceptor model for newly hired nurses employed in a long-term care facility. This Illinois project, Expanding the Teaching-Nursing Home Culture, improved RN recruitment and retention, reduced agency costs, eliminated the hiring of agency nurses to fill staffing gaps, and provided continuity of care for residents.

Courses Offered by Schools of Nursing

Preceptors are also used with undergraduate and graduate nursing students enrolled in academic courses (Rogan, 2009). In this setting, preceptors help nurses attain clinical objectives, develop knowledge and clinical leadership skills, and link theory with clinical practice. This preceptor arrangement is initiated by a course faculty member or clinical coordinator and assisted by a liaison from a clinical agency. The clinical liaison is responsible for identifying and recruiting qualified preceptors through discussions with nurse managers, NPDSs, and nursing staff. NPDSs or unit educators assume this role in some organizations.

Preceptors are usually partnered with students for the entire duration of the clinical practicum. Although preceptors, students, and faculty all participate in the student's evaluation process, faculty members maintain ultimate responsibility for the evaluation (Gaberson et al., 2015).

Many undergraduate programs use preceptors as clinical instructors for nursing students enrolled in upper-level clinical courses. These experiences usually occur in special clinical areas and are designed to help students transition from a student to a professional (Thomas, Bertram, & Allen, 2012).

While most authors have reported using preceptors during their students' final capstone courses, Stewart, Pope, and Hansen (2010) described their successful use of preceptors during 92% of the clinical hours required for students in an online accelerated second-degree nursing program. After a two-day on-campus orientation, students completed seven online credits followed by a two-week on-campus boot camp, where they engaged in lab exercises and a faculty-supervised clinical. The five remaining clinical courses were guided by preceptors who completed a faculty-designed training module. Student learning outcomes and stakeholder satisfaction reports were positive.

Graduate nursing programs also use preceptors in clinical courses in traditional and distance programs to help students develop competencies in advanced nursing practice roles, such as educator, administrator, clinical practitioner, and researcher (Link, 2009; Wilson, Bodin, Hoffman, & Vincent, 2009). In these courses, students are partnered with nurses who function in leadership roles within healthcare organizations.

Internships and Externships Sponsored by Healthcare Organizations

Preceptor programs have been used in hospital-sponsored internship and externship programs for students enrolled in prelicensure RN programs. Many of these programs are scheduled during the summer months when students usually are not enrolled in courses. These clinical programs often facilitate the subsequent recruitment and hiring of these students upon graduation.

Trends Supporting Preceptors in Clinical Teaching

Recent trends in health care and the nursing profession support the need for creative and cost-effective strategies to help nurses provide competent care to patients. Preceptor programs are one way to meet this goal.

The nation has been facing a current and future shortage of nurses, compounded by a turnover of experienced nurses employed in healthcare organizations (American Association of Colleges of Nursing [AACN], 2014). As a result, many organizations are actively recruiting nurses to fill vacant positions, retaining their own nurses, and cross-training or relocating experienced nurses to other patient care units. Some facilities have recruited foreign-educated nurses to fill vacancies (Thekdi, Wilson, & Xu, 2011). This trend may pose potential culture and communication issues in the workplace and increase the demand for experienced preceptors to assist with clinical teaching. Unfortunately, in some healthcare organizations the nursing shortage has resulted in inexperienced nurses functioning in preceptor roles.

Healthcare organizations have used innovative strategies to recruit new nurses and retain experienced nurses. Student internships are one approach to handle the nursing shortage and attract strong candidates for later employment (Letourneau, 2010). Unit-based preceptors are an important element in many of these initiatives.

Another trend is the shift from centralized to unit-based professional development. Many nursing professional development departments (NPDDs) in healthcare organizations were downsized or restructured over the past decades. This change has resulted in fewer NPDSs in some healthcare organizations and has shifted educational responsibilities from staff educators to nurses working on clinical units. These staff nurses, sometimes called *unit-based educators*, frequently assume responsibility for meeting the orientation needs of new employees and serving as preceptors. Some healthcare agencies include preceptorship as an expected behavior in position descriptions and promotions through clinical advancement programs. This shift suggests the need for experienced preceptors to help prepare other nurses to effectively perform this role.

Recent healthcare changes have also resulted in a decrease in length of hospital stays and an increase in acuity for patients. Nurses caring for these patients with complex needs have had to strengthen their competencies to deliver safe, quality care. Agencies that accredit healthcare organizations, such as the Joint Commission, focus on creating an environment in which patients receive safe nursing care (Joint Commission, 2015). Unit-based preceptors and NPDSs play significant roles toward achieving this goal through verifying and developing the clinical competencies of both new and experienced nursing staff.

The nursing shortage also has created the need for preceptors to help with the clinical learning of nursing students. Schools of nursing often collaborate with healthcare organizations who provide experienced staff nurses as preceptors for students in clinical settings (Schaubhut & Gentry, 2010). Using staff nurses as preceptors often leads to additional initiatives between these academic and service organizations. As an NPDS or unit educator, it is important for you to anticipate the increased demand for preceptor programs and prepare clinical nurses in your organization.

Changes in healthcare delivery also include a greater emphasis on accreditation and care quality. Hospitals seeking recognition for their nursing excellence through the American Nurses Credentialing Center (ANCC) Magnet Recognition Program® must provide evidence that their nurses are engaged in educational offerings within their work settings (ANCC, n.d.). Organizations also must have tangible evidence of a "development and mentoring program for staff preceptors for all levels of students (including students, new graduates, experienced nurses, etc.)" (ANCC, n.d., para. 13). Nurses should "serve as faculty and preceptors for students from a variety of academic programs" (ANCC, n.d., para. 13).

Advantages and Disadvantages of Preceptor Programs

Preceptor programs pose both benefits and challenges for healthcare organizations, schools of nursing, and nurses who are actively engaged in preceptorships. These individuals include preceptees, preceptors, NPDSs or staff educators, and faculty in schools of nursing. The partnering organizations and patients who are recipients of nursing care also experience advantages and disadvantages. Table 5-1 illustrates some of these advantages and disadvantages associated with preceptor programs. It is important for you to carefully weigh these factors in determining if preceptorships are appropriate for your staff and clinical units. Develop a proactive approach in handling the disadvantages posed by preceptorships while maximizing the benefits.

Preceptor programs allow preceptees to grow professionally (Lee, Tzeng, Lin, & Yeh, 2009) and develop their clinical competencies and critical-thinking skills (Kaddoura, 2013). These programs enhance quality of care by decreasing adverse events such as falls and medication errors (Lee et al., 2009). Preceptor programs also help students transition to a professional nursing role (Thomas et al., 2012), enabling them to be competitive applicants for positions upon graduation. Others view preceptorships as an effective mechanism to increase preceptees' self-confidence in their roles (Freiburger, 2002). The one-on-one nature of preceptorships

Table 5-1. Potential Advantages and Disadvantages of a Preceptor Program

Participant	Advantages	Disadvantages
Preceptor	Develops leadership, teaching, and clinical skills Provides opportunity to mentor and develop new nurses Maintains previously learned concepts Gives favorable status to serve as a preceptor Affords chance to network with school of nursing faculty	Limits time for patient care assignments Requires preparation in education and practice Becomes difficult if individuals are unprepared in the role or objectives are unclear
Preceptee	Helps with socialization to clinical unit Eases transition from student to staff role Provides one-on-one teaching experience on clinical unit Helps increase ability to function in organization	Hinders preceptee if poor match with preceptor Becomes difficult if individuals are unprepared in the role or objectives are unclear
Unit-based educator	Provides source of leadership development for staff Assists with task of orienting new staff	Limits time available for other duties because of selection, training, and evaluation needs
Patient	Ensures future care from competent nurses Limits potential mistakes with experienced nurses supervising care	Perceives care from preceptees as requiring supervision Permits role confusion with more nurses in contact with patient
Organization	Improves retention and recruitment Promotes staff development of colleagues on unit Encourages collaborative relationships between agency and school of nursing	Restricts direct patient care hours

offers nursing students an intense, consistent learning experience. Preceptorships have also been associated with decreased nurse turnover rates and increased retention (Baggot, Hensinger, Parry, Valdes, & Zaim, 2005; Goss, 2015).

Nurses who serve as preceptors also view this partnership as a step toward professional development and future leadership opportunities (Chang et al., 2013). Having the chance to be a preceptor can be viewed as an incentive for both experienced and inexperienced nurses. Preceptors may feel energized by the experience, view their work from a different perspective, and become motivated to strengthen their own nursing skills (Lawless, Demers, & Baker, 2002).

Experienced preceptors who assist with the educational needs of employees and nursing students can help healthcare organizations and unit-based educators attain their goal of employing competent nurses who provide safe, quality patient care. This outcome also can help organizations in meeting accreditation standards and marketing their services. Preceptor programs can improve an organization's recruitment efforts (Lawless et al., 2002), decrease turnover rates and costs (Lee et al., 2009), and strengthen collaborative partnerships with schools of nursing (Haas et al., 2002). NPDSs and staff educators can strengthen their leadership and educator skills by planning and coordinating preceptor programs.

The use of preceptors in clinical courses may assist faculty in schools of nursing in providing students with clinical experiences that resemble the day-to-day work of an RN, offering individualized teaching in a one-on-one arrangement, and networking with RNs who may serve as role models. In some instances, the use of preceptors can help extend clinical instruction with limited faculty and resources.

Although preceptor programs offer a variety of advantages, they also pose some negative features. Preceptorships can be a stressful experience for both preceptees (Marks-Maran et al., 2013) and preceptors, as both groups report role conflict, ambiguity, and overload (Omansky, 2010). Nurses who serve as preceptors may feel overwhelmed with a workload that includes both teaching and direct patient care roles (Hautala, Saylor, & O'Leary-Kelley, 2007; Omansky, 2010). They may also lack confidence in their preceptor role and perceive a lack of organizational support (Hautala et al., 2007). Some preceptors may become disappointed if they are paired with a preceptee who lacks the motivation to learn and demonstrates low levels of knowledge and skills (Hautala et al., 2007). Students who are unsafe in clinical practice present additional challenges and ethical dilemmas for preceptors (Earle-Foley, Myrick, Luhanga, & Yonge, 2012). Gaberson et al. (2015) noted that the use of clinical preceptors in academic courses does not decrease faculty responsibilities. Similar to traditional clinical models, a great deal of effort is spent on coordination and communication.

Healthcare organizations need to carefully weigh the costs of their preceptor programs against their benefits. NPDSs, unit educators, and faculty may find planning and coordinating a preceptor experience to be an overwhelming task. They may have difficulty recruiting experienced, qualified nurses to function as preceptors, especially in light of the nursing shortage. Available candidates may be experienced nurses who are new to the preceptor role and need training and guidance.

Assessing the Needs and Direction of the Preceptor Program

Before implementing a formal preceptor program at your workplace, carefully investigate resources available within your organization, other healthcare agencies, and the nursing literature. This information will lay the groundwork for your preceptor program and determine the direction and extent of your unit-based efforts. Although healthcare trends suggest the need for preceptor programs, only you can determine what is needed within your workplace. Your input is essential to the success of your preceptor program.

Gaining an Organizational Perspective

Start your investigation by meeting with the administrator and other specialists in your NPDD. If you are a unit educator, begin this conversation with the nurse manager or NPDS. The purpose of this meeting is to learn if the department already sponsors a preceptor program and, if it does, to learn more about it.

If a preceptor program does exist at your agency, review any policies and procedures available about the program. These documents may include reasons for using preceptors, eligibility criteria, the process used to select preceptors, how to match preceptors and preceptees, training programs available to prepare preceptors, methods used to evaluate preceptor and preceptee performance, and preceptor incentives and recognition programs. Remember to also find out what strategies are used to evaluate the long-term outcomes of the preceptor program.

Explore peak times when preceptors may be needed, such as the dates scheduled for hiring and orienting new employees. Confirm the amount of time preceptors usually commit to in an arrangement (e.g., two weeks, several months). Evaluate the human and financial resources available to you at the unit level and the process for requesting these resources. Uncover additional support that may be available to you for developing a unit-based preceptor program, such as secretarial or instructional services.

Use this opportunity to clarify how your unit-based efforts will blend with any centralized preceptor program or with informal preceptor programs sponsored by other clinical units within the organization. If a preceptor program does not exist on other units, meet with unit-based educators in the organization to explore collaborative opportunities.

Determine both immediate and long-term preceptor needs for your unit and the resources you will require to implement them.

Obtaining a Unit-Based Perspective

After meeting with key individuals at the department level in your organization, discuss your plans for developing a preceptor program with your nurse manager and staff on the clinical unit. Meeting with the nurse manager will help clarify unit-based goals and future preceptor needs. For example, if the nurse manager knows that your unit will merge with another next year or that it will increase the number of patient beds, qualified preceptors will be needed to orient newly hired or cross-trained staff.

Discuss your manager's expectations regarding a preceptor's workload, especially what patient care assignments the nurse will be expected to assume while serving as a preceptor. Taking inventory of available unit-based resources can help you determine the anticipated costs of implementing a unit-based preceptor program.

Meet with unit staff to gain their perspectives. Providing staff with an opportunity for input into the planning of a preceptor program may give them a sense of ownership and also encourage the program's success. Nurses who have been preceptors can provide personal insight on the learning needs of nurses in this role, feedback regarding ways to match preceptors with preceptees, details on the support that preceptors require, and ways to manage the program. It is important for unit staff to understand the roles and responsibilities of everyone involved in the program.

Benchmarking Preceptor Programs

Gain a perspective of existing national and regional preceptor programs in developing your own program. Search the nursing literature for recent articles that focus on preceptor programs. If your organization does not have a librarian to assist your search, contact faculty at an affiliated school of nursing for help. Retrieve articles and seek innovative approaches that may align with your organization. Pay attention to journals such as *Journal of Continuing Education in Nursing* (www.healio.com/nursing/journals/jcen) and *Journal for Nurses in Professional Development* (formerly known as *Journal for Nurses in Staff Development*) (http://journals.lww.com/jnsdonline/pages/default.aspx) that target readers in NPD roles. Many researchers have published personal accounts of preceptor programs from the perspectives of both preceptors and preceptees (e.g., Delfino, Williams, Wegener, & Homel, 2014; Kalischuk et al., 2013; Luhanga, Myrick, & Yonge, 2010; Madhavanprapha-karan et al., 2014; Marks-Maran et al., 2013; McCarthy & Murphy, 2010; Moore & Cagle, 2012). These may provide you with additional factors to consider when developing your program.

While the majority of preceptor programs focus on NPD, Bassendowski et al. (2010) described an interprofessional education (IPE) approach used for a preceptor orientation program (N = 80). This Canadian initiative not only supported the preceptors' preparation within the context of patient-centered IPE, but it also positively influenced the students' perspectives regarding IPE and the "inter-group processes of professionalism" (p. e-23). After this three-day program, preceptors reported a stronger understanding of their role in IPE and its value with students.

Using a different approach to develop preceptors, Schaubhut and Gentry (2010) designed nursing preceptor workshops through a collaboration between hospital nurse educators and school of nursing faculty. This initiative increased the number of preceptors, strengthened the academic–service partnership, and furthered the nursing community.

Additional ideas about preceptor programs can come from attending continuing education (CE) offerings at conferences sponsored by professional nursing organizations such as the Association for Nursing Professional Development (www.anpd.org) and the Professional Nurse Educators Group (www.pneg.org). Similarly, organizations that have a clinical specialty focus, such as the Oncology Nursing Society (www.ons.org) and the Academy of Medical-Surgical Nurses (www.amsn.org), also include nursing education topics at their conferences. Many organizations that sponsor these programs schedule roundtable sessions where clinical teaching topics, such as preceptor programs, are discussed among attendees who face similar challenges. If a preceptor program is not a topic on the agenda for these programs, request this learning need to the conference planning committee.

The American Academy for Preceptor Advancement (AAPA) is a web-based organization that provides a forum for nurses who serve in preceptor roles (AAPA, n.d.). Its website (www.preceptoracademy.com) includes various preceptor-related resources and opportunities for certification through portfolio development. AAPA has published *Core Curriculum for Preceptor Advancement* (Roth, 2015) and *Scope and Standards of Practice for Preceptor Advancement* (Roth, Figueroa, & Swihart, 2014) to guide nurse preceptors in developing their knowledge and skills.

Consult other NPDSs or unit-based educators at healthcare organizations within your local community about their preceptor programs. Start by negotiating this request with an agency with which you recently shared your clinical expertise. Also, consider contacting nursing faculty at affiliated schools of nursing (academic partners) for assistance with your preceptor program. In exchange for their involvement, consider sharing your expertise with students in their program.

Planning the Preceptor Program

After collecting information about preceptor programs from various sources, develop a detailed plan for your own unit-based preceptor program. Although designing such a plan may be a time-consuming task, this step will enable you to anticipate and manage potential problems before they pose barriers to program success. Careful planning will help your program run smoothly once implemented.

Recording this planning information in a personal notebook or an electronic file may be helpful for future reference, especially in developing policies and procedures and evaluating your program's success. Tracking resources, including time spent on each step of the planning phase, will help you determine cost-effectiveness (Allen, 2011). You must consider essential features in developing your unit-based preceptor program. Figure 5-3 provides you with a checklist to track each step of the planning process.

Figure 5-3. Checklist for Planning a Unit-Based Preceptor Program	
Program Tasks	**Comments**
1. Develop the purpose and objectives of your program.	
2. Clarify roles and responsibilities of key players.	
3. Develop criteria for preceptor selection.	
4. Prepare preceptors for their role.	
5. Provide support and incentives for preceptors.	
6. Develop key documents and a record-keeping system.	
7. Establish a communication system among players.	
8. Develop an evaluation plan.	
9. Clarify key steps in the process.	
10. Determine a timeline.	

Clarifying Purpose, Objectives, and Outcomes

Start the planning process by brainstorming the purpose of your program with colleagues who have experience with preceptor programs or will play a role in your proposed program. Be sure to include your manager and educators. You may decide, for example, that the purpose of your preceptor program will be to ease the transition of newly hired nurses at your organization to their role as professional RNs. You also want to develop their clinical competencies (i.e., knowledge, skills, and attitudes), critical-thinking and patient safety skills, and confidence. Clarifying your program's purpose will also determine how you prepare preceptors for their new role and where you can locate resources and support.

Decide who the learners or preceptees will be in your program. You may choose to focus on new graduates just hired into your organization, experienced RNs transferring to a new role or specialty unit, or nursing students enrolled in courses at your academic partners. Or, perhaps your learners will be other nurse educators or healthcare workers, such as physical therapists, pharmacists, assistive personnel, or unit secretaries.

After you have identified the program's purpose and targeted learners, develop specific objectives or outcomes based on its purpose (see Chapters 6 and 13). These objectives should be learner focused, measurable, and realistic. For example, Finn and Chesser-Smyth (2013) included "Discuss the roles, responsibilities, and competencies of the preceptor," "Discuss teaching and learning theories as they relate to student learning in clinical practice," and "Discuss the methods of assessing student competence in clinical practice" (p. 311) among eight total learning outcomes for their two-day preceptor program.

Once these elements are resolved, establish when the program will begin and conclude. Various factors in your organization may influence this time span. You may decide, for example, to match newly hired nurses with experienced staff nurses on the first day of a five-week orientation and end this formal arrangement on the last day of the orientation. On the other hand, you may decide to continue this relationship on an informal basis for an extended period of time after the formal orientation ends. The length of time that preceptors are matched with nursing students may be easier to predict because preceptorships usually end after a student fulfills the clinical objectives and credit hours required for the course.

If you serve as your agency's liaison for academic partners, communicate dates for clinical experiences with appropriate individuals in the NPDD and on your clinical unit. If you are not the liaison, obtain the information you will need to plan these arrangements. Determine hiring dates for new employees so that you may anticipate the need for preceptors. Representatives in your human resources department or NPDD may have this information. Work with NPDSs in scheduling nurses who need to participate in programs to prepare them for the preceptor role.

Determining the Roles and Responsibilities of Key Players

Collaboration and communication are essential when planning effective preceptor programs (Freiburger, 2002). After defining the goals and objectives of your preceptor program, identify key individuals who will be involved in the process. Although the preceptors and preceptees play key roles, be sure to consider others who function in supporting roles. These individuals include unit educators or liaisons, the nurse manager of the unit, unit staff, and other educators in your NPDD. If nursing students participate, involve course faculty from schools of nursing in this process.

Clarify each individual's roles and responsibilities to everyone involved in the program (Rogan, 2009). Make these duties explicit by developing written descriptions to include among your formal documents. Putting this information in writing will help identify roles, maintain consistency in performance, minimize confusion, and assist with performance evaluations. The roles and responsibilities of these individuals may vary depending on your organization and the associated school of nursing. Figure 5-4 provides examples of duties commonly assumed by preceptors, preceptees, NPDSs, unit-based educators, and faculty in schools of nursing.

Preceptors should meet with students before the program begins to discuss course objectives, clarify role expectations, and review organizational policies (Zimmermann, 2002). Preceptors should also meet with nursing faculty to discuss students' current competencies, specific learning needs, and organizational policies, such as accessing electronic records and medication administration. Similar to new employees, students need to be oriented to the organization, including mandatory training on emergency procedures, charting and medication policies, and reporting procedures (Zimmermann, 2002).

Although faculty are responsible for student performance and patient care assignments (Gaberson et al., 2014), preceptors assume responsibility for patient care.

Creating Key Documents and a Record-Keeping System

Key documents and a record-keeping system will help your program run smoothly and provide you with an easily accessible document retrieval system for accrediting agencies and other reviewers.

Before you attempt to develop a system to create, organize, and manage documents, discuss your plans with appropriate individuals in your agency. This will help you avoid duplicating documents that already exist and will prevent you from excluding features in documents

---

Figure 5-4. Responsibilities of Preceptors, Preceptees, Unit-Based Educators, and Nursing Faculty Involved in the Preceptorship Process

Preceptors
- Assist with competency verification, socialization, and role transition
- Provide psychosocial support for preceptee in role
- Understand objectives and outcomes of the learning experience (e.g., orientation, course)
- Communicate learning needs regarding preceptor role to unit-based educator
- Demonstrate self-direction in meeting learning needs related to role
- Evaluate performance of preceptees
- Provide ongoing (formative) and end-of-program (summative) feedback to preceptee
- Contribute to a positive learning environment

Preceptees
- Assume responsibility for self-learning needs
- Understand clinical objectives and expected outcomes
- Communicate learning needs to preceptor
- Conduct a self-evaluation of performance
- Provide feedback on preceptor process
- Contribute to a positive learning environment

Unit-Based Educators
- Coordinate the preceptor process
- Prepare preceptors to assume their role
- Provide support to preceptors in their role
- Select preceptors and match with preceptees
- Evaluate preceptor performance (or provide input)
- Evaluate preceptor process
- Contribute to a positive learning environment

Nursing Faculty
- Assist with the preparation of preceptors for their role
- Clarify the meaning of preceptors with students
- Maintain constant communication with preceptors
- Clarify clinical objectives and specific expectations of students
- Communicate with unit-based educator (liaison)
- Meet preceptor needs in a timely manner
- Assist with the selection and matching of preceptors with preceptees
- Provide feedback on the preceptor process
- Manage issues that develop during the course
- Facilitate the preceptor process
- Evaluate preceptor performance (or provide input)
- Compile final evaluation of students
- Evaluate overall preceptor program

---

that are applicable on a unit-based level. Find out how policies and procedures are reviewed and approved within your workplace. Clinical educators in the NPDD, unit managers, NPDSs, unit educators, and preceptors on other units and in other healthcare agencies can guide you in this process.

In addition to designing course materials for your program, you will need to develop policies, procedures, and forms that reflect the purpose, objectives, and outcomes of your preceptor program, the clinical unit, and the NPDD.

Policies and procedures are extremely important to the success of your preceptor program and should be communicated to all involved stakeholders. Policies can guide decision making and influence your preceptor program. Because policies are based on goals, they also help staff focus their efforts in a specific direction. A policy about criteria for selection of preceptors for new nurses or nursing students will guide you and others in this process.

Procedures help nurses implement policies, as they outline detailed, sequential steps included in the process. You might choose to develop a procedure for school of nursing faculty to follow when they request preceptors from your organization for their nursing students. Figure 5-5 lists examples of policies and procedures that may prove helpful for a unit-based preceptor program.

Figure 5-5. Suggested Policies and Procedures for a Preceptor Program

Policies
- Criteria for preceptors paired with agency personnel
- Criteria for preceptors paired with undergraduate nursing students
- Criteria for preceptors paired with graduate nursing students
- Roles and responsibilities of preceptors
- Roles and responsibilities of preceptees
- Roles and responsibilities of unit-based educators (liaison)
- Roles and responsibilities of school of nursing faculty
- Clinical workload of nurses serving as preceptors

Procedures
- Requesting preceptors for agency personnel
- Requesting preceptors for nursing students from schools of nursing
- Evaluation of preceptee performance
- Evaluation of preceptors

You will also need to develop forms that will help facilitate your work in the preceptor program. Figure 5-6 lists documents that you may consider. These documents can serve as templates for individuals who participate in the program and add consistency to your program.

Consider including the following documents as a start to your program: assessment of preceptees' learning needs, preceptorship schedule, daily clinical feedback form, final evaluation form, and daily preceptee logs.

If this is your first preceptor program, pilot these items before you begin the program and revise them accordingly after your first group of preceptors and preceptees. Keep your original file in a secure location and note changes while the process is still fresh in your mind.

If you do not have an existing record-keeping system tailored to your preceptor program, develop a secure one for your unit-based program. It is important to keep records related to your program for several reasons. First, you need to document performance progress for preceptees and preceptors. Second, having a record system allows you to critically evaluate the effectiveness of your unit-based efforts based on program goals. Finally, records provide you with evidence that may be shared with accreditation agencies or recognition programs.

Create your record-keeping system in a variety of ways, ranging from a box of file folders to a more sophisticated computerized database program. Before you start, investigate resources available to you within your agency to see how you can add your program files to an existing system.

Figure 5-6. Sample Documents and Forms for a Unit-Based Preceptor Program

- Preceptor and preceptee assignments
- Unit-based schedule
- Unit-based orientation plan and objectives
- Needs assessment
- Competency validation reports
- Daily anecdotes and checklists
- Summary evaluation of preceptee
- Summary evaluation of preceptor
- Self-evaluations

In most instances, you will need to organize three sets of documents: policies and procedures, original templates of documents used in the program, and documentation about the progress and performance of each preceptee and preceptor. Develop a system that is easily accessible and requires little energy to use and maintain. Documents, such as policies and procedures, can be kept in a notebook or posted on the hospital's intranet for easy reference. This same system can be used to maintain original templates of documents you frequently use during the preceptor program. Label separate files with the name and start date of each preceptee, and file the completed documentation in it. Include a copy of the preceptee's schedule in this file. Repeat this process for collecting evaluations and anecdotal notes regarding the performance of preceptors on the unit. You can use this same approach for nursing student preceptees on your unit, including a copy of the course profile and clinical objectives in their folders.

Be sure to keep confidential documents about employees or students in a secured location (e.g., locked file cabinet, dedicated secure electronic file). Determine who is permitted to access these files and how long they need to be maintained. Talk with your unit's nurse manager to determine when and if any of these documents, such as summary evaluations, should be forwarded to the employee's permanent personnel file.

Establishing and Maintaining Communication

Before you implement your preceptor program, establish communication with stakeholders in the program (see Chapter 3). Communication is essential to accomplish program goals and facilitates collaboration among all individuals involved. Schedule regular meetings with individuals involved in the preceptor program (Broadbent, Moxham, Sander, Walker, & Dwyer, 2014). These meetings can be held face-to-face or by telephone, Skype, or any other convenient means.

Start creating your communication system by identifying the key players. Along with the preceptor and preceptee, include the NPDSs for your unit, the nurse manager, and nursing staff on the clinical unit. You also may choose to include the human resources department that processes information on new employees and other unit-based educators in your organization. When the preceptorship includes nursing students, you will need to involve faculty assigned to the course and other contacts within both the school of nursing and your organization.

Investigate potential communication methods within your organization that you can use to accomplish this goal. In addition to using traditional communication methods, such as telephone calls, announcements at meetings, a unit communication book, or memos that are mailed or posted on unit bulletin boards, consider also using technology (e.g., social media sites, a secure hospital intranet system, electronic newsletters) to facilitate communication.

A solid strategy is to schedule a reception for new preceptees and their preceptors during the first week of orientation. Post photographs (with permission) of new nursing staff and their preceptors on the unit to enable staff who work other shifts to recognize them. Encourage existing staff to send a note to welcome preceptees to the clinical unit. These strategies help preceptees feel welcomed and valued on the unit and in the organization.

Determine what information about the program should be shared, with whom, and when. For example, two steps that occur early in most preceptor programs are obtaining a list of new employees with their start date and matching them with specific unit-based preceptors. This information would be of value to all people involved in the preceptor program before the new nurses arrive on the clinical unit. Think about the most effective way that this information can be communicated.

Developing Selection Criteria for Preceptors

After clarifying the responsibilities of key players, establish criteria to select potential preceptors from your clinical unit. In some organizations, nurse managers assume this responsibility; discover what the practice is at your workplace. If selection criteria are not already available at your workplace, develop them using the knowledge and resources you have obtained from the nursing literature, experts at your workplace, and other healthcare resources. If preceptors will be partnered with nursing students, contact faculty from academic partnerships.

Begin the preceptor selection process by compiling a list of personal and professional characteristics and skills that you think a preceptor should ideally possess. Be sure to include specific knowledge, skills, attitudes, and behaviors needed to fulfill this role, keeping targeted learners in mind. For example, Gurney (2002) recruited preceptors for an emergency department's transition program based on their knowledge of and commitment to competency-based learning and critical thinking.

After you have developed this list, prioritize the items along a continuum of most essential to least essential qualities. Keep in mind the characteristics and skills on your list that can be developed in your preceptors through CE offerings. Figure 5-7 lists some commonly identified criteria used when selecting preceptors.

Remember that criteria required of preceptors who orient staff nurses to a clinical unit may differ from the criteria of preceptors teamed with nursing students. Preceptors partnered with nursing students often need to meet specific criteria established by schools of nursing in response to mandates by regulatory and accreditation agencies. For example, the Commission on Collegiate Nursing Education (2013) states that preceptors who are used in academic programs need to be "academically and experientially qualified for their role in assisting in the achievement of the mission, goals, and expected student outcomes" (p. 10). Preceptors who work with undergraduate nursing students often need to hold a minimum of a bachelor's degree. Similarly, nurses precepting graduate students need to hold a minimum of a graduate degree in nursing. Some students enrolled in leadership and management courses may need to be matched with nursing staff who assume specific leadership positions, such as a charge nurse or staff educator, in your organization.

The process you use to select preceptors will depend on your organization's policies and procedures. In some agencies, nurses volunteer to serve as preceptors, whereas other organizations require that all nurses serve as preceptors, with preceptorship included as an expected behavior in job descriptions. Regardless of your agency's guidelines, begin your preceptor pro-

---

Figure 5-7. Common Criteria for Selection of Preceptors

- Education background (BSN, MSN)
- Clinical expertise in area of focus
- Effective communication skills
- Good interpersonal skills (i.e., listener)
- Professional leadership qualities and a role model
- Willingness to participate and an interest in helping new nurses
- Past experience in teaching
- Ability to create a positive learning environment

gram using nurses who you believe will be most effective in the preceptor role. This will help ensure your program's success and allow you to gradually develop a group of experienced preceptors who can mentor other nurses in the preceptor role.

Preparing Preceptors for Their Role

A nurse who serves as a preceptor for nursing staff and students assumes multiple roles: teacher, facilitator, mentor, colleague, role model, evaluator, coach, adviser, expert clinician, guide, consultant, tutor, and counselor. As an NPDS or unit-based educator, you are instrumental in selecting potential preceptors and ensuring they are prepared to function effectively in their role.

One way to prepare nurses as preceptors is to provide them with educational offerings designed to help them carry out their designated responsibilities. Envision a preceptor preparation program using throughputs mentioned within the scope of NPD (ANA & National Nursing Staff Development Organization, 2010). It is also important to provide preceptors with ongoing educational updates and preparation that will enable them to continually develop and advance in their role (Goss, 2015).

Another approach is to think of a preceptor preparation program as an orientation program for experienced nurses assuming preceptor roles on a clinical unit. It is a way to enhance the professional development of nurses through a series of unit-based in-service offerings scheduled over an extended period of time or in a CE program. Chapter 13 will also address the process and policies to follow in awarding contact hours for nurses who participate in a preceptor development program for the first time (ANCC, 2012).

You may use various levels of preceptor preparation programs, each one providing participants with higher levels of knowledge and skills. For example, your first program can help nurses develop basic skills as a preceptor, while a second or third offering might present advanced preceptor skills. You might start with a basic CE course to provide nurses with a foundation, followed by a series of in-service offerings or CE programs that gradually introduce new and more complex topics.

Depending on your workplace, you may be responsible for developing this program for your unit, or you might be asked to participate in a program sponsored by the centralized NPDD. In some settings, school of nursing faculty who request preceptors for their nursing students provide educational programs (face-to-face or online) or information to prepare preceptors for their roles. Faculty members also have the responsibility to prepare students for preceptee roles (Souers, 2002).

Several studies have identified characteristics and behaviors of preceptors that have contributed to preceptee learning (Finger & Pape, 2002). Figure 5-8 lists examples of topics that can be included in preceptor development programs. Although many topics are included in this list, it is important to recognize the influence of the preceptors' interpersonal skills in helping students transition to staff nursing roles. Gurney (2002) suggested the use of case studies to help novice preceptors effectively manage difficult situations in preceptorships. Preceptors also should understand which clinical responsibilities are appropriate to delegate to preceptees.

Preceptors need to develop a self-awareness of their verbal and nonverbal behaviors exhibited during preceptorship. A study in which perioperative preceptees evaluated the behaviors of their preceptors revealed that preceptors illustrated both positive, inviting behaviors and negative, disinviting behaviors when sharing their knowledge and skills (Finger & Pape, 2002). Preceptors who exhibit an inviting demeanor can increase recruitment efforts and decrease retention issues. Preceptors should work with educators to develop strategies to eliminate negative behaviors.

Figure 5-8. Common Content of Preceptor Development Programs

- Understanding the role and responsibilities of a unit-based preceptor
- Understanding the job description (expectations) of the preceptee
- Teaching effectively in the clinical setting (i.e., assessing learning needs)
- Working with healthcare professionals who are adult learners
- Understanding and working with various learning styles
- Maintaining effective communication skills in a preceptor role (i.e., constructive feedback)
- Evaluating clinical performance (validating clinical competencies)
- Documenting clinical performance (e.g., anecdotal notes, checklists, rubrics)
- Dealing with difficult situations (conflict) on the clinical unit
- Maintaining confidentiality and ethics as a preceptor
- Demonstrating an optimistic attitude in stressful situations
- Role modeling professional behaviors in difficult circumstances
- Understanding the influence of culture on learning
- Determining appropriate patient care assignments based on preceptee expertise

---

Many educators have reported using unique approaches in their preceptor programs. For example, in a preceptor program mentioned earlier, Finn and Chesser-Smyth (2013) provided their preceptors with "learning transfer principles" in a two-day preceptor preparation course to help them apply what they learned with preceptees in the clinical practice setting. The course included specific competencies, performance indicators, learning outcomes, case studies, and learning transfer logs. In addition to reviewing their specific roles and responsibilities, the preceptors focused on standards for nursing education programs, teaching-learning theories and strategies, assessment of competencies, and documentation related to instruction and learner performance (Finn & Chesser-Smyth, 2013).

Some authors have built upon the evidence reported by others to make their preceptor programs stronger and more efficient. In this respect, Bott, Mohide, and Lawlor (2011) described the "Five-Minute Preceptor" clinical teaching technique designed to help preceptors interact with students. This experiential technique included five steps: get the student to take a stand, probe for supporting evidence, teach general rules, reinforce the positives, and correct errors or misinterpretations (Bott et al., 2011). The authors recommended future research to validate the influence of this teaching technique.

When implementing your preceptor preparation program, use scheduling techniques that match the staffing needs for patient care on your clinical unit. The length of preceptor training programs may vary across healthcare organizations, with some programs lasting only one or two days and others lasting several weeks. Some programs consist of formal courses, whereas others employ a more informal approach with experienced preceptors serving as mentors to new preceptors.

Advances in technology have allowed preceptor preparation programs and ongoing support to be successfully delivered via self-paced, electronically delivered sessions rather than traditional face-to-face sessions. For example, Larsen and Zahner (2011) noted increased self-efficacy and knowledge scores in public health nurse preceptors after they completed a web-based preparation course. Their online course consisted of 10 modules that could be completed at the nurses' own pace and in any order. The preceptors' self-efficacy scores remained high three months following course completion.

Similarly, Myrick et al. (2010) created an extensive social e-learning space to prepare and support their preceptors. This online approach encouraged both interaction and dialogue over a five-month period.

Krampe, L'Ecuyer, and Palmer (2013) changed their face-to-face preceptor preparation course to an online format for their dedicated education unit (DEU). The authors emphasized that the nurse preceptor role on a DEU somewhat differs from the traditional role of orientees and students in instructor-led models.

Many hospitals and academic partners have collaborated to develop successful preceptor programs. For example, Burns and Northcutt (2009) created the Nursing Preceptor Program, targeted at community health and acute care nurses preceptors of undergraduate nursing students at an urban university. The program included an online course with six modules that learners could complete at their own pace, a common webpage for use by students and preceptors, and a relational database with search capabilities to locate preceptors and clinical sites. Evaluation data were positive, showing an increase in available qualified preceptors, clinical placements, and quality student learning outcomes. Contact hours were awarded to nurses who successfully completed the program.

Similarly, Horton, DePaoli, Hertach, and Bower (2012) described the Nurse Preceptor Academy, designed by academic and staff development educators who prepared more than 700 preceptors using this approach. The program helped preceptors feel supported in their new roles.

Because experienced preceptors have firsthand knowledge of the preceptor–preceptee relationship, be sure to include them in planning and implementing your program. They can be instrumental in role-playing difficult situations they may have encountered as preceptors and can provide effective ways to respond to these challenging scenarios. Be creative and use a variety of active teaching-learning strategies in your program (see Chapter 6).

Matching Learners With Appropriate Preceptors

The process of matching preceptees with preceptors begins when you, as the NPDS or unit-based educator, receive notification that new hires, transfers, or nursing students need to be oriented to the clinical unit. Discuss reasonable time frames for requests for clinical preceptorships with the human resources department or nursing school faculty so that you have adequate time to prepare.

Once you know how many preceptees you will have and their arrival dates, consider the preceptors who are prepared and available to work with the learners. If you do not have enough formally prepared preceptors, you might consider working informally on preceptor skills with staff nurses who show promise in performing the role. Other approaches include pairing novice preceptors with more experienced preceptors who can guide them as they work with a preceptee. Before you match preceptees with unit-based preceptors, obtain some background information about each. Start by reviewing their résumé, or curriculum vitae (CV) if appropriate, and note formal and informal educational backgrounds, prior work experience, and professional contributions. If you do not have an opportunity to meet with the new hires before your program begins, then schedule some time to talk with each preceptee within the first couple of days of the program to obtain this information.

During your interview with the preceptees, ask them questions that will help you match them with available preceptors on the clinical unit. For example, you might ask them how they best learn on the clinical unit, what they feel their strengths are, and what skills they hope to improve. Ask them to recall a positive experience they have had with a preceptor or clinical instructor. Listen to how they describe the characteristics or behaviors of the individual who facilitated their learning. You can also ask the preceptees how they problem-solved a difficult patient situation. This interview approach also may be helpful to implement with preceptors, especially if these nurses are unfamiliar to you.

Obtaining this information from preceptees will also help you design learning experiences that will strengthen their clinical competencies and highlight contributions that they can make to the unit through in-service educational offerings. You may discover that a new staff nurse has experience in caring for patients with a new type of IV catheter that will be introduced to your clinical unit next month. Asking this nurse to help with a future unit-based in-service educational offering on this topic may contribute to the individual's self-confidence and perception as a valued staff member.

A similar strategy can be used to match nursing students with preceptors on your clinical unit. School of nursing faculty should provide you with the criteria they require of preceptors paired with their students. Faculty can provide you with insight into the background and special learning needs of students so that you can match them with the most appropriate preceptor.

Organizations have used various strategies to pair preceptors with preceptees and ensure a positive experience. For example, some organizations match their preceptors with preceptees based on learning styles (Brunt & Kopp, 2007), leadership styles (Lockwood-Rayermann, 2003), or personality characteristics (Poradzisz, Kostovich, O'Connell, & Lefaiver, 2012).

Some schools of nursing expect their students, especially at the graduate level, to seek their own preceptors. Other organizations consider demographic factors. Regardless of the approach used, the priority is developing a team that is capable of understanding and learning through communication.

Developing a Teaching Plan for the Clinical Experience

After drafting a tentative plan to match preceptors with preceptees, create a teaching plan for the clinical preceptorship experience. One method of accomplishing this is to integrate the clinical preceptorship experience with the classroom teaching in an orientation program. Another approach is to combine both classroom teaching with clinical experience using a more informal, unit-based approach. Ask your NPDS, if applicable, which approach is used at your organization.

Regardless of your approach, the learning objectives or outcomes contained in the teaching plan should be relevant to the preceptees and aligned with their position description. Be sure to review the plan with appropriate individuals on your unit, especially the preceptees and their preceptors, and provide them with copies of the plan.

Teaching plans used with nursing students may differ from those used with newly hired nurses. When working with nursing students, ask faculty for a copy of the course syllabus, evaluation forms, and a course schedule. These documents will provide you and the preceptors with a general overview of the course, along with clinical objectives and expected competencies that nursing students need to demonstrate before the course ends (Sedgwick, Kellett, & Kalischuck, 2014). Clinical objectives and competencies may differ among courses and schools of nursing. Some students may be enrolled in customized courses called *directed* or *independent* studies that include a learning contract for the clinical experience. Be sure to maintain a copy of these items in your files.

Construct a schedule for your teaching plan, including the dates, hours, clinical focus (objective) for each day, and classes. Help preceptors select patient assignments that will enable preceptees to attain learning objectives. Similar to the lesson plan, the schedule may be integrated into a unit-based orientation program or separate.

According to Muir et al. (2013), preceptors often report that they lack sufficient time to meet their preceptees because of concurrent patient care responsibilities. When allotting time designated to direct patient care, also provide tranquil times during which preceptees and preceptors can reflect and evaluate performance either alone or together. Include time to meet with preceptors yourself and provide them with support and guidance.

Providing Preceptors With Support, Rewards, and Recognition

In addition to preparing nurses for the preceptor role, it is also important to provide preceptors with ongoing support and education, rewards, and recognition (Goss, 2015; Kalischuk et al., 2013; Modic & Schoessler, 2011). Preceptors play an essential role in the learning process of new nurses and student nurses and contribute to safe, quality patient care on the clinical unit. Therefore, it is vital that you develop a work environment that values this role and regards preceptorship as an honor, a privilege, and an integral step in leadership and NPD.

Evidence corroborates the need for preceptor support and recognition. A recent survey of 91 graduate-level clinical preceptors revealed that their commitment to the role was greater when they experienced rewards, benefits, and support (Donley et al., 2014). Increased commitment was also related to participating in preceptor programs and mentoring more than two students annually. Results also supported the need for preceptor roles to be more visible, recognized, and integrated between healthcare and academic organizations.

Nurses working as preceptors often are expected to assume additional roles, such as patient caregiver, on the clinical unit. Because these nurses may encounter multiple complex issues in an often hectic work environment, it is vital to explore and implement various strategies to prevent them from experiencing burnout (Blozen, 2010). It is important that preceptors have ongoing opportunities to share their concerns and receive assistance with their issues.

Be creative when developing strategies to support preceptors in your setting. One such approach is to pair new preceptors with experienced preceptors in a preceptor network. A second strategy is to develop a formal discussion group where preceptors from one or more clinical units gather together and share their experiences with each other. However, pay attention to the sharing of confidential information. Think about extending the preceptor group's discussions using technology such as Skype, email, or social media. Including experienced preceptors as faculty in CE programs to prepare preceptors also may serve as a source of support for nurses new to the role. Preceptors who work with nursing students may find ongoing communication and feedback from school of nursing faculty as an additional form of support. Regardless of the strategies you choose, it is important for you, the unit-based educator, to be available as a resource as well.

Beecroft, Hernandez, and Reid (2008) developed "team" preceptorships to minimize burnout in preceptors who repeatedly participated in extended pediatric residency programs for new nurses. In this team-based model, a novice preceptor mentors the resident during the basic instruction phase. At the same time, an expert preceptor "precepts" the novice preceptor and covers off days. After the resident obtains basic skills, the expert takes over for the novice preceptor. Positive evaluations supported this sequencing of preceptors, especially when residents were paired with novice preceptors, as these preceptors were recent graduates themselves and could easily identify with new nurses.

Blum (2014) used technology as a vehicle for stress reduction in preceptors. The study measured the influence of educational podcasts on preceptors' (N = 28) perceptions of support in learning how to manage difficult situations with newly hired nurses. In this correlational study, preceptors listened to four podcasts that demonstrated the use of caring behaviors in four hallmarks of unsafe practice identified by preceptors: attitude problems, poor communication skills, inability to demonstrate knowledge and skills, and unprofessional behavior (Blum, 2014). The use of podcasts revealed a statistically significant increase in preceptors' perceived support in their role from preintervention to postintervention. The least experienced preceptors reported the most support gained from the podcasts.

Providing preceptors with meaningful incentives or rewards for outstanding performance will not only motivate some nurses to become preceptors but also may serve to publicly recognize preceptor contributions to organizational success (Kalischuk et al., 2013). Because preceptor rewards may require agency resources or policy changes, be sure to discuss available opportunities with appropriate individuals within your organization. Because you know the nursing staff on your unit, think about what incentives and rewards they may perceive as important to them. Discuss this topic at a unit-based staff meeting, or ask your manager to discuss this issue with other managers at an administrative meeting.

Ask preceptors for feedback regarding what they value in return for serving in this capacity, as they may differ in what they perceive as an appropriate reward. This is an approach that Kalischuk et al. (2013) used in a Canadian liberal arts nursing program by surveying 331 preceptors regarding the perceived benefits, rewards, supports, challenges, and commitments involved in their role. In general, preceptors preferred nonmaterial rewards, such as having the opportunity to witness the professional development of a student, rather than material ones, such as a promotion. Modic and Schoessler (2011) differentiated recognition from rewards, referring to this phenomenon as *altruism* and a desire to "give back or pay forward" (p. 304). Conversely, preceptors have been discouraged by preceptees who are unsafe (Earle-Foley et al., 2012), poorly motivated, or unprofessional.

Although some preceptors value intrinsic rewards, other nurses may prefer extrinsic benefits. For example, serving as a preceptor is often among criteria for clinical advancement (see Chapter 10). Preceptor hours with nursing students are also included among the professional development requirements for nurses seeking recertification (ANCC, 2015). Some settings, according to a survey of nearly 300 preceptors in Canada, offer preceptors decreased patient assignments (Yonge, Krahn, Trojan, Reid, & Haase, 2002) or a different schedule to accommodate working with a preceptee. Some hospitals expect nurses to serve as preceptors and include this requirement in their position descriptions and performance evaluations.

Modic and Schoessler (2011) suggested that peers should take an active role in recognizing colleagues who serve as preceptors through verbal or written appreciation (e.g., email, written note) to the preceptors and their manager. Another suggestion involves collaborating with the shared governance council at an organization to propose creative recognition programs for nurses who make outstanding contributions.

Schools of nursing also acknowledge the clinical nurses who serve as preceptors for their students. Along with sending letters thanking preceptors for their unique contributions to the learning outcomes of their students, some schools, such as Western Kentucky University, award preceptors with a signed certificate of recognition, give them care baskets (Bryant & Williams, 2002) or small mementos (e.g., coffee mugs, mouse pads imprinted with the school's name or logo, pens), invite them to a campus celebration for preceptors (Bryant & Williams, 2002), or offer reduced-fee or free registration to educational programs or courses sponsored by the school (Gaberson et al., 2015). Other schools offer healthcare organizations assistance with their research projects or educational programs. Some confer titles, such as adjunct faculty, to preceptors (Gaberson et al., 2015), especially for those who go the extra mile to help students.

Select schools have invested a great deal of time and effort in defining appropriate rewards for preceptors. Dillon, Barga, and Goodin (2012) used a logic model approach at the Capital University Department of Nursing to design, implement, and evaluate a recognition program to thank clinical preceptors who mentored their nursing students. After studying the model's inputs, outputs, outcomes, assumptions, and external forces, the authors sponsored an evening reception that included a CE program to recognize the preceptors. Follow-up plans included the need to increase preceptors' attendance at the event.

Constructing an Evaluation Plan

Prior to the start of your unit-based preceptor program, develop a plan to evaluate key aspects of the program. This comprehensive evaluation plan should determine the effectiveness of your approach in attaining program goals. This plan also will provide you with the objective data needed to modify and improve your program.

An evaluation plan should provide you with feedback on the performance or behaviors of key individuals involved in the preceptorship program (e.g., preceptee, preceptor, unit-based educator, school of nursing faculty, nurse manager) and their overall satisfaction with the process and content of the preceptorship program (e.g., objectives, content, clinical teaching strategies, evaluation methods).

Although you are responsible for collecting evaluation data on preceptor programs sponsored by your organization, schools of nursing often use their own procedures and documents when evaluating preceptors paired with their nursing students in a clinical setting. Faculty course leaders ask preceptors to document a student's daily performance on the clinical unit and offer input in a final summary evaluation of the student. Some schools, such as Salisbury University School of Nursing, have collaborated with their preceptors to strengthen the quality and practicality of evaluation tools used to assess students' clinical performance (Walsh, Seldomridge, & Badros, 2008). Preceptors often are asked by faculty to provide feedback about the clinical course and the coordination efforts of faculty.

Because you select and develop unit-based preceptors, it is important to obtain feedback from faculty regarding your performance and the effectiveness of the clinical setting. This information can help you develop strategies to assist preceptors on your unit and to make improvements. Appendix 5-1 is an example of a clinical tool designed by a school of nursing for preceptors to evaluate students at periodic times throughout a semester. Specific guidelines that explain the tool's rating system are listed in Appendix 5-2, which also includes a final clinical evaluation tool that is completed by the student, preceptor, and faculty members. In addition to the preceptor's role in evaluation, nursing students are asked to evaluate their experience. These elements include their own clinical performance (see Appendix 5-3), the effectiveness of their preceptor in helping them attain clinical objectives and the clinical site (see Appendix 5-4), the coordination efforts of faculty, and the clinical course itself.

Because the evaluation process may be an overwhelming task, conceptualize this process using smaller components. First, decide which individuals in your program will need to be evaluated. Start by listing these individuals and names into a table, as illustrated in Table 5-2. Based on this matrix, decide what aspects should be evaluated within your organization and mark the appropriate block with an X. For example, preceptors should have not only an opportunity to evaluate their own performance but also a chance to evaluate the behaviors of their preceptees and the unit-based educator as the facilitator of the program. Likewise, preceptees should evaluate their own performance, along with the performances of their preceptor and unit-based educator. Finally, the unit-based educator should have input into the evaluation of both the preceptor and preceptee, along with themselves. Depending on your situation, you may choose to include the nurse manager and faculty in this process.

Table 5-2. Evaluation Map for Preceptor Program

	Preceptor	Preceptee	Unit-Based Educator	Nurse Manager
Preceptor	Self-evaluation	x	x	x
Preceptee	x	Self-evaluation	x	x
Unit-based educator	x	x	Self-evaluation	x
Nurse manager	x	x	x	Self-evaluation

Preceptees should receive feedback from their preceptors about their performance on a daily basis and at the conclusion of the clinical experience. Daily evaluation of the preceptor's performance, called *formative* evaluation, provides learners with feedback needed to help them shape their behaviors or competencies related to the objectives of the program or course (Oermann & Gaberson, 2014). To provide accurate feedback to preceptees regarding their performance, preceptors should consider recording daily notes that document the preceptees' learning activities and performance. This documentation also can help determine what learning experiences the preceptee will need in the future.

Evaluation that occurs at the conclusion of a clinical program, referred to as *summative* evaluation, helps determine if the preceptee attained the clinical objectives (Oermann & Gaberson, 2014). This evaluation provides learners with a summary regarding their behaviors compared to the clinical objectives for the program or course.

A variety of other methods can be used to conduct evaluations during your preceptor program. For example, consider conducting focus groups to obtain feedback about the preceptor program from preceptors and preceptees either during or at the conclusion of the program. Feedback obtained while the preceptor program is still in progress can be used to make immediate changes, if needed.

Implementing the Preceptor Program

Now that you have matched preceptees with preceptors and developed a teaching plan for the clinical experience, implement the program. If you are implementing your plan for the first time, be sure to note its positive features and those areas that need improvement.

Depending on the needs of your organization, consider pilot testing your preceptor program on a small scale before you implement a full-scale program. Piloting your program will enable you to determine the effectiveness of its policies, procedures, documents, and communication. It also will help you determine if preceptors need additional or different preparation. Evaluation comments received during pilot testing can help you revise the program before its next implementation.

Pilot testing can also provide you with data to calculate the cost of the program in light of its benefits. Track all expenses incurred in the program, such as time, materials, supplies, services, duplication costs, and staffing changes made to manage patient care. Ask your nurse manager for suggestions on how to best estimate these costs in your organization.

Use your star preceptors in the first program to maximize its success. Consider serving as a preceptor yourself to experience firsthand how the process works. Encourage a friendly, nonjudgmental learning environment on the clinical unit during the implementation of the program. Although some staff may occasionally experience a challenging day, be positive, encourage them to remain professional, and discuss their concerns in a private setting.

After the pilot preceptor program is completed, collect and analyze the evaluation data. Chapter 6 will provide you with an evaluation model and ways to collect evidence that supports future revisions. Discuss how the program progressed with unit staff and preceptors, and decide what changes need to be implemented before the next program is conducted. Obtain feedback about the preceptor program from the preceptees' perspectives immediately following the program, as well as at a later time (possibly six months or one year after their experience).

Moore (2009) described the initial development and validation of the Preceptor Evaluation Survey to be completed by newly hired nurses regarding their preceptor experience. Specific items were used to assess the performance of the preceptor, the support for the preceptor in the clinical setting, and the nurse's job satisfaction.

Consider designing and implementing a research study or quality improvement project to validate the effectiveness of your preceptor program on specific learning and organizational outcomes. Obtain assistance from NPDSs with research expertise or nurse researchers at academic partnerships, if needed (see Chapter 12). Disseminate your accomplishments through scholarship, such as publication in a journal (see Chapter 8) and oral podium or poster presentations (see Chapter 9).

Summary

Preceptor programs are used as a clinical teaching method by both healthcare organizations and schools of nursing. Nurses who assume the role of a preceptor require appropriate preparation and support in order to function effectively. The NPDS and unit-based educator play pivotal roles in coordinating unit-based preceptor programs and evaluating their overall effectiveness related to cost and delivery of safe, quality patient care. Disseminating successful outcomes of preceptor programs through presentations and publications is an essential role of the NPDS.

Helpful Websites

- American Academy for Preceptor Advancement: www.preceptoracademy.com
- Catholic University of America—Preceptor Guidelines: http://nursing.cua.edu/graduate/msn/preceptor-manual/preceptor-guidelines.cfm
- Michigan Center for Nursing—Faculty and Preceptor Tool Kits: https://michigancenterfornursing.org/education/preceptor-about
- Palm Healthcare Foundation—Podcasts: www.palmhealthcare.org/nursing-preceptor-podcasts

References

Aaron, C.S. (2011). The positive impact of preceptors on recruitment and retention of RNs in long-term care: A pilot project. *Journal of Gerontological Nursing, 37*(4), 48–54. doi:10.3928/00989134-20101112-01

Al-Hussami, M., Saleh, M.Y., Darawad, M., & Alramly, M. (2011). Evaluating the effectiveness of a clinical preceptorship program for registered nurses in Jordan. *Journal of Continuing Education in Nursing, 42,* 569–576. doi:10.3928/00220124-20110901-01

Allen, L. (2011). On the road to a meaningful, cost-effective orientation program. *Nursing Management, 42*(5), 10–12. doi:10.1097/01.NUMA.0000396498.38628.2d

American Academy for Preceptor Advancement. (n.d.). Home. Retrieved from http://www.preceptoracademy.com

American Association of Colleges of Nursing. (2014). Nursing shortage. Retrieved from http://www.aacn.nche.edu/media-relations/fact-sheets/nursing-shortage

American Nurses Association. (2000). *Scope and standards of practice for nursing professional development.* Washington, DC: Author.

American Nurses Association. (2015). *Nursing: Scope and standards of practice* (3rd ed.). Silver Spring, MD: Author.

American Nurses Association & National Nursing Staff Development Organization. (2010). *Nursing professional development: Scope and standards of practice.* Silver Spring, MD: American Nurses Association.

American Nurses Credentialing Center. (n.d.). Forces of Magnetism. Retrieved from http://www.nursecredentialing.org/Magnet/ProgramOverview/HistoryoftheMagnetProgram/ForcesofMagnetism.aspx

American Nurses Credentialing Center. (2012). *Educational design process: 2013 mini manual.* Silver Spring, MD: Author.

American Nurses Credentialing Center. (2015). 2015 certification renewal requirements. Retrieved from http://www.nursecredentialing.org/RenewalRequirements.aspx

Baggot, D., Hensinger, B., Parry, J., Valdes, M.S., & Zaim, S. (2005). The new hire/preceptor experience: Cost-benefit analysis of one retention strategy. *Journal of Nursing Administration, 35,* 138–145. doi:10.1097/00005110-200503000-00007

Bassendowski, S., Layne, J., Lee, L., & Hupaelo, T. (2010). Supporting clinical preceptors with interprofessional orientation sessions. *Journal of Allied Health, 39,* e23–e28.

Beecroft, P., Hernandez, A.M., & Reid, D. (2008). Team preceptorships: A new approach for precepting new nurses. *Journal for Nurses in Staff Development, 24,* 143–148. doi:10.1097/01.NND.0000320675.42953.7f

Blozen, B. (2010). Avoiding preceptor burnout. *American Nurse Today, 5*(11), 41–42. Retrieved from http://www.americannursetoday.com/avoiding-preceptor-burnout

Blum, C.A. (2014). Evaluating preceptor perception of support using educational podcasts. *International Journal of Nursing Education Scholarship, 11,* 47–54. doi:10.1515/ijnes-2013-0037

Bott, G., Mohide, E.A., & Lawlor, Y. (2011). A clinical technique for nurse preceptors: The five minute preceptor. *Journal of Professional Nursing, 27,* 35–42. doi:10.1016/j.profnurs.2010.09.009

Broadbent, M., Moxham, L., Sander, T., Walker, S., & Dwyer, T. (2014). Supporting bachelor of nursing students within the clinical environment: Perspectives of preceptors. *Nurse Education in Practice, 14,* 403–409. doi:10.1016/j.nepr.2013.12.003

Brunt, B.A., & Kopp, D.J. (2007). Impact of preceptor and orientee learning styles on satisfaction: A pilot study. *Journal for Nurses in Staff Development, 23,* 36–44. doi:10.1097/00124645-200701000-00008

Bryant, S.C., & Williams, D. (2002). The senior practicum. *Nurse Educator, 27,* 174–177. doi:10.1097/00006223-200207000-00010

Burns, H.K., & Northcutt, T. (2009). Supporting preceptors: A three-pronged approach for success. *Journal of Continuing Education in Nursing, 40,* 509–513. doi:10.3928/00220124-20091023-08

Carlson, E. (2013). Precepting and symbolic interactionism: A theoretical look at preceptorship during clinical practice. *Journal of Advanced Nursing, 69,* 457–464. doi:10.1111/j.1365-2648.2012.06047.x

Chang, A., Douglas, M., Breen-Reid, K., Gueorguieva, V., & Fleming-Carroll, B. (2013). Preceptors' perceptions of their role in a pediatric acute care setting. *Journal of Continuing Education in Nursing, 44,* 211–217. doi:10.3928/00220124-20130315-81

Commission on Collegiate Nursing Education. (2013). *Standards for accreditation of baccalaureate and graduate nursing programs.* Retrieved from http://www.aacn.nche.edu/ccne-accreditation/Standards-Amended-2013.pdf

Conley, S.B., Branowicki, P., & Hanley, D. (2007). Nursing leadership orientation: A competency and preceptor model to facilitate new leader success. *Journal of Nursing Administration, 37,* 491–498. doi:10.1097/01.NNA.0000295612.48065.ff

Delfino, P., Williams, J.L., Wegener, J.M., & Homel, P. (2014). The preceptor experience: The impact of the Vermont Nurse Internship Project/Partnership Model on nursing orientation. *Journal for Nurses in Professional Development, 30,* 122–126. doi:10.1097/NND.0000000000000060

Dillon, K.A., Barga, K.N., & Goodin, H.J. (2012). Use of a logic model framework to develop and implement a preceptor recognition program. *Journal for Nurses in Staff Development, 28,* 36–40. doi:10.1097/NND.0b013e3182417d94

Donley, R., Flaherty, M.J., Sarsfield, E., Burkhard, A., O'Brien, S., & Anderson, K.M. (2014). Graduate clinical nurse preceptors: Implications for improved intra-professional collaboration. *Online Journal of Issues in Nursing, 19.* Retrieved from http://www.nursingworld.org/MainMenuCategories/ANAMarketplace/ANAPeriodicals/OJIN/TableofContents/Vol-19-2014/No3-Sept-2014/Articles-Previous-Topics/Graduate-Clinical-Nurse-Preceptors.html

Duteau, J. (2012). Making a difference: The value of preceptorship programs in nursing education. *Journal of Continuing Education in Nursing, 43,* 37–43. doi:10.3928/00220124-20110615-01

Earle-Foley, V., Myrick, F., Luhanga, F., & Yonge, O. (2012). Preceptorship: Using an ethical lens to reflect on the unsafe student. *Journal of Professional Nursing, 28,* 27–33. doi:10.1016/j.profnurs.2011.06.005

Elmers, C.R. (2010). The role of preceptor and nurse leader in developing intensive care unit competency. *Critical Care Nursing Quarterly, 33,* 10–18. doi:10.1097/CNQ.0b013e3181c8e0a9

Finger, S.D., & Pape, T.M. (2002). Invitational theory and perioperative nursing preceptorships. *AORN Journal, 76,* 630–642. doi:10.1016/S0001-2092(06)60938-1

Finn, F.L., & Chesser-Smyth, P. (2013). Promoting learning transfer in preceptor preparation. *Journal for Nurses in Professional Development, 29,* 309–315. doi:10.1097/NND.0000000000000014

Freiburger, O.A. (2002). Preceptor programs: Increasing student self-confidence and competency. *Nurse Educator, 27,* 58–60. doi:10.1097/00006223-200203000-00004

Gaberson, K.B., Oermann, M.H., & Shellenbarger, T. (2015). *Clinical teaching strategies in nursing* (4th ed.). New York, NY: Springer.

Glynn, P., & Silva, S. (2013). Meeting the needs of new graduates in the emergency department: A qualitative study evaluating a new graduate internship program. *Journal of Emergency Nursing, 39,* 173–178. doi:10.1016/j.jen.2011.10.007

Goss, C.R. (2015). Systematic review building a preceptor support system. *Journal for Nurses in Professional Development, 31,* E7–E14. doi:10.1097/NND.0000000000000117

Gurney, D. (2002). Developing a successful 16-week "transition ED nursing" program: One busy community hospital's experience. *Journal of Emergency Nursing, 28,* 505–514. doi:10.1067/men.2002.129707

Haas, B.K., Deardorff, K.U., Klotz, L., Baker, B., Coleman, J., & DeWitt, A. (2002). Creating a collaborative partnership between academia and service. *Journal of Nursing Education, 41,* 518–523.

Hardin, S.R., & Kaplow, R. (Eds.). (2005). *Synergy for clinical excellence: The AACN synergy model for patient care.* Burlington, MA: Jones & Bartlett Learning.

Hautala, K.T., Saylor, C.R., & O'Leary-Kelley, C. (2007). Nurses' perceptions of stress and support in the preceptor role. *Journal for Nurses in Staff Development, 23,* 64–70. doi:10.1097/01.NND.0000266611.78315.08

Heffernan, C., Heffernan, E., Brosnan, M., & Brown, G. (2009). Evaluating a preceptorship programme in South West Ireland: Perceptions of preceptors and undergraduate students. *Journal of Nursing Management, 17,* 539–549. doi:10.1111/j.1365-2834.2008.00935.x

Horton, C.D., DePaoli, S., Hertach, M., & Bower, M. (2012). Enhancing the effectiveness of nurse preceptors. *Journal for Nurses in Staff Development, 28,* E1–E7. doi:10.1097/NND.0b013e31825dfb90

Joint Commission. (2015). Hospital 2015: National patient safety goals. Retrieved from http://www.jointcommission.org/standards_information/npsgs.aspx

Kaddoura, M.A. (2013). The effect of preceptor behavior on the critical thinking skills of new graduate nurses in the intensive care unit. *Journal of Continuing Education in Nursing, 44,* 488–495. doi:10.3928/00220124-20130816-21

Kalischuk, R.G., Vandenberg, H., & Awosoga, O. (2013). Nursing preceptors speak out: An empirical study. *Journal of Professional Nursing, 29,* 30–38. doi:10.1016/j.profnurs.2012.04.008

Krampe, J., L'Ecuyer, K., & Palmer, J.L. (2013). Development of an online orientation course for preceptors in a dedicated education unit program. *Journal of Continuing Education in Nursing, 44,* 352–356. doi:10.3928/00220124-20130617-44

Larsen, R., & Zahner, S.J. (2011). The impact of web-delivered education on preceptor role self-efficacy and knowledge in public health nurses. *Public Health Nursing, 28,* 349–356. doi:10.1111/j.1525-1446.2010.00933.x

Lawless, R.P., Demers, K.A., & Baker, L. (2002). Preceptor program boosts recruitment and retention. *Caring, 21*(9), 10–12.

Lee, T.Y., Tzeng, W.C., Lin, C.H., & Yeh, M.L. (2009). Effects of a preceptorship programme on turnover rate, cost, quality and professional development. *Journal of Clinical Nursing, 18,* 1217–1225. doi:10.1111/j.1365-2702.2008.02662.x

Letourneau, R.M. (2010). Attract the best and brightest with comprehensive internships. *Nursing Management, 41*(4), 12–16. doi:10.1097/01.NUMA.0000370872.17725.20

Link, D.G. (2009). The teaching-coaching role of the APN. *Journal of Perinatal and Neonatal Nursing, 23,* 279–283. doi:10.1097/JPN.0b013e3181b0b8d2

Lockwood-Rayermann, S. (2003). Preceptor leadership style and the nursing practicum. *Journal of Professional Nursing, 19,* 32–37. doi:10.1053/jpnu.2003.7

Luhanga, F., Myrick, F., & Yonge, O. (2010). The preceptor experience: An examination of ethical and accountability issues. *Journal of Professional Nursing, 26,* 264–271. doi:10.1016/j.profnurs.2009.12.008

Madhavanpraphakaran, G.K., Shukri, R.K., & Balachandran, S. (2014). Preceptors' perceptions of clinical nursing education. *Journal of Continuing Education in Nursing, 45,* 28–34. doi:10.3928/00220124-20131223-04

Marks-Maran, D., Ooms, A., Tapping, J., Muir, J., Phillips, S., & Burke, L. (2013). A preceptorship programme for newly qualified nurses: A study of preceptees' perceptions. *Nurse Education Today, 33,* 1428–1434. doi:10.1016/j.nedt.2012.11.013

McCarthy, B., & Murphy, S. (2010). Preceptors' experiences of clinically educating and assessing undergraduate nursing students: An Irish context. *Journal of Nursing Management, 18,* 234–244. doi:10.1111/j.1365-2834.2010.01050.x

Modic, M.B., & Schoessler, M. (2011). Recognition. *Journal for Nurses in Staff Development, 27,* 304–305. doi:10.1097/NND.0b013e318238654f

Moore, M.L. (2009). Developing the Preceptorship Evaluation Survey. *Journal for Nurses in Staff Development, 25,* 249–253. doi:10.1097/NND.0b013e3181ae2eba

Moore, P., & Cagle, C.S. (2012). The lived experience of new nurses: Importance of the clinical preceptor. *Journal of Continuing Education in Nursing, 43,* 555–565. doi:10.3928/00220124-20120904-29

Muir, J., Ooms, A., Tapping, J., Marks-Maran, D., Phillips, S., & Burke, L. (2013). Preceptors' perceptions of a preceptorship programme for newly qualified nurses. *Nurse Education Today, 33,* 633–638. doi:10.1016/j.nedt.2013.02.001

Myrick, F., Caplan, W., Smitten, J., & Rusk, K. (2010). Preceptor/mentor education: A world of possibilities through e-learning technology. *Nurse Education Today, 31,* 263–267. doi:10.1016/j.nedt.2010.10.026

Oermann, M.H., & Gaberson, K.B. (2014). *Evaluation and testing in nursing education* (4th ed.). New York, NY: Springer Publishing.

Omansky, G.L. (2010). Staff nurses' experience as preceptors and mentors: An integrative review. *Journal of Nursing Management, 18,* 697–703. doi:10.1111/j.1365-2834.2010.01145.x

Poradzisz, M., Kostovich, C.T., O'Connell, D., & Lefaiver, C.A. (2012). Preceptors and new graduate nurse orientees: Implications of psychological type compatibility. *Journal for Nurses in Staff Development, 28,* E9–E15. doi:10.1097/NND.0b013e31825515ec

Reilly, J.R., Collier, J., Edelstein, J., Vandenhouten, C., Hovarter, R., Hansen, J.M., … Turner, M.J. (2012). Collaborative design and use of an agency feedback form for student clinical practicum experience in community/public health nursing. *Public Health Nursing, 29,* 160–167. doi:10.1111/j.1525-1446.2011.00969.x

Rogan, E. (2009). Preparation of nurses who precept baccalaureate nursing students: A descriptive study. *Journal of Continuing Education in Nursing, 40,* 565–570. doi:10.3928/00220124-20091119-06

Roth, J.W. (Ed.). (2015). *Core curriculum for preceptor advancement: Preceptor specialty development.* Peyton, CO: American Academy for Preceptor Advancement.

Roth, J.W., Figueroa, S., & Swihart, D. (Eds.). (2014). *Scope and standards of practice for preceptor advancement.* Peyton, CO: American Academy for Preceptor Advancement.

Schaubhut, R.M., & Gentry, J.A. (2010). Nursing preceptor workshops: Partnership and collaboration between academia and practice. *Journal of Continuing Education in Nursing, 41,* 155–160. doi:10.3928/00220124-20100326-01

Sedgwick, M., Kellett, P., & Kalischuck, R.G. (2014). Exploring the acquisition of entry-to-practice competencies by second-degree nursing students during a preceptorship experience. *Nurse Education Today, 34,* 421–427. doi:10.1016/j.nedt.2013.04.012

Smedley, A., & Penney, D. (2009). A partnership approach to the preparation of preceptors. *Nursing Education Perspectives, 30,* 31–36.

Souers, C. (2002). Comprehensive performance review: Preparing students for a preceptor experience. *Nurse Educator, 27,* 9–12. doi:10.1097/00006223-200201000-00011

Stewart, S., Pope, D., & Hansen, T.S. (2010). Clinical preceptors enhance an online accelerated bachelor's degree to BSN program. *Nurse Educator, 35,* 37–40. doi:10.1097/NNE.0b013e3181c4210d

Thekdi, P., Wilson, B.L., & Xu, Y. (2011). Understanding post-hire transitional challenges of foreign-educated nurses. *Nursing Management, 42*(9), 8–14. doi:10.1097/01.NUMA.0000403285.34873.c7

Thomas, C.M., Bertram, E., & Allen, R.L. (2012). The transition from student to new registered nurse in professional practice. *Journal for Nurses in Staff Development, 28,* 243–249. doi:10.1097/NND.0b013e31826a009c

Walsh, C.M., Seldomridge, L.A., & Badros, K.K. (2008). Developing a practical evaluation tool for preceptor use. *Nurse Educator, 33,* 113–117. doi:10.1097/01.NNE.0000312185.43766.1e

Wilson, L.L. (2012). Redesigning OR orientation. *AORN Journal, 95,* 453–462. doi:10.1016/j.aorn.2012.01.022

Wilson, L.L., Bodin, M.B., Hoffman, J., & Vincent, J. (2009). Supporting and retaining preceptors for NNP programs: Results from a survey of NNP preceptors and program directors. *Journal of Perinatal and Neonatal Nursing, 23,* 284–292. doi:10.1097/JPN.0b013e3181b3075d

Yonge, O., Krahn, H., Trojan, L., Reid, D., & Haase, M. (2002). Being a preceptor is stressful! *Journal for Nurses in Staff Development, 18,* 22–27.

Zimmermann, P.G. (2002). So you're going to precept nursing students: One instructor's suggestions. *Journal of Emergency Nursing, 28,* 589–592. doi:10.1067/men.2002.128245

Appendix 5-1. Periodic Clinical Evaluation Tool Completed by Preceptors

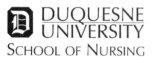
DUQUESNE
UNIVERSITY
SCHOOL OF NURSING

DUQUESNE UNIVERSITY SCHOOL OF NURSING
Periodic Clinical Progress Tool (CPT)
COURSE: UPNS 416 Synergy in Nursing Practice

Student _____

Semester/Year _____

Competency	Week _____	Week _____	Week _____
1. Integrates clinical judgment skills when implementing care for individuals, families, groups, and communities (Clinical Judgment*)	Independent_____ Supervised _____ Marginal_____ Dependent_____ Comments: _____ _____ _____	Independent_____ Supervised _____ Marginal_____ Dependent_____ Comments: _____ _____ _____	Independent_____ Supervised _____ Marginal_____ Dependent_____ Comments: _____ _____ _____
2. Justifies one's practice through the implementation of the role of being a moral agent (Advocacy and Moral Agency*)	Independent_____ Supervised _____ Marginal_____ Dependent_____ Comments: _____ _____ _____	Independent_____ Supervised _____ Marginal_____ Dependent_____ Comments: _____ _____ _____	Independent_____ Supervised _____ Marginal_____ Dependent_____ Comments: _____ _____ _____
3. Displays a caring attitude in all aspects of one's practice (Caring*)	Independent_____ Supervised _____ Marginal_____ Dependent_____ Comments: _____ _____ _____	Independent_____ Supervised _____ Marginal_____ Dependent_____ Comments: _____ _____ _____	Independent_____ Supervised _____ Marginal_____ Dependent_____ Comments: _____ _____ _____
4. Initiates collaborative efforts for the improvement of care to individuals and for improvement in the healthcare delivery systems (Collaboration*)	Independent_____ Supervised _____ Marginal_____ Dependent_____ Comments: _____ _____ _____	Independent_____ Supervised _____ Marginal_____ Dependent_____ Comments: _____ _____ _____	Independent_____ Supervised _____ Marginal_____ Dependent_____ Comments: _____ _____ _____
5. Demonstrates the ability to utilize integrated systems analysis for the personal and professional navigation of the healthcare delivery systems (Systems Thinking*)	Independent_____ Supervised _____ Marginal_____ Dependent_____ Comments: _____ _____ _____	Independent_____ Supervised _____ Marginal_____ Dependent_____ Comments: _____ _____ _____	Independent_____ Supervised _____ Marginal_____ Dependent_____ Comments: _____ _____ _____

(Continued on next page)

Appendix 5-1. Periodic Clinical Evaluation Tool Completed by Preceptors *(Continued)*

Competency	Week _____	Week _____	Week _____
6. Integrates cultural sensitivity in caring for individuals/families of diverse populations (Response to Diversity*)	Independent_____ Supervised _____ Marginal_____ Dependent_____ Comments: _____ _____ _____	Independent_____ Supervised _____ Marginal_____ Dependent_____ Comments: _____ _____ _____	Independent_____ Supervised _____ Marginal_____ Dependent_____ Comments: _____ _____ _____
7. Engages in evidence-based practice (Clinical Inquiry*)	Independent_____ Supervised _____ Marginal_____ Dependent_____ Comments: _____ _____ _____	Independent_____ Supervised _____ Marginal_____ Dependent_____ Comments: _____ _____ _____	Independent_____ Supervised _____ Marginal_____ Dependent_____ Comments: _____ _____ _____
8. Incorporates teaching into all aspects of one's practice (Facilitator of Learning*)	Independent_____ Supervised _____ Marginal_____ Dependent_____ Comments: _____ _____ _____	Independent_____ Supervised _____ Marginal_____ Dependent_____ Comments: _____ _____ _____	Independent_____ Supervised _____ Marginal_____ Dependent_____ Comments: _____ _____ _____
9. Evaluates the interrelationship of nurse competencies and the patient characteristics to patient outcomes	Independent_____ Supervised _____ Marginal_____ Dependent_____ Comments: _____ _____ _____	Independent_____ Supervised _____ Marginal_____ Dependent_____ Comments: _____ _____ _____	Independent_____ Supervised _____ Marginal_____ Dependent_____ Comments: _____ _____ _____
10. Demonstrates accountability for own nursing practice and professional growth	Independent_____ Supervised _____ Marginal_____ Dependent_____ Comments: _____ _____ _____	Independent_____ Supervised _____ Marginal_____ Dependent_____ Comments: _____ _____ _____	Independent_____ Supervised _____ Marginal_____ Dependent_____ Comments: _____ _____ _____

Comments: _____
_____
_____
_____
_____
_____
_____

Faculty/Preceptor Signature:_____Date_____

Student Signature:_____Date_____

* Competency from the AACN Synergy Model for Patient Care (Hardin & Kaplow, 2005).

Note. Figure courtesy of Duquesne University School of Nursing. Used with permission.

Appendix 5-2. Clinical Learning Indicator Tool Guidelines Used by Preceptor and Faculty

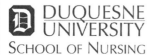

DUQUESNE UNIVERSITY SCHOOL OF NURSING
CLINICAL LEARNING INDICATORS
COURSE NAME: UPNS 413: Synergy in Nursing Practice

DIRECTIONS: Please indicate your rating of the student's performance on the Periodic Clinical Progress tool, using the learning indicators below.

Clinical Learning Indicators (Nurse Competencies):

1	Integrates clinical judgment skills when implementing care for individuals, families, and communities (Clinical Judgment*)
	1. Questions the limits of one's ability to make clinical decisions and seeks guidance from other clinicians 2. Follows algorithms, decision trees, and protocols with all populations 3. Integrates clinical judgments based on an understanding of the whole picture 4. Initiates multidisciplinary collaboration to solve patient problems 5. Identifies and/or demonstrates appropriate nursing actions during patient simulation scenarios 6. Successfully meets the math proficiency requirement
2	Justifies one's practice through the implementation of the role of being a moral agent (Advocacy and Moral Agency*)
	1. Analyzes ethical/legal issues within the healthcare setting 2. Incorporates patient values and rights in care, even when differing from personal values 3. Encourages the patient/family to speak for themselves when possible
3	Displays a caring attitude in all aspects of one's practice (Caring*)
	1. Creates a compassionate and therapeutic environment driven by the unique needs of the patient/family 2. Ensures patient and family safety 3. Ensures that the patient's/family's concerns surrounding issues of death and dying are met
4	Initiates collaborative efforts for the improvement of care to individuals and for the improvement in healthcare delivery systems (Collaboration*)
	1. Elicits others' advice and perspectives related to patient care delivery 2. Promotes collaboration among members of the healthcare team 3. Participates in team meetings and discussions regarding patient care and/or practice issues 4. Open to various team members' contributions
5	Demonstrates the ability to utilize integrated systems analysis for the personal and professional navigation of the healthcare delivery systems (Systems Thinking*)
	1. Utilizes a variety of strategies that are driven by the needs and strengths of the patient/family 2. Navigates through the healthcare system on behalf of the family 3. Develops a view of the patient and family's transition process back into the community

(Continued on next page)

	Appendix 5-2. Clinical Learning Indicator Tool Guidelines Used by Preceptor and Faculty (Continued)
6	**Integrates cultural sensitivity in caring for individuals/families of diverse populations (Response to Diversity*)**
	1. Assists patient/family to adapt to the culture of the healthcare environment 2. Anticipates cultural differences and their impact on patient/family care
7	**Engages in evidence-based practice (Clinical Inquiry*)**
	1. Individualizes standards and guidelines for particular patient situations 2. Utilizes nursing research findings to guide nursing practice 3. Responds to changing patient conditions (e.g., deterioration, crisis) 4. Seeks advice, resources or information to improve patient care
8	**Incorporates teaching into all aspects of one's practice (Facilitator of Learning*)**
	1. Incorporates input from other healthcare providers into the patient/family educational plan 2. Sees patients/families as having choices and consequences that are negotiated in relation to education
9	**Examines the interrelationship of nurse competencies and patient characteristics to patient outcomes**
	1. Evaluates the effectiveness of nursing interventions chosen to meet the needs of patients/families 2. Creates and implements a group community project based on the unique needs of the specific community 3. Implements the activities of the AMICI program according to the appropriate level consistent with the clinical course and established Student Guidelines 4. Submits an updated portfolio according to the specified guidelines
10	**Demonstrates accountability for own nursing practice and professional growth**
	1. Attends all clinical experiences regularly and punctually 2. Is prepared for all clinical experiences 3. Assumes responsibility for own learning, with faculty guidance, demonstrating motivation and self-directedness 4. Evaluates progress toward attainment of student and professional goals 5. Completes all clinical assignments within identified time frame 6. Demonstrates professional responsibility and accountability as well as peer accountability
	* Competency from the AACN Synergy Model for Patient Care (Hardin & Kaplow, 2005). *Note.* Figure courtesy of Duquesne University School of Nursing. Used with permission.

Appendix 5-3. Final Clinical Evaluation Tool Completed by Preceptor, Faculty, and Student

DUQUESNE UNIVERSITY
SCHOOL OF NURSING

____Faculty

FINAL CLINICAL EVALUATION ___Student

COURSE: UPNS 416 Synergy in Nursing Practice _____Preceptor

STUDENT:_____SEMESTER/YEAR:_____

Rating Scale: I – Independent   S – Supervised   M – Marginal   D – Dependent

(Rating of "Supervised" required for a passing grade in this course.)   DAYS ABSENT:_____

COMPETENCY	EXAMPLES OF BEHAVIORS
1. Integrates clinical judgment skills when implementing care for individuals, families, and communities (Clinical Judgment*)	
Rating: I S M D Comments:	1. Questions the limits of one's ability to make clinical decisions and seeks guidance from other clinicians 2. Follows algorithms, decision trees, and protocols with all populations 3. Integrates clinical judgments based on an understanding of the whole picture 4. Initiates multidisciplinary collaboration to solve patient problems 5. Identifies and/or demonstrates appropriate nursing actions during patient simulation scenarios 6. Successfully meets the math proficiency requirement
2. Justifies one's practice through the implementation of the role of being a moral agent (Advocacy and Moral Agency*)	
Rating: I S M D Comments:	1. Analyzes ethical/legal issues within the healthcare setting 2. Incorporates patient values and rights in care, even when differing from personal values 3. Encourages the patient/family to speak for themselves when possible

(Continued on next page)

Appendix 5-3. Final Clinical Evaluation Tool Completed by Preceptor, Faculty, and Student *(Continued)*

COMPETENCY	EXAMPLES OF BEHAVIORS
3. Displays a caring attitude in all aspects of one's practice (Caring*)	
Rating: I S M D	Comments:	1. Creates a compassionate and therapeutic environment driven by the unique needs of the patient/family 2. Ensures patient and family safety 3. Ensures that the patient's family concerns surrounding issues of death and dying are met
4. Initiates collaborative efforts for the improvement of care to individuals and for the improvement in health-care delivery systems (Collaboration*)	
Rating: I S M D	Comments:	1. Elicits others' advice and perspectives related to patient care delivery 2. Promotes collaboration among members of the healthcare team 3. Participates in team meetings and discussions regarding patient care and/or practice issues 4. Open to various team members' contributions
5. Demonstrates the ability to utilize integrated systems analysis for the personal and professional navigation of the healthcare delivery systems (Systems Thinking*)	
Rating: I S M D	Comments:	1. Utilizes a variety of strategies that are driven by the needs and strengths of the patient/family 2. Navigates through the healthcare system on behalf of the patient/family 3. Develops a view of the patient's and family's transition process back into the community

(Continued on next page)

Appendix 5-3. Final Clinical Evaluation Tool Completed by Preceptor, Faculty, and Student *(Continued)*

COMPETENCY	EXAMPLES OF BEHAVIORS
6. Integrates cultural sensitivity in caring for individuals/families of diverse populations (Response to Diversity*)	
Rating: I S M D Comments:	1. Assists patient/family to adapt to the culture of the healthcare environment 2. Anticipates cultural differences and their impact on patient/family care
7. Engages in evidence-based practice (Clinical Inquiry*)	
Rating: I S M D Comments:	1. Individualizes standards and guidelines for particular patient situations 2. Utilizes nursing research findings to guide nursing practice 3. Responds to changing patient conditions (e.g., deterioration, crisis) 4. Seeks advice, resources, or information to improve patient care
8. Incorporates teaching into all aspects of one's practice (Facilitator of Learning*)	
Rating: I S M D Comments:	1. Integrates input from other healthcare providers into the patient/family educational plan 2. Sees patients/families as having choices and consequences that are negotiated in relation to education
9. Evaluates the interrelationship of nurse competencies and the patient characteristics to patient outcomes	
Rating: I S M D Comments:	1. Evaluates the effectiveness of nursing interventions chosen to meet the needs of patients/families 2. Creates and implements a group community project based on the unique needs of the specific community 3. Implements the activities of the AMICI program according to the appropriate level consistent with the clinical course and established Student Guidelines 4. Submits an updated portfolio according to the specified guidelines

(Continued on next page)

Appendix 5-3. Final Clinical Evaluation Tool Completed by Preceptor, Faculty, and Student *(Continued)*

COMPETENCY	EXAMPLES OF BEHAVIORS
10. Demonstrates accountability for own nursing practice and professional growth	

| Rating:
I

S

M

D | Comments: | 1. Attends all clinical experiences regularly and punctually
2. Is prepared for all clinical experiences
3. Assumes responsibility for own learning, with faculty guidance, demonstrating motivation and self-directedness
4. Evaluates progress toward attainment of student and professional goals
5. Completes all clinical assignments within identified time frame and according to guidelines
6. Demonstrates professional responsibility and accountability as well as peer accountability |

Student Comments:_____

_____
_____
_____
_____
_____
_____
_____
_____
_____
_____
_____

Final Clinical Grade: (Pass/No Pass): _____

Faculty/Preceptor Signature:_____Date_____

Student Signature:_____Date_____

* Competency from the AACN Synergy Model for Patient Care (Hardin & Kaplow, 2005).

Note. Figure courtesy of Duquesne University School of Nursing. Used with permission.

Appendix 5-4. Evaluation of Preceptor and Clinical Site Completed by Student

DUQUESNE UNIVERSITY
SCHOOL OF NURSING

UPNS 416 Synergy in Nursing Practice
Clinical Preceptor Evaluation Form

Name (optional): _____   Date: _____

Semester: _____   Clinical Agency: _____

Please check the box in the most appropriate space below. Space is provided for any and all written comments you may have.

Please note that anonymity will be ensured with your responses.

	Quality	Seldom	Sometimes	Frequently	N/A	Comments
1	Is available to you during clinical time					
2	Demonstrates understanding of the role of the professional nurse					
3	In your opinion, is professional in appearance					
4	Demonstrates respect for clients of all cultural backgrounds					
5	Maintains an evidence-based practice					
6	Demonstrates research utilization in daily practice					
7	Is a positive role model to you					
8	Treats you with dignity and respect in the student role					

(Continued on next page)

Appendix 5-4. Evaluation of Preceptor and Clinical Site Completed by Student (*Continued*)

	Quality	Seldom	Sometimes	Frequently	N/A	Comments
9	Provides constructive feedback to you during clinical experience					
10	Has clinical expectations consistent with your specific course/clinical objectives					
11	Challenges and stimulates your critical thinking regarding client care					
12	In your opinion, is clinically competent and current in skills					
13	Reviews your charting on a daily basis					
14	Encourages questions					
15	Communicates his/her clinical knowledge well to you					
16	Utilizes an interdisciplinary approach to client care					
17	Provides you with feedback on your clinical evaluation tool at the completion of this experience					
18	Assigned clinical agency provided opportunities to meet course objectives					
19	Assigned clinical unit was flexible in assisting you to achieve required hours					
20	Assigned clinical unit fostered an atmosphere open to student learning					

Note. Figure courtesy of Duquesne University School of Nursing. Used with permission.

CHAPTER 6

Helping Clinical Nurses Develop Their Educator Role Through Unit-Based In-Service Educational Programs

A S mentioned in Chapter 1, responsibility for the professional development of clinical staff has been trending from NPDSs in a centralized department to unit-based nurses (e.g., staff educators, advanced practice nurses [APNs], unit managers, clinical nurses who provide or coordinate patient care). It is important for you, as an NPDS, to address the learning needs of these nurses related to not only patient care (standards of practice) but also staff education (standards of professional performance).

As explained in Chapters 1 and 2, the expectation for nurses to develop their skills and competencies in the educator role is advocated by the American Nurses Association (ANA) in *Nursing: Scope and Standards of Practice* (ANA, 2015); the Forces of Magnetism identified by the American Nurses Credentialing Center (ANCC) for Magnet® recognition (ANCC, n.d.); and the recommendation by the Institute of Medicine (IOM) for nurses to engage in lifelong learning in *The Future of Nursing: Leading Change, Advancing Health* (IOM, 2011).

Given these expectations, this chapter will illustrate how you, as an NPDS or unit-based educator, can use in-service educational programs to help clinical nurses acquire the skills they need to comfortably and confidently teach their peers. My 1996 work with Jane Bryce, RN, MSN, will provide an example of the process used to attain this goal. Although this example is dated, suggestions will be offered to increase its current application. A current example of a unit-based program will also be compared to this work.

In-Service Educational Programs

Chapter 2 introduced the NPDS practice model, which included several throughputs, including in-service education (ANA & National Nursing Staff Development Organization [NNSDO], 2010).

In-service educational programs are intended to develop the knowledge, skills, and values of nurses in their current job for a specific employer. Unlike typical CE programs, in-service educational activities are designated as facility-specific or organization-specific offerings and often are not eligible for contact hours (ANCC, 2012). However, if an in-service program provides content that learners can transfer to another work setting, that program may be eligible for contact hours (ANCC, 2012). It is important to clarify the eligibility of specific in-service educational programs with the appropriate CE nurse leaders at your healthcare facility.

As mentioned in Chapter 2, in-service educational activities are brief in practice, usually an hour or less. They often address mandatory topics that apply to a specific healthcare organization (ANA, 2000), such as fire, safety, and infection control; equipment updates; policies and procedures; resources; and documentation changes.

In-service education has been a key component of nursing staff development for several decades (ANA, 2000). However, its value as an appropriate and cost-effective vehicle during work hours was recently questioned by an APN employed in nursing education and research. Haggard (2011) described the complex demands placed upon nurses in the work setting and argued that in-service programs interrupt workflow and may increase the risk of errors. Rather than conducting face-to-face in-service programs, Haggard suggested that NPDSs investigate alternate delivery methods that meet the learning needs of nurses in the work setting.

Preparing Clinical Staff for Unit-Based Education

Although clinical nurses possess expertise as direct care providers, their experience in assessing, planning, directing, and evaluating the educational needs of other staff may be limited. Most RNs received formal instruction and experience with the teaching-learning process in their initial RN preparation; however, this educational content often focused on patients and the community as its learners. Therefore, it is likely that clinical nurses will need guidance to effectively assume a unit-based educator role. As with any new endeavor, it is important that clinical nurses are mentored by experienced educators such as NPDSs, APNs, and faculty at affiliated schools of nursing.

The unit-based educator role may vary among healthcare organizations. In some settings, a designated nurse or a group of nurses on a clinical unit may assume responsibility for staff education. Some organizations may rotate responsibility for staff education among several nurses on a clinical unit. Regardless of the approach, it is important to understand the responsibilities of a unit-based educator. These may include determining the learning needs of staff, coordinating and developing an education plan for the unit, implementing this plan, and evaluating its effectiveness. Figure 6-1 provides key steps that may be included in developing a unit-based education plan.

Having staff provide input and participate in an education plan can foster a sense of ownership in the plan and maximize its success. It may be advantageous to begin this process with an experienced staff nurse who can serve as a positive role model.

Determine the best times and locations for these unit-based efforts with staff on your unit. Decide if it is best to schedule a program in the early morning, at lunch, or at a shift change. If the unit has 12-hour shifts, then determine the best time to accommodate evening staff. Consider the number of times you will need to run the program to ensure that all staff have an opportunity to attend. Decide where the programs will be conducted, such as the unit's conference room or somewhere outside the unit. Also, plan to actively engage learners in the topic rather than presenting a traditional face-to-face lecture session. For example, if learning how to safely operate a new piece of IV equipment is the objective for an in-service activity, provide learners with the opportunity to gain hands-on experience manipulating the equipment using real IV supplies. Many of these details need to be discussed and finalized before an educational plan is implemented.

It is essential to provide a support system for staff if they are expected to serve as presenters of unit-based education programs. Some nurses may be experienced in preparing and present-

---

Figure 6-1. Key Steps for Developing a Unit-Based Educational Plan

- Assess the learning needs of staff.
  - Define the learners.
  - Conduct a needs assessment.
- Analyze the needs assessment data.
- Develop a master education plan for the unit.
  - Seek available resources.
  - Suggest a variety of teaching resources.
  - Anticipate return on investment.
- Implement the education plan.
  - Gain support from staff and administration.
  - Encourage staff input and participation.
  - Develop a support system for presenters.
  - Monitor program implementation and effectiveness.
- Evaluate the overall unit-based education plan.

---

ing educational programs, but this endeavor may be a new and uncomfortable one for others. Some staff may be at ease giving presentations at regional or national conferences but may fear sharing their expertise with peers at work. Therefore, it is important to determine the individual needs of each staff member and develop ways to create a nonthreatening environment on the unit. Remind staff to view this experience as part of the learning process related to professional development. Emphasize the added marketability of having effective presentation skills. Their comfort level will likely increase with repeated practice.

Before they begin presenting, advise staff to start with a comfortable teaching strategy. For example, rather than conducting an oral presentation, presenting a poster or demonstrating a clinical skill may make a staff nurse feel more at ease when conducting an in-service offering for the first time. Others may find presenting as part of a small group preferable to solo presentations at first. Suggest that staff present on topics with which they possess clinical expertise. If possible, try capturing these sessions on video. This approach not only provides staff with an opportunity to review their own presentation skills, but it also is a convenient way to give those unable to attend the program a chance to benefit from it at a later date. Be sure to provide guidance and constructive feedback for staff during this entire process.

A Model to Help Nurses Learn Basic Presentation Skills

In 1996, Jane Bryce and I developed a model that was effective in helping staff nurses learn how to develop and present in-service educational activities at the University of Pittsburgh Medical Center, a large, university-affiliated medical center. Although this model was reported two decades ago, the foundation of our approach still remains appropriate for helping nurses gain basic presentation skills (Lockhart & Bryce, 1996). This model included a 30-minute instructional session called *How to Develop a Unit-Based In-Service Offering* (UBIO). The primary purpose of the UBIO was to help staff nurses learn how to plan, implement, and evaluate an in-service program on their clinical unit. Content focused on the entire educational process, from assessing learning needs to evaluating learning outcomes. UBIO will provide the foundation for the remaining portion of this chapter.

In our project, unit-based clinical nurses completed the UBIO several months prior to the implementation of the unit's education plan (Lockhart & Bryce, 1996). This timing gave staff nurses an opportunity to use the information they learned in the UBIO when developing their own in-service educational program. It also minimized any anxiety they felt about presenting to their peers. In addition to providing nurses with this instructional session, we mentored them on an individual basis to develop their in-service educational programs. The UBIO was repeated at various times on several clinical units.

Handouts describing the key points of UBIO were instrumental to the model's success and learning outcomes (Lockhart & Bryce, 1996). Providing information in print form enabled the learners to focus on the content of the UBIO session. Learners could spend more time listening and interacting with other nurses who attended the session rather than concentrating on note-taking. These printed handouts enabled us to include a large amount of material within the 30 minutes allotted for the UBIO. We also could spend more time answering questions or discussing staff concerns (Lockhart & Bryce, 1996).

Because the majority of nurses who attended the session were scheduled to present their in-service educational programs at a later date, these handouts served as a useful resource. Staff could refer to the handouts when preparing their in-service offering or when they needed a refresher on specific details.

In addition to an outline that detailed the content of the instructional session, nurses who attended UBIO received the following materials: a tool called the 10-Step Checklist for Conducting a Unit-Based In-Service Offering (see Figure 6-2); a teaching plan for UBIO; a blank teaching plan that they could use when preparing their own session (see Figure 6-3); a list of action verbs to use when writing instructional objectives for their in-service program; and a learning activity, Choosing the Correct Educational Objective, which the group completed together during the UBIO.

10-Step Checklist for Conducting a Unit-Based In-Service Offering

The 10-Step Checklist for Conducting a Unit-Based In-Service Offering guided the instructional session and served as a worksheet for nurses as they developed their in-service educational offerings (Lockhart & Bryce, 1996). We limited the number of steps to 10 so that nurses would perceive this new endeavor as manageable. Although a few of the steps were complex and required more understanding and preparation time (e.g., Step 3: Clarify mutual goals), others were simple and easy to accomplish in a fairly brief time (e.g., Step 4: Schedule the date, time, place, and speaker).

The unit-based educators began each UBIO by asking participants to explain their understanding of the phrase *in-service educational offerings* (Lockhart & Bryce, 1996). This activity helped participants obtain a perspective of the NPD practice specialty. Participants also were asked to compare in-service educational activities to the other components of nursing staff development (e.g., orientation, CE programs).

Next, participants were asked to brainstorm and recall examples of nursing education programs they had attended at work and in the community over the past year (Lockhart & Bryce, 1996). This strategy enabled the group to compile a list of several educational offerings. Participants were asked to compare these offerings and designate each learning experience as part of their orientation, in-service education, or CE programs.

Participants benefited from this exercise in several ways. First, defining the boundaries of an in-service program helped them understand their charge. Second, it helped them clarify their roles as presenters and unit-based educators. Finally, it enabled them

---

Figure 6-2. The 10-Step Checklist for Conducting a Unit-Based In-Service Offering

1. Assess learning needs.

2. Select your topic.

3. Clarify mutual goals.

4. Schedule the following:
   Date:
   Time:
   Place:
   Speaker(s) if needed:

5. Advertise the program.

6. Develop a teaching plan.
   Develop objectives.
   Outline content and allot time.
   Choose teaching-learning strategies.
   Design audiovisuals and handouts.
   Develop evaluation process.

7. Conduct the in-service educational offering.
   Obtain audiovisuals and equipment.
   Ask participants to sign attendance sheet.
   Introduce yourself and participants.
   Share objectives.
   Present program using lesson plan as a guide.
   Allow time for questions and participation.

8. Evaluate the in-service offering.
   Participants:
   Program:
   Speaker(s):

9. Provide feedback to participants and speaker(s).

10. Revise in-service program for future presentations.

Note. From "A Comprehensive Plan to Meet the Unit-Based Education Needs of Nurses From Several Specialty Units," by J.S. Lockhart and J. Bryce, 1996, *Journal of Nursing Staff Development, 12,* p. 136. Copyright 1996 by Lippincott-Raven Publishers. Reprinted with permission.

---

to perceive the multiple dimensions of nursing staff development within the context of NPD.

Prior to this exercise, many nurses claimed that they had not previously understood what in-service educational offerings were, and only a few participants were familiar with the components of nursing staff development and how in-service offerings and these components were related. The nurses expressed feeling less anxious after learning the brief nature and core components of an in-service educational offering.

The 10 steps included in the checklist guided the content and sequence of the remaining portion of the UBIO (Lockhart & Bryce, 1996). To illustrate these 10 steps, we asked participants to identify a priority learning need (topic) on their unit. For example, nurses who worked on a head and neck oncology unit suggested "How to conduct a neurological assessment" as an example to use during the session (Lockhart & Bryce, 1996). Nursing staff from

Figure 6-3. Sample Teaching Plan Form

Program Title:_____

Presenter:_____

Location, Date, Time:_____

Objectives	Content (Time Allotted)	Teaching Strategies	Resources (Audiovisuals and Handouts)	Evaluation
1.				
2.				
3.				

other clinical units selected topics that were of interest to them, such as "Caring for central lines," "How to apply electrocardiogram leads properly," and "Maintaining chest tubes."

When discussing the model for NPD, include additional throughputs in addition to in-service education, orientation, and CE programs.

Step 1: Assess Learning Needs

The first step in the 10-Step Checklist for Conducting a Unit-Based In-Service Offering involves assessing the learning needs of staff on the clinical unit (see Chapter 13). In our 1996 project, we had already identified the learning needs of clinical staff, analyzed the data, and prioritized the needs. However, it was still important to remind staff to consider the assessment of learning needs before developing an in-service educational offering (Lockhart & Bryce, 1996).

When clarifying who the learners are, discover if they are limited to licensed nursing staff (e.g., RNs, licensed practical nurses [LPNs], licensed vocational nurses [LVNs]) or if they include assistive personnel (AP) and unit secretaries. Investigate if other healthcare professionals, such as social workers, nutritionists, or physical therapists, are considered among your learners (see Chapter 1).

Creative strategies have been developed to assess the learning needs of nurses in specialty care units. For example, Brixey and Mahon (2010) designed a self-assessment tool to help oncology nurses identify their learning needs and maintain their ongoing competence. The principles of adult learning (Knowles, 1990) and Benner's (1984) *From Novice to Expert: Excellence and Power in Clinical Nursing* provided the framework for the tool's development. After reviewing relevant oncology literature and standards of care and obtaining input from a team of interprofessional oncology experts, Brixey and Mahon (2010) organized the tool into 14 categories (e.g., chemotherapy, biotherapy, radiation therapy) with 139 items (e.g., patient teaching, community resources for support, follow protocols). Respondents were asked to rate their self-determined extent of experience for each oncology item using a four-point Likert-type scale from 1 (no experience) to 4 (highly experienced). This tool was recommended for use by professional development specialists in designing educational interventions, by managers in gauging ongoing staff performance, and by individual nurses in guiding their professional self-development.

Using a different approach in assessing the learning needs of nurses related to cancer care, Cannon, Watson, Roth, and LaVergne (2015) used an online survey approach through the Nurse Oncology Education Program (NOEP), a nonprofit state-level professional organization affiliated with the Texas Nurses Foundation. To provide current educational programs related to the prevention, detection, treatment, and survivorship of cancer for all nurses in Texas, NOEP surveyed 1,028 nurses (5% response rate) biannually across the United States (Cannon et al., 2015). The results concluded that 42% of nurses were employed in a hospital setting, 39% were working in an oncology setting, and 32% "provided direct care for patients currently undergoing cancer treatment or for patients who are cancer survivors" (Cannon et al., 2015, p. 578). Top learning needs identified by the study included management of cancer symptoms and treatment side effects; complementary, alternative, and integrative medicine; and recommendations for cancer screening (Cannon et al., 2015). Survey results are used by NOEP in offering targeted cancer-related CE programs for nurses regardless of practice specialty.

When designing self-assessment tools to capture the learning needs of nurses, it is essential to review the current curriculum and standards of practice related to your clinical practice specialty and incorporate them into your assessment tool. For example, an assessment tool for oncology nursing practice could include the *Core Curriculum for Oncology Nurses* (Itano, Brant, Conde, & Saria, 2016), *Chemotherapy and Biotherapy Guidelines and Recommendations for Practice* (Polovich, Olsen, & LeFebvre, 2014), and the oncology certified nurse (OCN®) test blueprint from the Oncology Nursing Certification Corporation (2014).

In addition to these resources, be alert for other current standards of practice, such as the "2013 Updated American Society of Clinical Oncology/Oncology Nursing Society Chemotherapy Administration Safety Standards Including Standards for the Safe Administration and Management of Oral Chemotherapy" (Neuss et al., 2013). As discussed in Chapter 1, you should familiarize yourself with the nursing care standards required by specialty accreditation bodies such as the American College of Surgeons Commission on Cancer (ACS CoC) and its publication *Cancer Program Standards 2012: Ensuring Patient-Centered Care* (ACS CoC, 2012). This voluntary program focuses on "improving survival and quality of life for cancer patients through standard-setting, prevention, research, education, and the monitoring of comprehensive quality care" (ACS CoC, 2012, p. 11). The standard that addresses nursing care indicates that care is "provided by nurses with specialized knowledge and skills" (ACS CoC, 2012, p. 27). The standard also specifies the documentation required to support the standard and compliance measures. Regardless of your specialty, these national standards need to be addressed by NPDSs in an education plan.

Step 2: Select Your Topic

For the second step of the checklist, select a topic from a list of learning needs identified in your unit's education plan. Some of these topics might be familiar to staff nurses, but others may pose new challenges. In our project, each nurse volunteered to present on a topic that was included in the unit's education plan. Mandatory education and competency verification programs also were scheduled (Lockhart & Bryce, 1996).

When planning a staff's unit-based educational needs, become familiar with the education programs that are mandated by your hospital's regulatory and accreditation agencies, such as the Joint Commission and the Occupational Safety and Health Administration. For example, according to *Joint Commission International Accreditation Standards for Hospitals*, staff should be able to demonstrate ongoing competence on critical skills such as cardiopulmonary resuscitation (CPR); emergency, fire, safety, and security policies and procedures; proper disposal of hazardous materials and wastes; and infection control policies (Joint Commission International, 2013). These topics should be included in each unit's education plan.

Step 3: Clarify Mutual (Learning) Goals

The third step of the checklist requires each presenter to validate that the learning needs identified by unit staff and that the participants' understanding of these needs are congruent with each other.

In our project, a learning need identified by staff was "How to change a laryngectomy tube" (Lockhart & Bryce, 1996). The nurse who was responsible to develop this topic as an in-service educational program discussed this learning need and clarified specific expectations with unit staff prior to developing a lesson plan. The nurse also determined the staff's current knowledge and skills on the topic. This included what the staff already knew about a total laryngectomy, the anatomic changes that result after this surgery, and the components of a laryngectomy tube. The nurse used this information to tailor the content of the in-service educational program to the learning needs of staff.

Because in-service educational sessions usually last a short time, knowing this information in advance is helpful. For instance, if staff had little prior knowledge on this topic, the nurse could have developed two separate in-service educational offerings. The nurse also could have designed a poster that reviewed the parts of a laryngectomy tube prior to the scheduled in-service.

It is common for educators to become confused with the terms often used in providing education activities: learning goals, learning outcomes, objectives, and competencies (Suskie, 2009). In Step 3 of the UBOI, the nurse educator clarified the intended goal of the in-service educational session regarding changing a patient's laryngectomy tube. *Learning goals* refer to what the educator intends to achieve by offering the session (Suskie, 2009). Similarly, *learning outcomes* are goals that convey the "destination rather than the path taken to get there—the end rather than the means, the outcome rather than the process" (Suskie, 2009, pp. 117–118). Both learning goals and outcomes convey the knowledge, skills, or attitudes that the learners will gain after participating in the educational program (Suskie, 2009).

Oermann and Gaberson (2014) identified several additional terms referring to the results that learners need to obtain in an education program: outcomes, objectives, competencies, and learning targets.

Step 4: Schedule the Date, Time, Place, and Speaker(s)

An in-service educational program should be scheduled well in advance so that all staff on the unit have an opportunity to attend it. Ask your nurse manager or NPDS to share successful strategies that have increased staff attendance at in-service programs on your clinical unit in the past. Clarify the best time to schedule the in-service offering and any alternative sessions to accommodate staff on all shifts. Remind staff that they can bring lunch or dinner, especially if you are presenting the in-service as a brown-bag session.

Reserve a room for the program. If you are not familiar with the location, visit the room before the scheduled date of the in-service offering to check its design, seating capacity, audio-visual accommodations, and lighting. It is much easier to plan and adapt your program around a physical environment if you have this information in advance. Regardless of your preference for the time and location of your in-service offering, check with your unit manager for these details. Also make sure that the room is free of clutter with seating, equipment, and resources appropriately arranged based on the program's purpose.

If you need a clinical laboratory setting or simulation equipment, check the feasibility of using a clinical skills laboratory at your worksite or at a local school of nursing. This setting is ideal for practicing psychomotor skills, such as CPR, or for videotaping participants' performances during a mock emergency code. If this option is not available, consider conducting the in-service educational session in an unoccupied patient room.

Maximize available resources by collaborating with staff from other clinical units within your organization. If physical space is limited, try sharing conference rooms and displays for in-service presentations that are of interest to other units. For example, in my work with Bryce (1996), we displayed a drug update bulletin board that was used by two separate patient care units on a rotating basis.

If you are inviting a guest speaker to present the in-service educational program, such as faculty from an affiliated school of nursing or a vendor, confirm the correct date and time of the presentation with the speaker. Check with your nurse manager to determine if a procedure exists for allowing guests from outside organizations into your institution, especially commercial vendors. These individuals may need organizational clearance before they visit a clinical unit. Various individuals from your agency, such as staff nurses, clinical nurse specialists, clinical instructors, and other members of the interdisciplinary healthcare team, can be targeted as potential presenters.

If nursing students use your unit for their clinical practicum, remember to include both faculty and students as potential speakers. Students often need to conduct an educational session as a course requirement. Nursing faculty can help update staff on topics pertaining to teaching, researching, or publishing.

Investigate educational services available from representatives of pharmaceutical and supply companies. Many purchasing agreements include these services and provide printed materials and samples free of charge. Consider contacting your vendors for teaching materials and supplies for these programs.

Reserve any equipment (e.g., LCD projector, screen, flip chart, markers, erasers, a laptop or notebook) that you may need for your program well in advance. Clarify the procedure and timelines that need to be followed to duplicate program handouts. Identify resources that exist within the workplace to meet these needs. Although some organizations allocate money in a clinical unit's budget for staff education purposes, these funds may be limited or restricted to CE programs.

Given the controversy presented earlier in this chapter questioning the value and effectiveness of delivering face-to-face in-service educational programs for nurses who work in intense clinical settings (Haggard, 2011), be sure to explore this issue with leaders and colleagues at your own clinical setting. Discuss this concern with the manager of your unit and gain input from staff regarding their expectations and preferences. Consider introducing a variety of delivery methods, especially those using technology, to address nurses' learning needs and work schedules rather than relying on traditional face-to-face sessions.

Step 5: Advertise the Program

After you have completed the first four steps of the checklist, you can begin to market your program to staff. Consider a communication method that is effective at your institution. This may involve posting a printed flyer on the unit or advertising the program through emails, staff mailboxes, meetings, the hospital's intranet, or a closed-circuit television. Submit information about the program to your organization's newsletter, if appropriate.

When creating a flyer, be creative in preparing an attention-getting, colorful presentation with eye-catching graphics. Include the title of the program; the speaker's name and credentials; the date, time, and location of the program; and the program's objectives on the flyer. Remind staff about the program frequently before it begins.

Explore how other programs achieve good attendance and how these programs are communicated to targeted learners at your organization. Inquire how you can gain access to your organization's secure intranet or an email list to invite participants, share documents, and conduct any preassessments or postassessments. Gain support from nurse managers who can set aside protected time for staff to attend.

Step 6: Develop a Teaching Plan

The sixth step of the checklist focuses on developing a teaching plan that serves as the presenter's blueprint, map, or worksheet of the in-service educational program. The plan can also help presenters be fairly consistent when repeating multiple sessions on the same topic.

Step 6 comprised a major portion of the UBIO session that Bryce and I implemented. Because most participants in our project were not familiar with teaching plans, we made an analogy between the teaching plan and a familiar nursing care plan (Lockhart & Bryce, 1996). A sample of a teaching plan was distributed along with a teaching plan template that participants could duplicate for their future presentations (see Figure 6-3). Participants were advised to limit their plan to one or two pages and to use it to guide them during their presentation.

Because this organization had a clinical advancement program, participants planned on including their teaching plans in their professional portfolios (see Chapter 10). Participants commented that these written plans accurately reflected the content, organization, and depth of their unit-based in-service programs (Lockhart & Bryce, 1996).

The teaching plan portion of the UBIO session focused on five topics: developing instructional objectives, outlining specific content, choosing appropriate teaching-learning strategies, designing audiovisuals and handouts, and developing an evaluation process or plan (Lockhart & Bryce, 1996). These topics headed each column in the sample teaching plan that was distributed to participants.

Many different formats for teaching plans or lesson plans exist. Although experienced nurses may present brief in-service educational programs without explicitly drafting a written teaching plan, novice presenters can benefit from carefully considering the plan's key elements. Carefully thought-out learning outcomes and objectives will guide the content, teaching methods, learning strategies, and assessment methods of the plan (McDonald, 2013).

Create Learning Objectives

Learning to construct realistic learner-centered instructional objectives is an important step in designing a teaching plan for a unit-based in-service educational program (Lockhart

& Bryce, 1996). Most nurses already have experience in writing patient-centered objectives. Building upon similarities that exist between patients and peers can help participants develop objectives.

Objectives serve several purposes that benefit both presenters and learners. For example, objectives help presenters focus on the specific learning outcomes they expect of participants (McDonald, 2013). This benefit is especially helpful for presenters who have a tendency to include more content than can logically be reviewed within the time allotted for an in-service program. Focusing on the purpose of the session using one or two objectives keeps presenters and succinct and prevents them from covering too much on a topic.

Because instructional objectives denote the learning outcomes of an education program, they help learners understand what the presenter will expect of them after the program concludes (McDonald, 2013). With this purpose in mind, remember to share the session's objectives with learners before it begins.

Objectives guide presenters in designing the education program's content, selecting appropriate teaching-learning strategies, and choosing assessment methods that enable learners to attain intended outcomes (McDonald, 2013). Clearly stated objectives help presenters determine if learners were able to demonstrate expected outcomes. Because objectives are instrumental in evaluating the performance of learners, they need to be clearly written, learner-oriented, and measurable. They also must begin with an action verb and focus on higher-order cognitive skills and abilities (Suskie, 2009). It is important to develop objectives and outcomes appropriate to the experiences of the learners. Some educators use the terms *competencies* or *proficiencies* when referring to learning outcomes or objectives (Suskie, 2009).

Standards used to develop education objectives in nursing have evolved over recent years from specific to general, allowing educators to modify their teaching strategies and assessment methods (McDonald, 2013; Oermann & Gaberson, 2014). The following sections will review the processes used in developing objectives in nursing.

Traditional objectives are quite specific and include four key elements: a description of the learner, a description of the behavior the learner needs to exhibit to demonstrate a new competence, a description of conditions under which the learner will demonstrate this competence, and a statement regarding the standard of performance or criterion expected to indicate excellence (Mager, 1984; McMillan, 2001).

An example of these objectives in action could be the following: After the in-service program on laryngectomy care (condition), the staff nurse (learner) will follow hospital policy and procedures (criterion) when changing a laryngectomy tube on a five-day postoperative total laryngectomy patient (behavior).

When developing specific objectives, first focus on the learners of your in-service educational session. Determine their knowledge, skills, and attitudes on the topic. Keep these factors in mind when developing realistic learner outcomes.

Defining who the learners are for an education program is often an easy task for presenters. However, objectives may vary based on the knowledge and skill level of the learners. For example, you may need to develop different objectives for an in-service educational program when presenting it to novice nurses compared to the objectives you would create for more experienced nurses.

Adapt your objectives appropriately when teaching a group of learners with diverse knowledge and skill levels, such as a group consisting of RNs, LPNs, LVNs, AP, and vocational nurses. In the sample objective on laryngectomy care, the learners are RNs new to a head and neck oncology unit.

The second step in developing objectives focuses on what learners can perform as a result of attending the education program (Mager, 1984). In your program, state exactly what you expect learners to do at its completion. Use action verbs to describe this performance, such as those used in developing patient-centered objectives. Examples of action-oriented verbs can be retrieved from the websites of university teaching centers, such as Indiana University–Purdue University Indianapolis (IUPUI) (http://ctl.iupui.edu/OnlineTeachingCourse-Organization--Planning/Learning-Outcomes-Goals-and-Objectives/Objectives). This website lists verbs that can be used in developing objectives and provides a helpful categorization of domain and level. It also offers model questions and instructional strategies that align with domain and level. Another helpful IUPUI website features a learning activity in which learners must match verbs with appropriate domain levels (http://ctl.iupui.edu/OnlineTeaching/Course-Organization--Planning/Learning-Outcomes-Goals-and-Objectives/Blooms-Taxonomy-Activity). The third step in developing objectives requires you, the presenter, to describe the conditions or circumstances that you will impose upon learners as they perform outcomes (Mager, 1984). In the objective example, learners were asked to demonstrate the behavior (changing a laryngectomy tube) after they had attended the in-service educational program on laryngectomy care. They were also asked to change the laryngectomy tube on an actual patient who had undergone a total laryngectomy five days prior. As an alternative, the learners could have been asked to change the tube on a mannequin in a clinical skills laboratory.

The final step in developing objectives requires you to determine how the learners must perform the outcome (Mager, 1984). This step requires you to think about how you will assess the outcome or the learner's performance based on each objective of the in-service educational session. In the objective example, nurses were expected to change the laryngectomy tube according to the procedure approved by the healthcare organization. This procedure lists critical behaviors that nurses need to demonstrate when changing the tube.

As mentioned in Chapter 4, this psychomotor skill (changing a laryngectomy tube) may be one of your unit's ongoing competency requirements. New nurses could be asked to demonstrate changing a laryngectomy tube during their orientation, whereas experienced nurses could perform this skill during the unit's annual competency review.

General Objectives

Evaluation experts advise nurse educators to use general instructional objectives rather than traditional, specific ones (McDonald, 2013; Oermann & Gaberson, 2014). General objectives are beneficial because they are less restrictive and allow educators more freedom in selecting their teaching activities and assessment methods for learners (Oermann & Gaberson, 2014). In fact, McDonald (2013) referred to general objectives as being content-free, as they omit procedure descriptions and instructional strategies.

According to Oermann and Gaberson (2014), quality objectives have four basic elements: they denote expected learner outcomes, are measurable, are broad enough for use within courses with multiple content areas, and exclude teaching strategies. Given this information, the previous specific objective on laryngectomy care reworded as a general objective might look like this: The staff nurse (learner) will demonstrate (behavior) safe performance of laryngectomy procedures (content).

Domains and Levels of Objectives

Similar to objectives that are used in clinical practice, those developed for educational programs are categorized into three domains of learning according to the type of behavior they reflect: cognitive, psychomotor, or affective (Oermann & Gaberson, 2014). Each domain is further divided into levels that increase in complexity. This classic framework, called Bloom's taxonomy (Bloom, Englehart, Furst, Hill, & Krathwohl, 1956), was updated in 2000 by Anderson and Krathwohl. The updates included labeling the levels using verbs and reversing the names of the two highest cognitive levels (Anderson & Krathwohl, 2000). A pictorial comparison of these two taxonomy versions can be found at http://ww2.odu.edu/educ/roverbau/Bloom/blooms_taxonomy.htm.

An objective written in the cognitive domain focuses on outcomes that deal with the learner's knowledge or intellectual outcomes (Oermann & Gaberson, 2014). For example, in the specific objective that was presented earlier, you could have asked a staff nurse to verbally explain the procedure for changing a laryngectomy tube or to describe this procedure in writing.

Psychomotor objectives relate to learners' motor skills and competencies using equipment or technology (Oermann & Gaberson, 2014). In the objective example, nurses were asked to demonstrate their psychomotor skills by changing a laryngectomy tube. The educator would be able to observe their coordination in performing this motor skill and to assess or validate this skill.

Objectives written in the affective domain focus on the learner's values, attitudes, or beliefs as a professional nurse (Oermann & Gaberson, 2014). The objective could have focused on the attitude or reaction that nurses experienced when changing the laryngectomy tube in the example, as nurses may be uncomfortable the first time they view a laryngectomy stoma.

Regardless of the objective's domain, it is important that you match the domain of each objective with the intended purpose of the in-service educational program. You also need to use teaching-learning strategies that are appropriate for the objective's domain. For example, the sample objective on laryngectomy care is in the psychomotor domain because the learner is asked to demonstrate manual skills. Teaching strategies during the in-service program could include practice in changing a tube on a mannequin. Matching teaching-learning strategies with the domain of objectives will be discussed later in this chapter.

Objectives also can vary based on their level of complexity within each of the three domains (Oermann & Gaberson, 2014). A section of the IUPUI website previously mentioned (http://ctl.iupui.edu/OnlineTeaching/Course-Organization--Planning/Learning-Outcomes-Goals-and-Objectives/Blooms-Taxonomy) illustrates the various levels that exist within the cognitive domain. Consider including objectives written at an appropriate level of difficulty for learners who participate in your program. For example, when developing objectives in the cognitive domain, ask learners to apply or relate the concepts they learned using a case study rather than merely having them verbally recite what you presented.

When developing a UBIO, choose the teaching-learning strategies that you use in your in-service program based on the characteristics of your objectives (Oermann & Gaberson, 2014). When asking learners to perform a complex behavior, you will use teaching strategies that appropriately match. For example, if your goal is to have learners evaluate the effectiveness of interventions used to relieve postoperative pain in a patient, your teaching strategy may include the use of a case study and group discussion.

In our project, Bryce and I used a learning activity in the UBIO to help participants learn more about developing objectives. In this exercise, we asked nurses who were given a pair of objectives to select the correctly written one (Lockhart & Bryce, 1996). Consider using this approach with a group of learners to help them develop their objectives. Ask them to test their knowledge by identifying the domain in which an objective belongs. Active learning exercises such as this one can help nurses increase their understanding and develop their confidence in developing and refining objectives.

Outline Program Content and Allot Time

After identifying the key objectives for your in-service educational program, outline the content that will help learners meet objectives and attain outcomes. Contact the librarian at your organization or nearby school of nursing to help you locate resources for developing the content of your program or for conducting a literature search. Think about organizing a session with the librarian or visits to the library so that other nursing staff can learn these skills.

Your content outline should be brief, consistent, and directly related to the objectives and learning outcomes that you have identified. Organize your outline using a format that is familiar, such as a standard outline or a list of bulleted items. Once you have drafted the content, estimate how much time you will dedicate to each of the major sections. Because keeping on schedule is vital during a unit-based in-service program, estimating small segments of time will help you determine a realistic amount of content. Avoid overwhelming learners with vast amounts of information within a short period of time.

Allow sufficient time during the in-service program for introductions, questions, discussion, and demonstrations or return demonstrations of skills. As mentioned earlier, keep your in-service program within the prescribed allotted time to accommodate work schedules.

Choose Teaching-Learning Strategies

After you have developed the objectives and content for your in-service educational program, choose teaching strategies that will best communicate this information to your learners. View teaching strategies as methods to help learners understand the content of the program and attain objectives and expected outcomes. When choosing a teaching strategy for your educational program, consider factors such as the program's objectives, intended outcomes, content, characteristics of learners, your own preferences as a presenter, and available resources.

When planning your in-service educational program, include evidence-based teaching strategies that actively engage participants in learning and strengthen their ability to think critically in clinical practice (Clark, 2007). Evidence-based teaching (see Chapter 12) involves reading published research studies that investigate a specific educational topic, reviewing the results in concert with the opinions of experts and other sources of evidence, evaluating these sources of evidence, and determining their applicability to your own practice situation (Oermann, 2013). Be sure to consider cost, safety, fidelity, and completeness when choosing a strategy for your program (Clark, 2007).

NPDSs are expected to incorporate technology in their practice (ANA & NNSDO, 2010). In fact, recent advances in educational technology (e.g., Internet-based resources, patient portals, mobile applications, social media) have greatly expanded the pool of teaching strategies for NPDSs (see Chapter 1) (Conn, 2013).

Despite these advances, the results of a survey of 1,304 Association for Nursing Professional Development (ANPD) members revealed that they did not use technology (e.g., learning management systems, podcasts, webcasts, telecommunication, simulation) to its greatest potential (Harper et al., 2014). Although NPDSs expressed an interest in these technologies, barriers included lack of knowledge, time, exposure, resources, and comfort. The authors advised NPDSs to assume personal responsibility for developing their competence in technology (Harper et al., 2014).

Similar findings from an earlier Springer Publishing Company (2011) survey revealed that the majority of the 1,106 nurses who responded owned a smartphone (74.9%), downloaded applications related to nursing or medicine (54.6%), did not own an e-book reader (58.5%), and had not yet bought nursing or medical e-books. NPDSs need to be alert for current technology assessments and use these data to advance the use of learning technologies by learners within their healthcare organizations.

Thompson (2015a) urged nurses, especially those assuming APN roles, to incorporate technology, such as mobile applications, in their daily clinical practice to support the need for making fast, evidence-based decisions. According to Thompson (2015a), the "ability to search, retrieve, interpret, and use information effectively" (p. 115) is a core competency for nurses when using health-related resources. It also reminds them to carefully evaluate their reliability and practice application prior to adoption in practice (Thompson, 2013, 2015a). Thompson (2015a, 2015b) also offered lists of evidence-based applications grouped by category, cost, and platforms for use by APNs with smartphones and tablet devices.

Choosing teaching strategies that align with the objectives and content of your in-service educational offering should be a priority (Clark & Kwinn, 2007; Hagler & Morris, 2013). For example, suppose you are planning an in-service educational program on how to provide safe, quality nursing care for patients with a central IV line. One of your objectives for this session is "Following the in-service session, the learner will change a central line dressing on a patient according to hospital procedure."

Because this objective reflects behaviors from the psychomotor domain (changing a dressing), you dedicate a portion of your program to learners practicing this skill on a mannequin. Table 6-1 illustrates a basic example of teaching strategies matched according to objectives stated in the cognitive, psychomotor, and affective domains. Additional examples of aligning learning objectives, student assessments, and teaching strategies are provided at the Carnegie Mellon University website (www.cmu.edu/teaching/assessment/basics/alignment .html).

If you used an objective from a cognitive domain for the same in-service session, it might look like this: "Following the in-service educational session, the learner will correctly state the steps used in applying a central line dressing based on hospital procedure."

In this case, you may choose discussion as a teaching strategy, allowing time for learners to verbally state the steps they would follow in applying a central line dressing rather than actually having them perform the procedure. You could also ask learners to complete brief pretests and post-tests focused on these steps.

If your goal is to explore and possibly change the attitudes of nurses toward caring for patients from diverse cultural backgrounds, your teaching method might include the use of experiential approaches, such as role-play or game strategies. These options provide learners opportunities to experience a situation firsthand within a traditional teaching-learning setting.

Another thing to consider when choosing a teaching strategy for your education program is the characteristics of the learners (Clark & Kwinn, 2007; Hagler & Morris, 2013). Use these characteristics to help you determine learners' preferred teaching-learning strategies and their degree of competency and experience regarding topics. Consider the number of learners who will attend your program and their educational and clinical experiences. Be ready to adjust your teaching method if the number of participants is larger than what you originally had expected. Consider scheduling multiple sessions of your program if a hands-on learning exercise is involved.

Table 6-1. Sample Teaching Strategies by Objective Domains for In-Service Educational Programs

Objective Domain	Suggested Teaching Strategies
Cognitive	Lecture, group discussion, nursing rounds, self-learning modules, case studies, critical incidents
Psychomotor	Demonstration, return demonstration, simulation, checklists
Affective	Role-play, debate, games, simulations, role modeling

If your group of learners is composed of nurses who vary in clinical expertise, consider presenting two separate sessions—one designed for new graduates at a beginning level and another session targeting experienced nurses. Use the clinical strength of the expert nurses to assist you with educating the novice nurses. This strategy can foster a mentor–mentee relationship among the nursing staff on a clinical unit.

Regardless of the approach you use, it is important that you use controls for various learner characteristics that you are able to modify, if needed. Careful assessment of learners can help you make the necessary changes in your in-service educational session to maximize learning.

Reflect on your own preferences and abilities as a presenter when choosing a teaching strategy for your program (Hagler & Morris, 2013). If you are new to conducting in-service sessions, select a teaching method that matches the program's objectives and learners and one that you feel comfortable using. As you gain more experience in presenting programs, experiment with other teaching strategies. Ask an experienced educator at your workplace to help you master these skills, or attend CE programs on the topic. Be creative when developing teaching strategies for your in-service educational offering. Figure 6-4 illustrates various teaching strategies to meet the learning needs of staff on a clinical unit. It is important to note that some of these strategies engage participants in their learning to a greater extent than others. The University of New Mexico College of Nursing has a webpage (http://nursing.unm.edu/resources/teaching-and-learning-strategies.html) that provides a few examples of teaching strategies designed to promote learners' critical-thinking skills (e.g., analogy, case study, concept map, debate, jigsaw, problem-based learning, role-play, simulation, journal articles). This valuable resource also includes strategy definitions, examples, implementation, advantages, and disadvantages.

Be realistic when selecting teaching strategies that are available in your work setting (Hagler & Morris, 2013). Consider issues such as conference room and laboratory space, available equipment and supplies, cost, and allotted time for in-service sessions.

In the ANPD survey previously discussed, 750 (97.2%) of the total 772 NPD respondents reported that they used learning management systems to deliver mandatory education programs to their staff (Harper et al., 2014). However, some staff educators have shared other cre-

---

Figure 6-4. Possible Teaching Strategies for Unit-Based Educational Programs

- Lecture and group discussion
- Case presentations/grand rounds
- Posters and bulletin boards
- Education fairs
- Role-play, drama
- Reflections
- Concept mapping
- Demonstration/return demonstration
- Clinical unit and clinical simulations
- Self-learning modules, self-paced
- Problem-based learning
- Journal article review (journal club)
- Audiovisuals (videos, slide presentations)
- Written or electronic materials (pamphlets, books)
- Games and simulations
- Computer-assisted instruction, web-based programs, videoconferences
- Social media
- Flipped classroom (classroom time spent problem-solving with studying out-of-class time) (Bergmann & Sams, 2012)

ative, cost-effective strategies that they have used to engage participants in mandatory learning, capture their attention, and make learning fun. While some of these examples may be dated, they continue to offer current NPDSs interesting options in educational technology.

For example, Thurber and Asselin (1999) organized a three-day educational fair with interactive stations, questions, and posters to enable hospital staff to receive information on 25 mandatory organizationwide topics. Their approach was not only cost-effective but was also successful in providing 93% of hospital staff with education, on-site feedback, and testing.

A similar approach was later used by Stokamer and Soccio (2000), who developed a one-week theme-based program to provide mandatory safety training for all hospital personnel. Participants had the opportunity to interact in their learning with hands-on experiences at their own pace.

Finally, Peterson (2002) created a gaming strategy to address mandatory education training in safety, infection, and biohazard-related topics for long-term care staff by modeling a program after the *Wheel of Fortune* television show. This alternative, the Wheel of Disaster program, actively engaged 75 staff members as they learned.

Design Audiovisuals and Other Resources

After you have determined the objectives, content, and teaching strategies for your in-service educational program, consider the audiovisuals and other resources you may need to convey your message and help participants attain learning outcomes. When added to your verbal presentation, visual material (e.g., handouts) can increase both the retention and learning of material by participants. Select your audiovisuals like teaching strategies: based on your objectives and their domains. Become proficient with any equipment that you plan on using during your presentation in advance of your program. Table 6-2 provides examples of audiovisuals that vary in style, preparation, and cost.

Be cost-conscious when supplementing your presentation with printed handouts; try to keep them at a minimum. Consider placing copies of your handouts on the bulletin board of each unit's conference room for staff to duplicate if desired, posting them on the hospital's intranet site, or emailing them to participants.

Develop an Evaluation Process or Plan

After you have confirmed the program's objectives, learning outcomes, content, and teaching strategies, determine how you will assess participants' learning. Basically, formulate a method to determine how effective the in-service educational program was on the participants' ability to attain objectives and meet learning outcomes. As mentioned earlier in this chapter, this task is facilitated with detailed and objectively stated goals.

Select an assessment method that aligns with each objective and its domain (Oermann & Gaberson, 2014). In the example regarding a laryngectomy tube, a possible assessment method would be to observe the learners while they changed a laryngectomy tube on a mannequin, model, or patient.

Evidence regarding the participants' performance can be collected using direct or indirect assessment methods (Suskie, 2009). Direct assessment methods are "tangible, visible, self-explanatory, compelling evidence of exactly what students have or have not learned" (Suskie, 2009, p. 20), while indirect methods are "proxy signs that students are probably learning . . . less clear and less convincing than direct evidence" (Suskie, 2009, p. 20). Based on these two definitions, direct assessment methods are valued as being stronger sources of evidence regarding learning outcomes. However, the use of multiple measures of assessment is recommended (Suskie, 2009). Table 6-3 illustrates a few examples of direct and indirect assessment methods that may be helpful in NPD activities, including in-service educational sessions.

Table 6-2. Sample Audiovisual Resources for In-Service Educational Programs

Category	Examples
Audiotapes and podcasts	Breath sounds, heart sounds, presentations, music files
Writing surfaces	Chalkboard, whiteboard with dry markers, flip chart, presentation board with overhead projector, flash cards
Posters	Diagram of venous access in the arm for IV use
Slide presentations	Main points of presentation, graphics, tables, figures, photographs
Printed or electronic materials	Books, chapters, journal articles, handouts (e.g., case study, chart form), pamphlets, commercially produced literature on drugs and products
Simulation (low to high fidelity)	Low- to high-fidelity mannequins, torso models for cardiopulmonary resuscitation, automated defibrillator device, selected body parts (e.g., eye, ear, larynx, kidney), arms equipped with veins for IV insertion practice, breasts with lumps used for palpation, medical equipment (e.g., nasogastric tubes, suction catheters, sutures)
Movies, television, film clips, video	Videotapes, reenactments of situations, online media (e.g., YouTube), live broadcasts (e.g., conferences, surgeries)
Web-based programs, computer software, learning management systems	Audio or visual reenactments of clinical scenarios focusing on decision making, review of core curriculum, web pages of specialty nursing organizations, databases used to conduct literature searches, social media, blogs, wikis
Live study participants, standardized patients	Volunteer patient or clinical staff upon which to demonstrate clinical procedures, such as physical assessment skills, proper application of electrocardiogram leads, central line dressing changes, and pulse and blood pressure readings

In addition to assessing the learning of participants, obtain feedback from them at the end of the program about the in-service education and your performance as a presenter. Ask learners about their ability to meet the stated objectives of the in-service session. Include responses about your teaching effectiveness and skills as a presenter, quality of the content presented, teaching strategies used, and other items, such as the audiovisual materials used in the session. Ask learners to evaluate the learning environment, such as the space and accommodations. Include an area at the end of the evaluation form for participants to suggest future programs.

Feedback obtained through the evaluation process can strengthen your education plan and promote the professional development of presenters. To obtain additional feedback on your performance, ask a peer, manager, or mentor to observe your presentation. Consider video recording your presentation for future review.

An example of a short evaluation form that can be adapted for any in-service educational session is illustrated in Figure 6-5. Your organization may already have an evaluation form for this purpose. Consider administering the evaluation electronically, if possible, using survey software that can also provide you with quick analysis and a visual display of results.

Suskie (2009) recommended using Kirkpatrick's Four-Level Evaluation Model (Kirkpatrick, 1998; Kirkpatrick & Kirkpatrick, 2006) to better understand the use of direct and indirect

---

Table 6-3. Direct and Indirect Assessment Methods for
Nursing Professional Development

Assessment Method	Examples
Direct	Ratings of physical skills as observed by educator or preceptor
	Responses to questions posed using a classroom response system (clickers)
	Written assignments scored using a rubric
	Role-play
	Feedback from computer-simulated tasks
	Reflections on values, attitudes, and beliefs
	Multiple-choice or essay items on examinations developed using a test blueprint
	Portfolios
	Observation of behaviors
	Scores and pass rates on licensure or certification examinations
	Think-alouds, in which students verbalize their thoughts while working on a problem
Indirect	Assignments without a rubric
	Self-reported satisfaction ratings (after an educational session)
	Self-reports regarding objectives or skills learned after instruction
	Staff retention rates
	Honors, awards, and recognition
	Participation rates in research, publications, and conference presentations
	Perceptions of satisfaction
	Questions on end-of-course evaluation forms

Note. Based on information from Suskie, 2009.

evidence in assessing learning outcomes of education programs. Kirkpatrick's model describes four levels of outcomes, which will be described here in the context of an in-service program. Level 1 (Reaction) captures participants' responses to the program, such as how satisfied they were with the presenter, the content, or the teaching-learning strategies. Level 2 (Learning) reflects what participants learned from attending the in-service program, as assessed by the knowledge or skills that they gained or the attitudes that changed. Level 3 (Behavior/Transfer) captures any changes that occurred in the participants' behavior based on the program. Level 4 (Results) reflects outcomes that result in the clinical practice setting over time as a result of learning (Kirkpatrick, 1998; Kirkpatrick & Kirkpatrick, 2006). According to Suskie (2009), levels 1, 3, and 4 comprise indirect evidence of learning.

Step 7: Conduct the In-Service Educational Offering

Now that you have completed the first six steps of the checklist, you are ready to present your program. Use the 10-Step Checklist for Conducting a Unit-Based In-Service Offering to keep track of the things you need to complete. Arrive earlier than the scheduled start time of the in-service session. This will not only give you time to handle last-minute changes but also will minimize a rushed appearance on your part.

Prior to the start of the program, either obtain audiovisuals and equipment yourself or have them delivered by someone else. Practice with the equipment and make sure that you can operate it with ease. Take time to make the room conducive to learning. For example, if you are using a conference room, be sure that it is clean and presentable and that the temperature and lighting are adjusted as needed.

Figure 6-5. Sample Evaluation Form

HEALTHCARE-UNIVERSITY MEDICAL CENTER HOSPITAL
In-Service Educational Program

Name (Optional): _____

Program: _____ Speaker: _____

Date and time: _____ Location: _____

Title of program: _____

Directions: Please provide us with your feedback regarding this in-service session. Circle the number that best represents your response. Provide comments if desired.

5 = Excellent; 4 = Above Average; 3 = Average; 2 = Below Average; 1 = Poor

1. Your ability to meet the stated objectives (list them here) Comments:	5	4	3	2	1
2. The quality and relevance of the content presented Comments:	5	4	3	2	1
3. The overall effectiveness of the speaker Comments:	5	4	3	2	1
4. The teaching strategies used by the speaker Comments:	5	4	3	2	1
5. Audiovisuals/handouts used in this session Comments:	5	4	3	2	1
6. The teaching-learning environment Comments:	5	4	3	2	1
7. Your overall rating of the in-service offering Comments:	5	4	3	2	1

Please provide suggestions for future programs and speakers:

Ask participants to sign an attendance sheet to verify their presence. Placing this form on a clipboard will prevent it from getting lost during the session. If your institution does not have a standard form, adapt the one presented in Figure 6-6.

Before you start your presentation, take a few minutes to introduce yourself. Share with participants the reasons why you are presenting the session and the benefits it offers to them. If you have not done so earlier, obtain information about the participants, such as their names, assigned unit, and previous experience with the topic. All of these things will create a more relaxed learning environment, placing you and the learners at ease. This is especially important because in-service educational programs usually are scheduled during work time. It often takes participants a while to shift their thinking from the caregiver role in a hurried clinical atmosphere to that of a learner in a classroom setting. Give the participants time to focus on the session.

As mentioned earlier in this chapter, explain the program objectives with the learners. Do this at the start of the session so that learners will understand what will be expected of them.

Present your in-service educational program as you planned. Using your teaching plan as a blueprint for your presentation may be helpful. You may also choose to rely on note cards or other cues to keep you on track. Consider assigning a colleague as a timekeeper to stay on schedule. Although you have carefully planned your program, be attentive to learners' needs and flexible to changes that may occur during the presentation. Observe both verbal and non-verbal cues from your learners.

Figure 6-6. Sample Attendance Record

HEALTHCARE-UNIVERSITY MEDICAL CENTER HOSPITAL
Program Attendance Record

Program: _____

Speaker: _____

Date and time: _____

Location: _____

Name (Print first and last name)	Position	Identification Number	Unit	Shift
1.				
2.				
3.				
4.				
5.				
6.				
7.				
8.				
9.				
10.				
11.				
12.				
13.				
14.				
15.				

Allow time for questions and participation. Inform learners in advance when you will welcome questions from them. You may decide to entertain questions during your session, at the conclusion of the session, or both. Allow for this additional time when planning your session. If you run out of time or encounter an unusual number of questions, consider scheduling an additional session when you can continue this discussion.

Welcome, rather than fear, questions posed by participants. Although you have researched your topic, you are not expected to have all the answers. Rely on other learners who may be able to answer questions, or tell the participants that you will investigate their questions and get back to them. Be sure to thank the participants for their questions.

If your plan included learner participation during the program, such as demonstration and return demonstration of psychomotor skills, then allot time for this activity. Be flexible in case you need to adjust your plan at the last minute.

Step 8: Evaluate the In-Service Educational Offering

Evaluation is an essential component of any educational offering. Use the strategies discussed earlier in this chapter to conduct the assessment of participants' learning. Also, conduct an evaluation of the program's components and speakers.

Step 9: Provide Feedback to Participants and Speaker(s)

Provide both learners and speakers with feedback regarding their performances. For example, you can provide learners with feedback during the program while observing them perform a dressing change or as they verbally discuss the steps involved in changing a sterile dressing. You can conduct evaluations following the program. Use the objectives to evaluate learners' performances and include both formal and informal feedback.

Step 10: Revise the In-Service Program for Future Presentations

While the in-service session is still fresh in your mind, reflect on your teaching plan and determine what went well and what areas need improvement for next time. For example, you may conclude that learning activities took longer than expected or you prepared way too much content for the time allotted.

Use evaluation comments provided by learners as well as your own personal insight. Determine if learners were able to meet objectives. Consider changing your teaching plan when you repeat this presentation, such as sequencing the content in a different order or developing additional handouts to expedite the session. Each time you present your program, you will see ways to make it more effective.

Regardless of the revisions, congratulate yourself on completing a carefully planned in-service educational program!

While evaluating the program, be sure to monitor for changes in quality indicators collected and monitored by the clinical unit, including patient and staff satisfaction surveys, quality assurance outcomes, competency testing of nursing staff, and employee performance appraisals. Although these measures can reflect a variety of changes that have occurred on the clinical unit, they can still be used to understand the influence of in-service educational programs. Regardless of the indices you use, it is important to obtain a complete picture of the process.

Be sure to evaluate the unit's overall education plan at regular intervals before the end of the year. Figure 6-7 offers suggestions that can be used by NPDSs to evaluate the education plan process—from assessing and analyzing staff learning needs to developing and implementing the plan on the clinical unit.

Putting It All Together in a Unit-Based Educational Program

Now that you have reviewed the 10-Step Checklist for Conducting a Unit-Based In-Service Offering (Lockhart & Bryce, 1996), it may be helpful to apply these steps through published accounts of unit-based programs (see Chapter 13). A helpful example is an article published by Fischer-Cartlidge and Mahon (2014) that describes the results of a unit-based study course that was designed to prepare oncology nurses to pass the certified breast care nurse (CBCN®) certification examination offered by the Oncology Nursing Certification Corporation. (Certification and its importance will be described later in Chapter 14 when reviewing career planning.) Table 6-4 compares the authors' description of the project with the steps outlined in the 10-Step Checklist for Conducting a Unit-Based In-Service Offering. Although Fischer-Cartlidge and Mahon's unit-based program could be categorized as a CE program rather than an in-service educational program, their assessment, planning, implementation, and evaluation steps may help NPDSs and unit-based clinical educators plan their own unit-based in-service educational programs.

Figure 6-7. Evaluating the Overall Education Plan: Key Components

Assessing the Learning Needs of Staff
• Were the learning needs of staff captured accurately?
• Were the data representative of all staff?
• Were data collected in an efficient and timely manner?

Analyzing the Data
• Did the data analysis results reflect the overall learning needs of staff?
• How could the data analysis process be expedited?
• How can this process be facilitated in the future?

Developing a Master Education Plan
• Was limiting the plan to a six-month time period manageable?
• Did the staff feel actively involved in the development process?
• Was the plan realistic?
• Was the plan flexible enough to permit the inclusion of new needs or changes?

Implementing the Education Plan
• Were staff prepared adequately to present unit-based programs?
• What teaching strategies did presenters use?
• Was the approach used cost-effective? What was its return on investment?
• What was the response of clinical staff involved?

Evaluating the Process and Outcomes
• Did the staff feel prepared to present unit-based in-service programs?
• How did the staff respond to their new roles as providers of education?
• Could some programs be marketed to the community?
• How much individual assistance did staff need to present programs?

Table 6-4. Example of Applying the 10-Step Checklist for a Unit-Based Educational Program

Step	Implementation in Example
1. Assess learning needs.	Obtained organizational and anecdotal reports from nurses regarding learning needs. Data included the low certification rates of oncology nurses at the cancer center, low motivation to take the exam, and reported barriers regarding taking the certification exam (e.g., test cost, no employer reimbursement, fear of failure, unsure how to prepare for the test, unaware of the certified breast care nurse [CBCN®] certification).
2. Select your topic.	The topic related to the organization's need to increase certification rates among these nurses. In this example, the topic involved breast care as outlined in the Oncology Nursing Certification Corporation's (ONCC's) test blueprint available for the certification exam, the focus of this review and preparation course.
3. Clarify mutual goals.	The goal of the project was to increase nurses' knowledge and confidence and to motivate more nurses to increase their knowledge of breast care and successfully pass the certification exam. Other goals were to educate nurses about the CBCN® exam, raise awareness of possible preparation resources, and provide education aimed at preparing for the examination. The course was first pilot-tested.
4. Schedule the date, time, place, and speaker(s).	Scheduled one-hour didactic sessions offered during the first hour of the workday once a week for 16 weeks. The course was repeated two times each year, and protected time was obtained from the nurse manager. The course was taught on the unit (breast center) and included only those nurses for the first offering; later, the program was expanded. (No details about the setting were located in the article.) The speaker (first author) was a clinical nurse specialist who had previously passed the CBCN® exam, was prepared at the graduate level in nursing education, and possessed expertise in breast care.
5. Advertise the program.	Course was advertised using email, by word-of-mouth via participants, and by nurse managers at meetings and staff performance reviews.
6. Develop a teaching plan. • Develop objectives. • Outline content and time. • Choose teaching-learning strategies. • Design audiovisuals and resources. • Develop evaluation process.	(Specific learning-focused objectives were not located in the article, but can be implied from the CBCN® test blueprint by topic.) The content was based on the topics included in the ONCC test blueprint and references for the CBCN® exam. Topics were presented in a "progressive sequential manner" beginning with risk assessment and ending with survivor care. (The amount of time dedicated to each topic was not located in the article, but content was delivered over 16 weeks, one hour each week.) Teaching-learning strategies, audiovisuals, and handouts included didactic lecture, self-learning modules, and practice questions. Copies of the lecture and practice questions were provided. Nurses were taught how to access web-based oncology guidelines, tables, and charts that supplemented the lecture.

(Continued on next page)

Table 6-4. Example of Applying the 10-Step Checklist for a Unit-Based Educational Program *(Continued)*

Step	Implementation in Example
7. Conduct the in-service educational offering. • Obtain audiovisuals and equipment. • Ask participants to sign attendance sheet. • Introduce yourself and participants. • Share objectives. • Present program using lesson plan as a guide. • Allow time for questions and participation.	(The logistics of the actual implementation of the unit-based course were not located in the article, but we know that the course was implemented and repeated.) Because contact hours via the American Nurses Credentialing Center were provided to nurses who attended each session, they would be required to document their attendance and completion of evaluation forms. The speaker would also be required to provide a formal lesson plan and evaluation (see Chapter 14).
8. Evaluate the in-service offering.	**Participant Evaluation** • Outcomes that were tracked prior to and after the course were related to the project goals: CBCN® certification exam pass rates; anecdotal comments; self-reports of knowledge level and confidence; certification rates in breast medical oncology, surgery, and chemotherapy. **Program Evaluation** • Course scheduling conflicts (e.g., lack of protected time, attendance issues, session scheduled on days off) were resolved by rotating class days. • Lack of incentives (i.e., not paid for course attendance or test-taking) was addressed, with certification being included in clinical advancement program with pay increase if passed, contact hours being awarded for attendance, and some hours being applied toward exam eligibility. • Nurses reported barriers to not taking the exam after completing the course (e.g., cost, already certified, plans to take other exams, life issues, lack of sufficient practice hours to be eligible). • Anecdotal information from author, managers, and staff included increased staff morale on the unit, increased certification rates by experienced nurses, and new relationships among participants. • Reported "little or no budget impact while meeting the needs of the nurse seeking certification" (Fischer-Cartlidge & Mahon, 2014, p. 220). **Speaker Evaluation:** Not indicated in article.
9. Provide feedback to participants and speaker(s).	Feedback provided to participants was not located in the article.
10. Revise in-service program for future presentations.	Over time, the course was expanded institutionwide and included nurses who worked in the institution's satellite locations using web conferencing (both audio and visual) in the classroom. Sessions were recorded for nurses to sustain the program and for those unable to attend a session and/or needed a review. The course was continually updated as the test plan changed or new resources were available. The authors provided a three-year summary of the unit-based project and offered suggestions for expanding the course content in various educational venues, such as orientations.

Note. Based on information from Fischer-Cartlidge & Mahon, 2014; Lockhart & Bryce, 1996.

Summary

Many clinical nurses have taken on unit-based educational responsibilities previously assumed by clinical instructors in centralized NPD departments, such as conducting in-service educational activities. It is helpful for nurses to use a model to assist them in planning, implementing, and evaluating unit-based in-service educational activities. A 10-step checklist can serve as a practical tool that can guide nurses in developing a unit-based program.

Helpful Websites

- Carnegie Mellon University—The Simon Initiative: www.cmu.edu/simon
- Indiana University–Purdue University Indianapolis: The Center for Teaching and Learning—Learning Outcomes, Goals, and Objectives: http://ctl.iupui.edu/OnlineTeaching/Course-Organization--Planning/Learning-Outcomes-Goals-and-Objectives/Definitions
- Old Dominion University—Bloom's Taxonomy: ww2.odu.edu/educ/roverbau/Bloom/blooms_taxonomy.htm
- University of Connecticut—Assessment: http://assessment.uconn.edu/why/index.html
- University of New Mexico College of Nursing—Teaching and Learning Strategies: http://nursing.unm.edu/resources/teaching-and-learning-strategies.html

References

American College of Surgeons Commission on Cancer. (2012). *Cancer program standards 2012: Ensuring patient-centered care* [v.1.2.1, released January 2014]. Retrieved from https://www.facs.org/~/media/files/quality%20programs/cancer/coc/programstandards2012.ashx

American Nurses Association. (2000). *Scope and standards of practice for nursing professional development.* Washington, DC: Author.

American Nurses Association. (2015). *Nursing: Scope and standards of practice* (3rd ed.). Silver Spring, MD: Author.

American Nurses Association & National Nursing Staff Development Organization. (2010). *Nursing professional development: Scope and standards of practice.* Silver Spring, MD: American Nurses Association.

American Nurses Credentialing Center. (n.d.). Forces of Magnetism. Retrieved from http://www.nursecredentialing.org/Magnet/ProgramOverview/HistoryoftheMagnetProgram/ForcesofMagnetism

American Nurses Credentialing Center. (2012). *Educational design process: 2013 mini manual.* Silver Spring, MD: Author.

Anderson, L., & Krathwohl, D.R. (Eds.). (2000). *A taxonomy for learning, teaching, and assessing. A revision of Bloom's taxonomy of educational objectives.* New York, NY: Pearson.

Benner, P. (1984). *From novice to expert: Excellence and power in clinical nursing practice.* Menlo Park, CA: Addison-Wesley.

Bergmann, J., & Sams, A. (2012). *Flip your classroom: Reach every student in every class every day.* Washington, DC: International Society of Technology in Education.

Bloom, B.S., Englehart, M.D., Furst, E.J., Hill, W.H., & Krathwohl, D.R. (1956). *Taxonomy of educational objectives: The classification of educational goals: Handbook I: Cognitive domain.* White Plains, NY: Longman Publishers.

Brixey, M.J., & Mahon, S.M. (2010). A self-assessment tool for oncology nurses: Preliminary implementation and evaluation. *Clinical Journal of Oncology Nursing, 14,* 474–480. doi:10.1188/10.CJON.474-480

Cannon, C.A., Watson, L.K., Roth, M.T., & LaVergne, S. (2015). Assessing the learning needs of oncology nurses. *Clinical Journal of Oncology Nursing, 18,* 577–580. doi:10.1188/14.CJON.577-580

Clark, C.C. (2007). *Classroom skills for nurse educators.* Burlington, MA: Jones & Bartlett Learning.

Clark, R.C., & Kwinn, A. (2007). *The new virtual classroom: Evidence-based guidelines for synchronous e-learning.* San Francisco, CA: Pfeiffer.

Conn, J. (2013, December 14). No longer a novelty, medical apps are increasingly valuable to clinicians and patients. *Modern Healthcare.* Retrieved from http://www.modernhealthcare.com/article/20131214/MAGAZINE/312149983

Fischer-Cartlidge, E., & Mahon, S. (2014). Increasing certification through unit-based education. *Clinical Journal of Oncology Nursing, 18,* 215–220. doi:10.1188/14.CJON.215-220

Haggard, A. (2011). Unit inservice classes—Are they obsolete? *Journal for Nurses in Staff Development, 27,* 301–303. doi:10.1097/NND.0b013e31823864e5

Hagler, D., & Morris, B. (2013). Teaching methods. In M.H. Oermann (Ed.), *Teaching in nursing and role of the educator: The complete guide to best practice in teaching, evaluation, and curriculum development* (pp. 35–59). New York, NY: Springer.

Harper, M.G., Durkin, G., Orthoefer, D.K., Kilcoyne, D., Powers, R., & Tassinari, R.M. (2014). ANPD technology survey: The state of NPD practice. *Journal for Nurses in Professional Development, 30,* 242–247. doi:10.1097/NNP.0000000000000106

Institute of Medicine. (2011). *The future of nursing: Leading change, advancing health.* Washington, DC: National Academies Press.

Itano, J.K., Brant, J.M., Conde, F.A., & Saria, M.G. (Eds.). (2016). *Core curriculum for oncology nursing* (5th ed.). St. Louis, MO: Elsevier.

Joint Commission International. (2013). *Joint Commission International accreditation standards for hospitals* (5th ed.). Retrieved from http://www.jointcommissioninternational.org/assets/3/7/Hospital-5E-Standards-Only-Mar2014.pdf

Kirkpatrick, D.L. (1998). *Evaluating training programs: The four levels* (2nd ed.). San Francisco, CA: Berrett-Koehler.

Kirkpatrick, D.L., & Kirkpatrick, J.D. (2006). *Evaluating training programs: The four levels* (3rd ed.). San Francisco, CA: Berrett-Koehler.

Knowles, M.S. (1990). *The adult learner: A neglected species* (4th ed.). Houston, TX: Gulf Publishing Co.

Lockhart, J.S., & Bryce, J. (1996). A comprehensive plan to meet the unit-based education needs of nurses from several specialty units. *Journal of Nursing Staff Development, 12,* 135–138.

Mager, R.F. (1984). *Preparing instructional objectives: A critical tool in the development of effective instruction.* Atlanta, GA: Center for Effective Performance.

McDonald, M.E. (2013). *The nurse educator's guide to assessing learning outcomes* (3rd ed.). Burlington, MA: Jones & Bartlett Learning.

McMillan, J.H. (2001). *Essential assessment concepts for teachers and administrators.* Thousand Oaks, CA: Corwin Press.

Neuss, M.N., Polovich, M., McNiff, K., Esper, P., Gilmore, T.R., LeFebvre, K.B., … Jacobson, J.O. (2013). 2013 updated American Society of Clinical Oncology/Oncology Nursing Society chemotherapy administration safety standards including standards for the safe administration and management of oral chemotherapy. *Oncology Nursing Forum, 40,* 225–233. doi:10.1188/13.ONF.40-03AP2

Oermann, M.H. (2013). Module 15: Evidence-based teaching in nursing. In M.H. Oermann (Ed.), *Teaching in nursing and role of the educator: The complete guide to best practice in teaching, evaluation, and curriculum development* (pp. 303–316). New York, NY: Springer.

Oermann, M.H., & Gaberson, K.B. (2014). *Evaluation and testing in nursing education* (4th ed.). New York, NY: Springer.

Oncology Nursing Certification Corporation. (2014). OCN® test blueprint. Retrieved from http://www.oncc.org/files/ocn_blueprint.pdf

Peterson, R. (2002). W-H-E-E-L of disaster. *Journal for Nurses in Staff Development, 18,* 210–212. doi:10.1097/00124645-200207000-00009

Polovich, M., Olsen, M., & LeFebvre, K.B. (Eds.). (2014). *Chemotherapy and biotherapy guidelines and recommendations for practice* (4th ed.). Pittsburgh, PA: Oncology Nursing Society.

Springer Publishing Company. (2011). *The Springer Publishing 2011 nursing ebook and smartphone survey.* Retrieved from http://nicolaziady.com/wp-content/uploads/2011/11/Springer-Publishing_2011_Nursing_eBook-Smartphone_Survey.pdf

Stokamer, C.L., & Soccio, D.A. (2000). Reinvigorating mandatory safety training: A case example. *Journal of Continuing Education in Nursing, 31,* 169–173.

Suskie, L. (2009). *Assessing student learning: A common sense guide* (2nd ed.). San Francisco, CA: Jossey-Bass.

Thompson, C.J. (2013). Graduate nursing education in the 21st century: There's an app for that! *Clinical Nurse Specialist, 27,* 332–335. doi:10.1097/NUR.0b013e3182a8bf51

Thompson, C.J. (2015a). Clinical practice in CNS education: There's an app for that! Part 1: Apps for evidence-based practice. *Clinical Nurse Specialist, 29,* 115–118. doi:10.1097/NUR.0000000000000112

Thompson, C.J. (2015b). Clinical practice in CNS education: There's an app for that! Part 2: Apps for general reference, specialty practice, and patient education. *Clinical Nurse Specialist, 29,* 181–185. doi:10.1097/NUR.0000000000000119

Thurber, R.F., & Asselin, M.E. (1999). An educational fair and poster approach to organization-wide mandatory education. *Journal of Continuing Education in Nursing, 30,* 25–29.

CHAPTER 7

Getting Involved in Professional Nursing Organizations and the Community

AS mentioned in Chapter 2, professional development is a lifelong, continuous process expected of nurses (American Nurses Association [ANA], 2015; ANA & National Nursing Staff Development Organization [NNSDO], 2010). Although nurses need to assume primary responsibility for their professional development, NPDSs, unit-based educators, and employers also have a responsibility to assist nurses in this process (ANA & NNSDO, 2010). The professional development of nurses and their involvement in professional organizations and the community are among the 14 Forces of Magnetism identified by the American Nurses Credentialing Center (ANCC, n.d.). These forces represent organizational "outcomes that exemplify nursing excellence" (ANCC, n.d., para. 2) and serve as the basis for Magnet® recognition.

With the advent of social media and the Internet, nurses can find and participate in a variety of professional and community-based activities at the local, regional, national, and international levels. This chapter will highlight the benefits of becoming involved in these activities as an NPDS or unit-based educator.

Benefits of Involvement

Why should I become involved in professional organizations or community activities?

Isn't my performance as a professional nurse at work enough?

I do not have time to do anything besides go to work every day and take care of my personal responsibilities at home. I have a life besides nursing!

These questions and comments may be commonly heard at your workplace, especially in light of the changes in nursing and health care over recent decades.

As an NPDS or unit-based educator, you need to be able to effectively respond to such questions and comments and clarify your own issues regarding the expectations of nurses in the professional development process.

Being an active professional nurse offers a variety of advantages to you, the recipients of your efforts, the nursing profession, and any affiliated organizations. Armed with this information, you need to determine how to prioritize these groups at this crucial time in your professional career.

Professional Rewards

Nurses can benefit professionally by engaging in activities at their own workplace, within the nursing profession, and in the community. Although some of these professional rewards meet job-related expectations or specific personal needs, others relate to overall development as a professional nurse.

Job and Professional Advancement

Whether you are an experienced nurse or have just passed the licensure examination, your participation in various nursing and community organizations can give you an advantage over other applicants when seeking employment or promotion opportunities. This is true whether you are seeking your first nursing position, moving to a new clinical unit, or changing jobs to work at another healthcare agency.

If you are in the process of finding a job, your participation in these organizations sends a positive message to prospective employers. It shows that even though you have not found a nursing position to date, you have become involved in professionally related activities. This behavior tells prospective employers that you have assumed a leadership role in your professional development. As a prospective employee, you have the potential to support team-building efforts and promote a positive professional attitude. Your activities also reflect your concern about the community. Employers may make the assumption that, if hired, you will continue this professional behavior to the benefit of patient care and the successful operation of the healthcare organization.

Being active in professional nursing and community associations may be an expectation for promotion within institutions that offer clinical advancement programs. This is viewed as an example of a professional behavior. These behaviors require active involvement, the use of leadership skills, and a sense of personal responsibility. Possessing these skills may set you apart from others who have not yet assumed the same level of professional development.

If you are currently employed in the profession, remember to use your participation in nursing organizations and activities within the community as a strategy to maintain or secure your present position. Your success in using this tactic depends greatly upon the value that your organization places on these professional behaviors. With this in mind, you may need to help your employer understand the benefits and importance of professional involvement. Your explanation is vital in an era of organizational mergers and restructuring, especially at a time when nurses need to be perceived as valuable and indispensable healthcare leaders.

Funding Opportunities, Resources, and Certification

Belonging to a professional organization can help you meet specific developmental needs as a professional nurse. Many nursing organizations offer benefits that reflect their missions, goals, and purposes. As a result, various opportunities are made available to active members, including research and literature review grants and scholarships for pursuing formal education (i.e., nursing degree) or informal education (i.e., continuing education programs). Many organizations sponsor financial awards that support certification examinations and opportunities to members who meet specific educational and clinical requirements. Some organizations also offer travel grants for members to attend national conventions or regional conferences.

Personal and Professional Development

Professional rewards offered by nursing organizations can positively influence your career development. Involvement in professional and community organizations can help you develop a professional career plan and attain professional goals (see Chapter 14). Benefits include working on an assigned project, interacting with other members, or leading the work of a committee or task force. Such activities provide you with opportunities to learn and practice leadership skills and mentor others in these skills.

Participating in professional organizations enables you to network with experienced nurses who possess leadership qualities and allows you to demonstrate your professional management skills. Through active involvement, clinical nurses have an opportunity to develop their own leadership skills. Figure 7-1 provides a partial list of the leadership skills that can be obtained through this process.

Shekleton, Preston, and Good (2010) piloted a leadership development program aimed to prepare newly elected American Association of Nurse Anesthetists (AANA) members for leadership roles in their state anesthesiology associations. Three nurses who were AANA president-elects at the state level participated in a three-day leadership development boot camp to gain the skills necessary to succeed in their new roles. Because of its positive outcomes, the program was included in AANA's infrastructure of ongoing professional development programs.

> **Figure 7-1. Examples of Leadership Skills Developed Through Participation in Professional Nursing Organizations**
>
> - Communication (oral and written)
> - Managing time
> - Being a group or team member
> - Managing conflict
> - Negotiating
> - Running a productive meeting
> - Defining a mission
> - Goal setting
> - Strategic planning
> - Organizing projects
> - Allocating resources effectively
> - Budget planning
> - Conference or program planning
> - Developing creativity
> - Motivating others

Although many behaviors can be observed in members of nursing organizations, it may be unrealistic to assume that all of these behaviors are positive. It is important for you to recognize the differences in these behaviors and learn from them. Negative behaviors, such as those exhibited with incivility, usually serve a member's personal interests or goals, but they often pose barriers to meeting organizational goals. Try to use the less-than-admirable qualities you may observe as examples of what not to do.

Members of professional nursing organizations also can serve as a professional support system for nurses, forming a link or network among individual members inside and outside an organization. Networking can help you learn more about your professional role, solve issues, develop collaborations, and establish your career plan. For example, networking can help you acquire a mentor who can assist you in developing expertise identified in your professional career plan. This mechanism can help members form nursing groups that share common interests such as clinical teaching, health promotion, or research.

Being active in a professional organization or community agency also provides you with current information related to its focus. Members usually receive some form of communication (often via email) about other members, upcoming events, and career opportunities at the local, regional, national, or international level. For example, you might be able to join an email list that will notify you about upcoming workshops, new products, or special services exclusive to members.

Most organizations also provide members with access to valuable networking platforms housed on their websites and on various forms of social media (e.g., Facebook, Twitter, blogs). Having access to this information will help you keep abreast of knowledge and updates within a specialty and will enable you to share ideas with other professionals with similar interests.

Professional Recognition

Being an active and productive member in professional nursing organizations and community associations can bring professional recognition to your employer, school of nursing, and any other associated organizations. Your success sends a positive message to the public about you and your affiliations. This, in turn, adds to the positive reputation of your workplace or school within the community.

Serving as an officer of a national nursing organization is a professional accomplishment that can bring prestige to your school of nursing. The success of a school's alumni has the potential to add to its national status and marketability to future applicants.

Many groups recognize and reward members who demonstrate outstanding overall leadership in nursing, provide outstanding service to their mission and goals, or display exceptional performance in specific areas such as clinical practice, teaching, research, or community service. Other nursing associations have writing contests or offer competitive awards to local chapters.

Professional Image, Identity, and Voice

Visibility of nurses within a community creates a positive image and identity for the profession. It demonstrates concern for a community's health and welfare and unites nurses under a common goal. This positive image also encourages recruitment of individuals into the nursing profession.

Dedicated members can advocate for the nursing profession and for the best interests of society (Matthews, 2012). Collectively, nurses can support changes that are in the best interest of the nursing organization, the profession, and the quality and safety of patient care. For example, members of a professional nursing organization can lobby legislators who influence laws or regulations that govern the nursing profession. Nurses also can form alliances with other organizations or groups and function as a powerful team to influence decisions about the profession. Updates regarding current legislation, professional nursing issues, and healthcare changes enable members to have a voice and influence outcomes in the best interests of the profession.

Supporting Consumers

Consumers can benefit directly and indirectly from nurses' involvement in professional and community organizations. The knowledge and skills gained by nurses through their participation in professional nursing organizations can influence the quality of nursing care that consumers receive. For example, results of unit-based research, quality improvement, or evidence-based projects supported by a nursing organization can be used in patient care protocols on a clinical unit. Journal publications and presentations at conferences enable nurses to consider changes to their own nursing practices. Nurses also can prepare evidence-based patient education materials and share their expertise through consumer education. Consumers can reap the benefits of healthcare resources gained through the lobbying efforts of professional nursing organizations.

As mentioned in Chapter 1, growing interest and advances in patient-centered technology, such as patient portals, mobile technology applications, and social media, have created a demand for nursing expertise in clinical practice, education, research, and administration. Unfortunately, limited evidence exists supporting the efficacy of such technology in improving consumers' participation in their health, fostering community building (Househ, Borycki, & Kushniruk, 2014), and offering quality content (Conn, 2013). These gaps offer nurses opportunities to lead future efforts in evaluating the quality of existing consumer technology resources, designing new patient resources, and investigating patients' perspectives regarding the acceptability, affordability, and availability of these resources.

Other nurses and assistive personnel (AP) can benefit from professional and community organizations by modeling their professional skills after colleagues involved in these organizations. They also can enhance their clinical performance through mentor relationships and attendance at educational offerings sponsored by nurses within these professional organizations.

Personal Benefits

Playing an active role in community and professional organizations can be personally rewarding. For instance, working on a specific task force with set goals can provide you with a sense of belonging to that group. Being an active member of a group can help you learn skills and overcome personal challenges. Participating in these activities can help you realize that your professional and personal qualities are valued, adding to your self-esteem. You may obtain personal satisfaction in knowing that you made a difference in the lives of others, your organization, and the nursing profession. You can apply the leadership skills you developed to your personal life or to your work setting by mentoring other nurses.

Ways to Share Your Professional Expertise

Although nurses can function in community groups as laypeople, it is important that they offer their special talents and expertise as professionals. Nurses can use their much-needed and valued knowledge and skills in community and professional organizations.

Speaker at Educational Programs

One way to share your professional expertise with your local community is to volunteer to present an educational program. For example, if your expertise is cardiovascular nursing, contact a local church's representatives and explore their learning needs. Offer to sponsor a program on cardiopulmonary resuscitation (CPR) or on the risk factors associated with heart attacks. Share your talents with your own organization, its outreach agencies, or schools of nursing. Consider presenting a unit-based in-service educational program, coordinating a learning activity such as grand rounds on your clinical unit, or volunteering to sponsor a booth on smoking cessation at your hospital's annual health fair. Be sure to include other healthcare workers as learners, such as AP, physical and occupational therapists, physicians, nutritionists, and social workers. Volunteer to teach educational programs for your professional nursing organization, exploring local, regional, and national opportunities. Help develop a continuing education program for nurses through the local chapter of your nursing organization (see Chapter 13). Be sure to consider a variety of potential learners in your community who could benefit from your expertise as a professional nurse.

Expert Consultant

Think about offering your professional nursing knowledge as an expert consultant. Start this process by taking an inventory of your strongest professional talents (e.g., clinical expertise in a specialty, such as oncology; advanced skills in trauma nursing; experience in designing ambulatory care units). Once you have identified your strengths, brainstorm groups or individuals who need your services. Ask your colleagues for help with this step. Many law firms use experienced nurses as expert witnesses in legal cases that involve questions related to patient care. Many local chapters of community organizations, such as the American Cancer Society (ACS), sponsor professional educational programs that use the expertise of experienced oncology nurses. For example, members of the Oncology Nursing Society (ONS) volunteered their expertise as researchers, educators, and clinicians to help develop the ONS Educator Resource Center, a website designed to support academic and clinical educators in preparing students and staff nurses to care for cancer survivors (ONS, n.d.-b). You may also consider helping at a local homeless shelter or with activities at your local division of the American Heart Association (AHA).

Investigate ways to market your expertise to your target audience and develop a plan to implement your services. If being an expert nurse witness interests you, research ways to connect with law firms in your community. Contact professional organizations, such as the American Association of Legal Nurse Consultants, for guidance regarding this role. If you are interested in assisting community organizations, contact your local chapters and inquire about opportunities. Consider appearing on a local television program or radio station to discuss timely topics related to health care. Offer to write a column on a health topic for a local newspaper or community publication. Some nurses choose to start their own for-profit businesses and market their services in this manner.

Mentor or Coach

Some nurses have been fortunate to have a mentor or role model, a person who helps with decisions regarding professional development. Even if you have never experienced such a relationship, think about becoming a mentor or career coach for a less-experienced nurse.

Start by volunteering to serve as a preceptor for a nursing student or a new nurse on your unit or by joining the membership committee of your local professional nursing organization. Sometimes mentoring relationships develop informally through working with others on projects within professional organizations, community agencies, or affiliations. For example, Vioral (2011) described a successful oncology nurse immersion program designed and implemented by members of an ONS chapter and funded by the ONS Foundation. This mentoring program was a collaborative effort among the chapter members, senior nursing students enrolled at local schools of nursing, and healthcare organizations. Its aim was to engage students in various professional development activities related to oncology nursing under the direction of a chapter member who served as a mentor. Activities included clinical experience in oncology nursing, participation at chapter meetings, attendance at continuing education programs, writing for a newsletter, and networking. Program outcomes revealed interest in professional nursing organizations, the oncology nursing specialty, and lifelong mentoring.

Community Volunteer Activities

Consider volunteering your services to organizations within your community such as the American Red Cross, AHA, or ACS. You may choose to focus your volunteer efforts on a community agency with a focus similar to your professional nursing organizations or one that personally appeals to you. Offer to speak about various health needs and concerns at schools, prisons, or community clinics.

Approach this goal using a well-developed plan. Start by making a list of community agencies that relate to your career goals, your clinical specialty expertise, or to your professional strengths. Perhaps you pride yourself on being an effective teacher, a compassionate listener, or a productive group leader. Focus on these strengths.

You can find a list of community agencies online or through your local library. For example, if you are interested in pediatrics, select several community organizations that reflect this interest. Be sure to investigate available opportunities for professional nurses within each organization. Even if an organization does not have a defined role for nurses, explore the possibility of developing a unique position. Select the organization that best matches your goals. Examples of some professional activities appropriate for a professional nurse include organizing a community support group, teaching CPR or childbirth classes, providing instruction in parenting, and coordinating public and professional educational programs.

Getting Started: Possible Sources for Involvement

What is the best way to start getting involved in professional nursing and community organizations? In reality, there is no wrong way. In fact, sometimes an individual's involvement begins purely by accident. For example, a colleague asks you to attend a program sponsored by the local chapter of a professional nursing organization. You belong to this organization but have not been active. At this meeting, you are asked to serve on a committee. Before you know it, the group elects you to chair the committee. The satisfaction you gain from your involvement influences you to run for an elected office the following year. Later, you serve on a task force for the organization at its national level. Keep in mind that all of these events occurred without planning them from the start.

But what if you choose to be active in an organization from the start? Simply join the organization and indicate that you would like to explore volunteer opportunities. Attend meetings and educational programs to gain a better understanding of the organization and meet other members.

When planning your involvement in a professional nursing organization, consider several factors. First, try to match your choice of organizations with the goals you identified in your career plan (see Chapter 14). Next, choose the pace at which you want to become involved within the organization. Decide where you want to be within that organization using a specific time frame. For example, is your goal to chair a committee by next year? Do you want to master the role of a committee member first before you decide to run for office two or three years down the road?

Then, select your desired level of involvement within the organization. Do you want to be active as a general member, a committee member, a chair of a committee, or an elected officer? Determine if you are interested in being active at the local, regional, national, or international levels of the organization. Consult other nurses who hold positions to which you aspire. Ask for their perspective on what position to seek and how to prepare for that role. In the meantime, observe their leadership skills and take detailed notes. Incorporate their advice into your career plan.

Finally, think about your overall involvement in professional nursing organizations. Because it is highly likely that there may be more than one organization that matches your professional interests, decide which ones to join and at what level you plan on participating in each. Although it is common practice to belong to several different organizations at the same time, you will need to carefully plan your time among them to avoid feeling overwhelmed with commitments you cannot keep. Regardless of your decision, be sure that the quality of your performance does not suffer by the quantity of your involvement. Think about being just a "card-carrying member" in some organizations for a while as you rotate your participation among them.

Recent advances in technology and social media have allowed nurses to become more engaged in professional nursing organizations despite potential barriers such as time, distance, or funds. For example, members of ONS can easily network and communicate with other oncology nurses with similar interests using various social media, such as Facebook, Twitter, Pinterest, YouTube, and LinkedIn (ONS, n.d.-c).

Professional Nursing Organizations

Nurses can belong to a variety of professional nursing organizations. The Helpful Websites section at the end of this chapter provides links to lists of the more than 100 professional nursing organizations currently available. These websites regularly update their information and provide links to each organization's home page. Although most of these organizations are national or international associations, many have regional or local chapters in which nurses can become actively involved. For example, ONS reports more than 225 chapters in which members can network on cancer care topics on a regional level (ONS, n.d.-a).

How does one go about choosing an organization for membership? Although professional nursing associations can be organized in a variety of ways and have overlapping purposes, Matthews (2012) arranged them into six categories (see Table 7-1). Examples of professional nursing organizations that may belong in each category with links to their websites are included next to Matthew's six groupings.

As an NPDS or unit-based educator, consider joining the Association for Nursing Professional Development (ANPD), formerly NNSDO (www.anpd.org). Listed under Matthew's sixth category of "Educational-level specific and graduate and professional development," ANPD is dedicated to meeting the needs of educators and offers members various opportunities to learn more about their role in NPD through ongoing educational events, publications, and resources. As a member, you can network with other ANPD members to discuss issues and seek solutions through collaboration.

Of course, some professional nursing organizations may be included in more than one of Matthew's categories (2012), for example, the Association of Pediatric Hematology/Oncology Nurses (www.aphon.org) (age periods along the continuum of life; system-specific disorders or conditions) and the National Association of Pediatric Nurse Practitioners (www.napnap.org) (graduate level and advanced practice nurse specialties; age periods along the continuum of life). ONS, like many other specialty organizations, offers members the opportunity to participate in professional communities that link members to others with similar areas of professional interest.

According to Matthews (2012), ANA (www.nursingworld.org) and the International Council of Nurses (ICN) (www.icn.ch) are two large professional nursing organizations that support the needs of nurses and the profession across all categories, irrespective of clinical specialty or other categories. In fact, ANA serves as a member organization within ICN. Similarly, Sigma Theta Tau International Honor Society of Nursing (STTI) (www.nursingsociety.org) is an international organization focused on "advancing world health and celebrating nursing excellence in scholarship, leadership, and service" (STTI, n.d.).

Nursing alumni associations can be conceptualized as an additional type of professional nursing organization. These associations mostly limit membership to graduates from their respective schools of nursing. Although specific goals vary among alumni associations, they often foster the needs of their members, current students, and the school. These associations provide excellent opportunities to develop mentor relationships between alumni and students, offering alumni opportunities to shape the future direction of their alma mater and its graduates.

Regardless of category, explore organizations with a mission, vision, and purpose that match your current or future professional career interests. Although you can belong to many

Table 7-1. Categories of Professional Nursing Organizations and Examples

Category	Related Professional Nursing Organizations
Setting-specific nursing	Association of periOperative Registered Nurses (AORN): www.aorn.org Emergency Nurses Association (ENA): www.ena.org/pages/default.aspx Home Healthcare Nurses Association (HHNA): www.hhna.org National Association of School Nurses (NASN): www.nasn.org
System-specific disorders or conditions	Academy of Medical-Surgical Nurses (AMSN): www.amsn.org American Association of Critical-Care Nurses (AACN): www.aacn.org Association of Pediatric Hematology/Oncology Nurses: (APHON): www.aphon.org Association of Women's Health, Obstetric and Neonatal Nurses (AWHONN): www.awhonn.org/awhonn Hospice and Palliative Nurses Association (HPNA): http://hpna.advancingexpertcare.org International Transplant Nurses Society (ITNS): www.itns.org Oncology Nursing Society (ONS): www.ons.org Society of Otorhinolaryngology and Head-Neck Nurses (SOHN): http://sohnnurse.com Society of Trauma Nurses (STN): www.traumanurses.org
Age periods along the continuum of life	Academy of Neonatal Nursing (ANN): www.academyonline.org Association of Pediatric Hematology/Oncology Nurses (APHON): www.aphon.org National Association of Pediatric Nurse Practitioners (NAPNAP): www.napnap.org National Gerontological Nursing Association (NGNA): www.ngna.org Society of Pediatric Nurses (SPN): www.pedsnurses.org
Ethnic and cultural-specific	American Assembly for Men in Nursing (AAMN): www.aamn.org National Association of Hispanic Nurses (NAHN): www.nahnnet.org National Black Nurses Association (NBNA): www.nbna.org Transcultural Nursing Society (TCN): www.tcns.org
Graduate level and advanced practice nurse specialties	American Association of Nurse Anesthetists (AANA): www.aana.com/aboutus/pages/default.aspx American Association of Nurse Practitioners (AANP): www.aanp.org American Organization of Nurse Executives (AONE): www.aone.org National Association of Clinical Nurse Specialists (NACNS): www.nacns.org National Association of Pediatric Nurse Practitioners (NAPNAP): www.napnap.org
Educational-level specific and graduate and professional development	American Association of Colleges of Nursing (AACN): www.aacn.nche.edu Association for Nursing Professional Development (ANPD): www.anpd.org National League for Nursing (NLN): www.nln.org Organization for Associate Degree Nursing (OADN): www.oadn.org

Note. Based on information from Matthews, 2012.

organizations at one time, review the fees and eligibility criteria for national and local chapter membership for those that appeal to you. Consider prioritizing organizations based on information from their websites or from conversations with current members. Decide what organizations you will dedicate your time and contributions to over the next one to three years. Refer to your career plan goals to help you make these decisions.

Employer Affiliations in the Community

Investigate potential opportunities for involvement with community organizations affiliated with your workplace, including community wellness clinics, nurse-managed centers, homecare settings, urgent care centers, or daycare centers for seniors and children.

Neighborhood and Religious Organizations

Your community may need the expertise of a professional nurse. Various neighborhood citizen associations, religious groups, homeless shelters, and school districts can benefit from your knowledge and skills as a nurse. For example, initiate health screenings, health education, and referrals for a parish nurse group if your goal is to work within a faith community. If you are unsure what opportunities exist in your area, conduct a community assessment with the help of your local librarian or community leader.

Maximizing Your Involvement

Regardless of your choice of professional involvement, be sure to communicate your participation in professional and community organizations with others. Sharing this information creates an awareness that may encourage similar behaviors in other nurses and results in recognition for you, your colleagues, your workplace, and your school.

Be sure to communicate your involvement using both oral and written methods. Record your involvement appropriately in your professional files through your portfolio and résumé. Write about your experiences in your local community or nursing newspaper, school newsletter, or employer's newsletter. Share the details of your involvement in a manuscript for publication or present it as a poster at a nursing conference. Share your efforts with your colleagues in a unit-based in-service program or informal roundtable presentation. Communicate your accomplishments in an interview with the public relations representative at your workplace.

Summary

Nurses can benefit from becoming actively involved in professional nursing organizations and community activities that pique their professional and personal interests. Among the many professional rewards are opportunities for advancement, funding and resources, recognition, advocacy, and supporting consumers. Nurses can share their expertise as speakers at educational programs, consultants in their area of expertise, mentors or coaches for nurses and consumers, and community volunteers. Professional nursing organizations, employer-affiliated community groups, and local neighborhood and religious organizations allow numerous opportunities for nurses to become engaged.

Helpful Websites

- American Nurses Association—Organizational Affiliates: www.nursingworld.org/affiliated organizations
- Nurse.org—Nursing Organizations: http://nurse.org/orgs.shtml
- Sigma Theta Tau International Honor Society of Nursing—Professional Nursing Organizations: www.nursingsociety.org/connect-engage/our-global-impact/professional-nursing -organizations

References

American Nurses Association. (2015). *Nursing: Scope and standards of practice* (3rd ed.). Silver Spring, MD: Author.

American Nurses Association & National Nursing Staff Development Organization. (2010). *Nursing professional development: Scope and standards of practice*. Silver Spring, MD: American Nurses Association.

American Nurses Credentialing Center. (n.d.). Forces of Magnetism. Retrieved from http://www.nursecredentialing. org/ForcesofMagnetism.aspx

Conn, J. (2013, December 14). No longer a novelty, medical apps are increasingly valuable to clinicians and patients. *Modern Healthcare*. Retrieved from http://www.modernhealthcare.com/article/20131214/MAGAZINE/312149983

Househ, M., Borycki, E., & Kushniruk, A. (2014). Empowering patients through social media: The benefits and challenges. *Health Informatics Journal, 20,* 50–58. doi:10.1177/1460458213476969

Matthews, J.H. (2012). Role of professional organizations in advocating for the nursing profession. *Online Journal of Issues in Nursing, 17*(1). Retrieved from http://nursingworld.org/MainMenuCategories/ANAMarketplace/ ANAPeriodicals/OJIN/TableofContents/Vol-17-2012/No1-Jan-2012/Professional-Organizations-and -Advocating.html

Oncology Nursing Society. (n.d.-a). Chapters. Retrieved from https://www.ons.org/member-center/chapters

Oncology Nursing Society. (n.d.-b). Educator Resource Center. Retrieved from https://erc.ons.org

Oncology Nursing Society. (n.d.-c). Social media. Retrieved from https://www.ons.org/newsroom/social-media

Shekleton, M.E., Preston, J.C., & Good, L.E. (2010). Growing leaders in a professional membership organization. *Journal of Nursing Management, 18,* 662–668. doi:10.1111/j.1365-2834.2010.01152.x

Sigma Theta Tau International Honor Society of Nursing. (n.d.). Sigma Theta Tau International organizational fact sheet. Retrieved from http://www.nursingsociety.org/aboutus/mission/Pages/factsheet.aspx

Vioral, A.N. (2011). Filling the gaps: Immersing student nurses in specialty nursing and professional associations. *Journal of Continuing Education in Nursing, 42,* 415–420. doi:10.3928/00220124-20110601-01

CHAPTER 8

Sharing Your Expertise Through Publishing

SHARING clinical expertise with others through publishing is one way that nurses can develop themselves as professionals. Nurses often assume they are not capable of being good writers. It is always that "other" nurse with special talents who gets articles published in journals.

Maybe you are just the opposite. Perhaps after reading an article related to your clinical area you thought: *I could have written that! We had a more effective approach to that clinical problem than the one published in that article!*

Most nurses think of journal articles, book chapters, or textbooks when they hear the phrase "writing for publication." However, nurses can participate in the publishing process in many other ways. In fact, most nurses have been involved in publishing without even realizing it. For example, think about the ways you use your writing skills at work. Your contributions to your organization's standards of care, patient teaching materials, and policies and procedures can be seen as a beginning form of professional writing. Think about courses or educational programs you have conducted, the articles you have published in your organization's newsletter or a community newspaper, or the poster presentations you have developed. In some way, you have gained experience in professional writing.

As leaders, NPDSs have an opportunity to shape the future of nursing by supporting nurses in unfamiliar and challenging pursuits, such as publishing and public speaking (Ashton, 2012). As an NPDS, you may be asked by your employer to not only publish your own work through the nursing literature but also to mentor clinical nurses in publishing their successes in research (Carlson, Masters, & Pfadt, 2008), clinical practice, education, and other areas (see Chapter 2) (American Nurses Association [ANA] & National Nursing Staff Development Organization, 2010). Regardless of your employer's expectations, it is important to understand the publication process to become a strong mentor and advance your professional career.

Why Should Nurses Publish?

So, why should clinical nurses like yourself publish? You will be glad to know that this is a common question asked by those in the profession. A major reason nurses should publish is because of their clinical expertise and educational background that provide valuable firsthand knowledge and insight into what is important for patients and colleagues. You have most likely been involved in research or evidence-based practice projects on your clinical unit and have witnessed the influence of these projects on patients and their families. These experiences prepare you to contribute valuable information to the nursing literature. In addition to your clinical expertise, other reasons to publish involve the needs of your patients, the profession, your employer, and yourself.

Positive Influence on Patient Outcomes

Publishing your work concerning best practices in a clinical specialty or details of your clinical experiences can help shape the nursing practice of others. Whether you are a new graduate nurse just beginning your professional role or an experienced nurse with specialty knowledge and skills, your published work can help nurses provide safe, quality patient care.

Think about questions you ask yourself in the clinical setting: *How should I teach my patients to care for their new appliance? What is the best way to handle that new procedure? What is considered safe clinical practice?*

You, as an expert practitioner in your clinical specialty, have a responsibility to answer these questions for other nurses.

Think about the resources you have read as a nursing student while learning to care for patients. In addition to your nursing textbook, you probably searched journal articles that gave you current information about meeting the needs of patients and their families. Remember how helpful those articles were in developing your current clinical competencies, and recall how you relied upon information presented in the articles to understand how to care for your patients. Realize the influence that these references have had on your current skills. As an experienced nurse, you are in a prime position to help novice nurses learn about patient care.

Experienced nurses also may rely on the nursing literature to maintain or develop clinical competencies. The merging and restructuring of many healthcare organizations has often led to the closing of clinical units and departments (see Chapter 1). These changes required many nurses to relocate to unfamiliar clinical units and care for patients with new health-related needs. Articles written by nurses with expertise in a particular area can help these relocated nurses to develop the knowledge and skills they need in order to function in their new role or setting.

It is important for you to publish articles that may be helpful to assistive personnel, as they need your expertise and leadership to guide them through many of the complex patient situations they encounter. They also need published resources that will help them understand how to function as a team member in a restructured healthcare environment.

Patients can benefit directly from your clinical expertise by reading your articles on topics that explain medications and procedures, the illness experience, and health promotion practices. Lay caregivers, such as spouses and significant others, need your help as they assume more responsibilities at home with their loved ones. Resources you publish specifically for them can support their expectations as caregivers.

Consider publishing articles that focus on controversies in practice with current healthcare trends. Offer other nurses and consumers an opportunity to view multiple perspectives of an issue so they can make informed decisions regarding their health care.

Positive Influence on the Nursing Profession

Publishing can also be viewed as a professional responsibility of nurses by disseminating best practices that add to existing nursing knowledge. It would not have been easy for you to become a nurse without having access to the current evidence-based nursing literature. How would your nursing faculty have gained information about what or how to teach without this literature? Nurses often take for granted that someone else created the knowledge base for the profession.

Publishing strengthens the history of the nursing profession. Without the printed word, only oral accounts would be available to preserve nursing's knowledge base, practices, and traditions. There would be no documentation describing the evolution of the profession and no research to support nursing practice. Nurses would not realize the best ways to provide care and teach patients and families. Publishing is an excellent way to document these historical landmarks and events.

Benefits for Your Employer and School of Nursing

Your employer also benefits from your publishing efforts in the nursing literature. Nursing journals and books typically include authors' places of employment with the authorship listing. This information is free publicity for your employer and offers a great deal of prestige for your organization. It also credits past employers that may have given you the knowledge and the content needed to publish your efforts. Readers interested in the topic may also gain a positive opinion of your organization. Your organization may be viewed as having an environment that is innovative and offers the latest advances to its patients and employees. Because both you and your institution are recognized in publications, your success is also your employer's success.

Your publishing efforts will also be valued by your healthcare organization if it is seeking American Nurses Credentialing Center (ANCC) Magnet® Recognition for its "quality patient care, nursing excellence, and innovations in professional nursing practice" (ANCC, n.d., para. 1). Such publications may focus on evidence-based practice, clinical innovations, or research outcomes.

Publishing also benefits the school of nursing in which you are currently enrolled or have previously attended. Evidence of scholarship is one of several program outcomes tracked by schools through alumni surveys. Evidence of ongoing scholarship produced by nurses is also valued by the schools of nursing from which they graduated or are currently enrolled.

Personal and Professional Rewards

Publishing provides personal and professional rewards for you as the author (Oermann & Hays, 2016). It is rewarding to see your article and name while browsing through a prestigious nursing journal. You may receive compliments from colleagues who see your article in the recent issue of their specialty journal. Nursing students assigned to your clinical unit might use your article as a guide to prepare for their patient plan of care. A nurse living in another country might read your article and contact you for help with managing a clinical situation. A concerned family member also might contact you requesting guidance for a loved one who is about to undergo a surgical procedure discussed in your article.

Writing also can be a personal outlet. Morgan (2014) advocated using expressive writing as a tool for nurses to cope with stressful situations that arise in either their personal or professional lives. This form of self-help writing involves expressing your inner thoughts and feelings on paper in an attempt to minimize emotional discomfort or stressful situations (Morgan, 2014). Conversely, writing about a happy, more positive situation can also help reduce stress. Morgan (2014) suggested that nurses create a positive work environment by organizing ongoing group writing sessions for colleagues.

Publishing builds upon your professional expertise and positively influences your career. Others who read your publications will assume you are an expert on a particular topic. As a result, other publishers may contact you to write for them, colleagues may invite you to speak at a chapter meeting, or a law firm may ask you to serve as an expert witness in a legal case or to provide your professional opinion on a case related to an article you wrote. You also may be asked by nurses at other hospitals for advice on a clinical tool that you shared in a recent publication. Publications can also support a promotion or advancement at your workplace, especially if publishing is among the criteria for the clinical advancement program at your organization.

The experience of preparing a manuscript for publication can be rewarding in itself. Although you may choose to write on a familiar topic, additional research can expand your knowledge and strengthen your competency on that topic (Oermann & Hays, 2016). In fact, your ongoing writing efforts can eventually lead to developing a chapter for a book or similar work.

Publishing with colleagues can result in lasting friendships and networking options. Rather than simply being a consumer of the nursing literature, you become a contributor to the nursing profession on a particular topic, progressing your lifelong professional development and career plan (see Chapter 14).

Overcoming Barriers to Publishing

Before you start teaching other nurses about the publishing process, consider some common reasons why nurses may choose not to publish. Develop strategies aimed at minimizing or overcoming these barriers. Motivation is one of the most important issues to consider when helping nurses write for publication (Fowler, 2010a).

Lack of Time

Many nurses cite lack of time as a reason why they do not publish (Oermann & Hays, 2016). They claim that their job, family, and personal lives consume most of their day. Some nurses feel that someone else can publish because it is too much work for them. Do these comments sound familiar? Sometimes, it is too easy to talk yourself out of devoting time to writing.

Assuming that you and your colleagues are interested in professional writing and want to make it a priority in your nursing careers, think of creative ways to incorporate writing into your existing schedule, either at home or at work. This task is essential if publishing is among your professional goals. Gennaro (2014) recommended identifying a day or days each week that you will dedicate to writing. The author also suggested refraining from emails, phone calls, and housework during these days. Also, ask colleagues and family members to avoid interrupting you unless an emergency arises.

If you plan to write alone, first decide what day or what portion of a day you typically feel most creative (Oermann & Hays, 2016). Maybe your best time is the early morning hours before work, or maybe weekend afternoons. Lunchtime at work can also provide a productive time for writing. For others, writing flows best in the evening or late at night. Regardless of the time you choose to write, set aside a time that works for you.

Next, determine how much time you can dedicate to publishing on those days. Whether it is one hour or two, any block of time dedicated to your writing project will help you progress in the right direction. For example, a couple of hours of writing on the weekend can accumulate significantly over time. Try to record something on paper, even on days when you are not feeling particularly creative. You will be surprised how much progress you can make with small, continuous additions to your project. Establish a time schedule with a mentor or former teacher in which small portions of a manuscript are due by specific dates. This approach may help you get past small hurdles or delays in writing that you may encounter.

Another way to find time to publish is to coauthor a manuscript with a colleague. Although this approach may take a little more coordination with schedules, working with a partner also has benefits. Besides having to contribute to only part of the total manuscript, writing with a partner may encourage you to meet deadlines. You may not want to disappoint your colleague or embarrass yourself with your lack of productivity. If coauthoring a paper, be sure to establish authorship order and expectations at the start of your collaboration. If you prefer to author a manuscript by yourself, try bouncing your publishing ideas off colleagues or friends, as they can serve as preliminary editors of your work and provide encouragement.

Another strategy is to develop a small writing group with colleagues on your clinical unit. Identify preexisting formal or informal work groups on your unit and encourage them to publish using their clinical projects as examples. For example, you may approach members of a patient education committee to transform their recent success with patient-focused critical pathways into a journal article. You might also encourage members of a staffing work group to document the novel approach they devised to meet staffing needs of several specialty units. Nurses who have firsthand experience with new events, such as restructuring, can provide leadership and insight so that others may avoid their pitfalls. Sharing the challenges faced and the strategies used to manage these activities is vital.

You can also introduce writing for publication as part of your professional nursing organization's local chapter activities. This strategy can not only develop your skills in publication but also can assist others within your organization in meeting their publishing goals. Because nurses who participate in these organizations most likely will have interests similar to yours, this strategy can help nurses quickly develop ideas and gain support. For example, suppose a group of RNs just returned from presenting a clinical project on critical pathways at a national nursing conference. Develop a plan that will take advantage of the current excitement of this group. Suggest that they turn their presentation into a manuscript. If you have an opportunity to talk with them before they present, ask them to record their presentation. Once they have transcribed the tape, they will have a draft of their manuscript. Because their abstract was accepted for a national presentation, there probably is an audience that would like to have access to it in a published form. Even if they did not get a chance to record their presentation on site, suggest they record it as they repeat it at a unit-based conference or at a local chapter meeting of a professional nursing organization. Or, as a way to develop your own skills in publishing, capture the essence of a recent poster presentation in a manuscript. The work that you already put into organizing your poster will help you develop an outline to structure your paper draft.

Horstman and Theeke (2012) consulted with a former editor to sponsor a one-day writing retreat aimed at helping staff nurses and nurse leaders at a Magnet-designated medical center learn how to prepare a journal article to disseminate best practices, create a professional poster presentation, and design research. Their program offered continuing education (CE) contact hours and included face-to-face small group learning, hands-on experience with a group project, and ongoing communication that included a teleconference and electronic progress reports. Outcomes were positive, with four of nine submitted manuscripts accepted for publication one year after the retreat.

Fear of Failure

Nurses may delay or avoid writing for publication because they fear they will fail (Oermann & Hays, 2016). Some may worry their manuscript will be rejected by a journal editor. Others may dread receiving constructive criticism or feedback about their work from manuscript reviewers or may perceive preparing a manuscript as an overwhelming task.

You can manage these fears of failing by focusing on the skills you possess that will make your future publication successful, such as your content expertise as a professional nurse or your ability to solve complex problems at work. Imagine the worst-case scenarios that can happen during the publishing process and plan strategies to minimize these fears. For example, it is possible that an editor may reject your manuscript. Even the most experienced, successful authors have had their share of rejections and have survived. Turn negative thoughts into positive opportunities. Consider the feedback you received during the review process as valuable expert advice that you can use when revising your manuscript. An editor should provide you with specific reasons why your manuscript was rejected so that you can strengthen it for your next submission. You article might have been rejected for reasons other than your writing style. For instance, an editor may say your topic was not appropriate for a journal's readership or that your idea was already published in a previous article.

A journal's editor will be the only other person to know that your manuscript was rejected and the reasons why it was rejected. Because with most journals, your name is removed from the manuscript for the review (*blind review*), peer reviewers do not know your identity. It is your prerogative to tell others about your rejection or to keep it private. It is important to remember that you have control over this situation.

Writing for publication takes practice and faith in oneself. You needed many hours of practicing and mentoring to become the competent practitioner that you are today. This process of practice and guidance applies to writing for healthcare publications. Before, you were a novice nurse; now, you are a novice author. Allow yourself some time, lots of practice, and the encouragement of others. Believe in yourself and give yourself credit for trying and heading in the right direction.

Share your paper with colleagues before submitting it. Ask for their honest opinions about the importance of the topic, the way you organized the content, and your writing style and grammar. Also, ask them if additional tables or figures would help clarify the content. Their feedback will help you make changes before you submit your work to a journal. This strategy also may provide you with the self-confidence needed to complete the document.

Some authors deal with their fear of failure by teaming up with an experienced author, especially for their first manuscript. This approach can give you that extra assurance to move forward. Consider existing networks in your personal and professional life when finding a suitable coauthor. For instance, you could approach a clinical nurse specialist who has a successful publishing record and inquire about collaborating. Because faculty in university-based schools of nursing usually are experienced in the publishing process, ask a former nursing instructor to join you in coauthoring your manuscript.

Limited Skills or Resources

Some nurses are worried that they may not have access to resources needed for producing a manuscript. Earlier, this chapter described ways to obtain additional human resources for your project and plan time to fit writing into your schedule. Use this advice to rectify any problems you may have with lack of resources.

Preparing a manuscript may entail some costs depending on the resources available to you at your workplace or at your school (if you are a student). Most often, conducting a literature search may be a free service offered by your employer. However, you may encounter costs associated with printing and duplicating articles to review, obtaining permission to reuse copyrighted material, acquiring Internet access and typing services to prepare your paper, and having an experienced writer edit your paper before submission. If you need help in creating figures, illustrations, or photographs to enhance your final paper, the services of an expert with these skills, such as an illustrator, may also involve a fee. Most journals request an electronic version of your documents, so paying for the cost of duplicating and mailing multiple manuscript copies to an editor is unusual. Although these costs may vary depending on your project, they often can be minimized if you do them yourself, share them with coauthors, or combine them with your other projects.

If typing is not your strongest skill, consider creating a manuscript draft and contracting with a professional typist who can prepare your final product. This strategy especially holds true with any pictures, images, or computer-generated tables you may need to develop. Consider asking clerical staff at your workplace if they are interested in completing this task on their own time for a negotiated fee. Perhaps they can connect you with someone who may be interested in the job. When recruiting typists, ask for references to gauge the quality of their services.

Most journals have implemented web-based management systems for submitting manuscripts. These systems require potential authors to submit their manuscript materials online using a specific website and password. This approach not only facilitates the submission process for authors, but it also allows them to track the progress of their manuscript as it proceeds through the peer-review process. This system also enables peer reviewers to access assigned manuscripts and allows them to submit comments and recommendations online.

Difficulty Generating Ideas

Finding a specific topic or idea to write about is a barrier for some nurses, especially when under pressure to publish. A good way to avoid this obstacle is to create a file folder of writing ideas. As you think of topics, write them down on a piece of paper and store them in this folder. You can also develop this system electronically on your computer or smartphone. You will be surprised how these ideas come in handy when you are ready to write. As time passes, you may opt to organize your ideas into a publishing binder that contains several file folders, each labeled with a different topic. You may also want to store your general references on publishing or some sample articles from various journals here. Additionally, this is a good place to keep your writing style manual or similar resources so that they can be easily retrieved.

Record ideas for articles as soon as you think of them. Sometimes ideas come to you in the strangest situations, such as when you are driving, waiting for a doctor's appointment, or listening to a speaker at a nursing conference. If preferred, consider voice recording your ideas as they come to you. Remember, the more details you record about your proposed article, the easier you will be able to recall them. Later, this chapter will present creative methods you can use to capture your publishable ideas.

Journal clubs may offer strategies that nurses can implement on the clinical unit to get others involved in publishing. Usually, these clubs involve a group of clinical nurses who meet on a regular basis to discuss research articles on topics that interest them in their practice (Polit & Beck, 2012). Reviewing research articles may help nurses become more familiar with not only the research process but also how articles are organized in a manuscript format. Consider using a journal club approach to help you and coauthors prepare a particular type of manuscript, such as a CE article, by reviewing the content and format of similar articles.

Unfamiliar With the Publishing Process

I don't know how to get published! If this is your claim, then approach this problem in a similar fashion as with other skills you have tried to master. Seek sources of instruction that can help you with various aspects of the publishing process. If writing is not your strength, then enroll in a creative writing class for adults at a local community college. Ask a local bookstore or librarian to locate available "how-to" books on publishing or other web-based resources that can help you get started. In the same vein, consider enrolling in a writing-for-publication course offered by a school of nursing. I described the successful implementation of such a course conducted through a partnership between Allegheny General Hospital and Duquesne University School of Nursing in Pittsburgh, Pennsylvania (Lockhart, 2000). Several graduate nursing students and clinical nurse managers enrolled in the course were able to get articles published after course completion. This project also enabled both organizations to attain additional goals related to recruitment and professional development.

If you are still unsure how to proceed after sharpening your writing skills, seek various writing opportunities either inside or outside your healthcare organization. Writing retreats sponsored by employers for their novice nurse authors have reported successful outcomes (Horstman & Theeke, 2012; Jackson, 2009). For example, Stone, Levett-Jones, Harris, and Sinclair (2010) developed the Neophytes Writers' Group, which was created through a collaboration between nurse academics and clinical nurses. Strategies employed within this writing support group were guided by Bandura's (1977) Theory of Self-Efficacy and focused on participants' self-confidence, motivation, capacity, and self-efficacy in writing for publication. Investigate writing retreats or sessions sponsored by professional nursing organizations either as stand-alone, for-fee programs or as writing sessions at annual conferences.

Another way to familiarize yourself with the writing process is to invite a published nurse to speak to a group of interested colleagues at work or to nurse members at a chapter meeting of a professional nursing organization. Richardson and Carrick-Sen (2011) conducted a successful development program in which 50 nurses, midwives, and allied health professionals learned how to write for publication under the leadership of two experienced authors. Outcomes at one year revealed that 25% of participants had submitted manuscripts to a journal.

Learn more about publishing on your own by reading many of the available "how-to" books, articles, and web-based resources that focus on the basics of publishing and are targeted to novice authors (Driscoll & Aquilina, 2011; Happell, 2012; Morton, 2013a, 2013b). Other literature provides helpful suggestions on publishing particular types of papers, such as case studies (Harrison, 2012), clinical narratives (Heinrich, Tafas, & Jackson, 2011), literature reviews (Kable, Pich, Maslin-Prothero, & Sian, 2012; Wright, 2010), project reports (Fowler, 2011c), quality improvement and patient safety reports (Holzmueller, & Pronovost, 2013), research (Benton, 2014; Berkey & Moore, 2012; Price, 2014, 2015), and continuing professional development articles (Price, 2008).

Web-based modules related to publishing are also available. For example, Knievel (2008) detailed an online tutorial on publishing that was developed for faculty and graduate students by librarians at the University of Colorado (www.publishnotperish.org).

Few Incentives to Publish

Because publishing can be considered a change in behavior for some nurses, try relying on the approach you usually use when implementing a new policy or piece of equipment to staff on your unit. For example, start by identifying the positives and negatives that nurses might encounter regarding publishing. Positives may include a group's desire to publish or the benefits that publishing can have on advancing up the career ladder. On the other hand, negatives might include a lack of time or fear of failure. Develop a plan for nurses on your clinical unit that emphasizes the benefits of publishing and minimizes its negative factors. Continue to provide nurses with ongoing support throughout this process.

Include strategies that will help you meet your goal, including publicly recognizing the work of colleagues. Appeal to your colleagues' sense of reason by promoting all of the positive aspects related to having their article published; or try a different approach by reminding colleagues that publishing is a criterion for advancement up the clinical ladder at your organization. You can also use your organization's newsletter to showcase a group that has been successful at publishing. Once a few nurses on your unit start publishing, those who do not may feel out of place. Over time and with the right support systems in place, these nurses may be encouraged to participate.

In a qualitative study conducted by Moos (2009), certified RN anesthetists cited several barriers to publishing: lack of time, preparation, motivation, institutional support, and mentorship, and limited outlets for dissemination. Strategies to remedy some of these barriers included the provision of adequate education, time, mentorship, professional or institutional support, and motivation. The need for institutions to identify writing for publication as a professional expectation was seen among organizational-level solutions. Failure to hold publishing as an expectation had the potential to negatively influence nurses both personally and professionally.

Understanding the Publication Process: The 10-Step Approach

Once you overcome some of the emotional and logistical barriers to publishing, you will need to focus on the practical aspects of writing for publication. If you have never published before, it is likely that you may not know how to begin. It is important to spend time developing a plan to accomplish your goal of producing a manuscript for publication (Morton, 2013b). This section reviews the publishing process using my 10-Step Approach to Publishing as an example (Lockhart, 2000). Figure 8-1 displays the details of this model. Although authors may begin at any step, this model is most helpful for beginning authors who start at step 1. Do not become discouraged with this process along the way, as the writing experiences of each individual who uses this model may differ.

Step 1: Identify a Topic or Idea

Step 1 of the 10-Step Approach to Publishing (Lockhart, 2000) involves identifying a topic or idea for your paper. If you have not yet identified a topic, review your notes in your publishing files, if available. Carefully explore a topic before deciding to discard the idea.

You can use various strategies to identify a topic that you can develop into a manuscript. For instance, write on a topic on which you struggled to find substantial examples in the nursing literature. Or, reflect upon your professional experiences with patients, families, or colleagues. Recall a critical incident or patient situation that stands out in your mind, such as clinical exemplars or clinical narratives required for many clinical advancement programs. For example, Heinrich et al. (2011) created a 12-step program to help nurses reduce pressure when writing clinical narratives for advancement within healthcare settings. You could also develop a case study from your experiences that you feel would be helpful to other nurses (Fowler, 2011b).

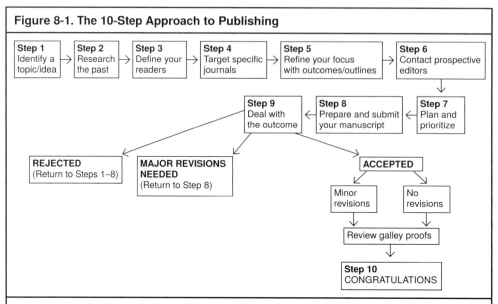

Figure 8-1. The 10-Step Approach to Publishing

Note. From "Writing for Health Care Publications: A Partnership Between Service and Education," by J.S. Lockhart, 2000, *Nurse Educator, 25,* p. 197. Copyright 2000 by Lippincott Williams & Wilkins. Reprinted with permission.

Gately (2011) advised nurse authors to share the human drama they encounter on a daily basis in clinical practice. For example, you could write about how you successfully addressed a patient's cultural needs during preoperative teaching. Or, you could describe a situation in which your patient avoided developing a postoperative complication because of your astute nursing assessment skills. Consider sharing a successful teaching tool you developed for patients to help them remember to take their medications at home or the process you followed to interview families on your clinical unit for a research project on caregivers. Developing a narrative of these accounts can help other nurses manage similar clinical situations or prevent future problems. When using clinical examples, follow your organization's privacy policies, obtain appropriate approvals before sharing your stories in print, and remove any identifiers for patients, colleagues, or family members.

A third method you can use to identify a publishable topic is to reflect on best practices at your organization (Price, 2010) or your own clinical strengths. Do nurses from other clinical units call you for advice when learning how to care for patients with tracheotomies? Do colleagues contact you when they need help preparing a poster presentation? Do you have a unique role (e.g., case manager, unit-based educator, resource nurse) on your clinical unit?

Consider sharing information about your role and any transition you had to make to your role. Sharing successes like these in print may help other nurses in their ongoing professional development and career planning.

School papers or projects can serve as a fourth strategy to identify a publishable topic. For example, consider adapting a manuscript on the debate you presented on the advantages and disadvantages of obtaining a nursing specialty certification. Share how you juggled multiple personal and professional roles while finishing your RN to BSN degree. Although your actual school paper in its original format should not be submitted as a manuscript, it can certainly serve as a beginning draft that you can adapt to a journal's readership.

Another source for a manuscript idea may come from your involvement in community projects or professional nursing organizations. You could share how you used technology to develop a cost-effective electronic newsletter for local chapter members, the outcomes of a child immunization project that you led in an underdeveloped country, or the vision screening program you designed for school-age children in your local neighborhood. Consider sharing your nursing expertise with your community by writing for your local newspaper (Smith, 2010).

Although most of these ideas focus on your role as a professional nurse, contemplate sharing your personal experience as a patient or family caregiver. For example, write about how you overcame challenges in being a caregiver for your elderly parent with a debilitating illness. Or, share your experience in making a decision regarding life support for a loved one. From your perspective as a patient, detail how you coped with a diagnosis and how nurses helped you recover. These stories can benefit others facing similar situations.

Write about strategies that your clinical unit developed to cope with organizational changes or national trends and issues (see Chapter 1). For example, describe the innovative ways in which nurses on your clinical unit have dealt with the nursing shortage. Write about the novel patient education approach you recently implemented to help nurses deal with shorter lengths of stay in the hospital after surgery. Discuss the critical pathways you developed or the creative staffing approach you created. Share the quality improvement project that reduced the patient falls on your unit and informed nursing practice changes.

Transform the presentation that you gave at a nursing conference into a publishable paper (Alspach, 2010; Happell, 2008). Use your slides as a basis for developing an outline for your manuscript. Feedback received can help shape your paper. Investigate whether the conference is associated with a journal that could potentially showcase your work. In some cases, conference organizers require that presenters first submit any future manuscripts to the journal associated with the conference.

Consider recruiting the help of colleagues to generate additional ideas. For example, maybe colleagues commented on your exemplary conflict resolution with a physician. Or, perhaps they admired the teaching strategies you used as a preceptor with a senior nursing student last semester. Their perspectives of events such as these can be invaluable when brainstorming ideas.

If you are familiar with some of the journals that publish in your clinical specialty, you may be able to gain a snapshot of current published topics by accessing each journal's table of contents online. Examine not only the topics but also the perspectives used by the authors and the types of published papers. This may help identify what topics have already been published or ones that have not yet been addressed. While this strategy is not a substitute for a systematic review of the literature, it can help you identify ideas and become familiar with what journals publish.

Types of Manuscripts

As you explore a topic for your paper, decide what type of manuscript you would like to produce. Table 8-1 lists some common types of manuscripts and examples of published articles in each category. Although these options are presented as single manuscripts, many of the examples can be categorized into multiple options. Review some of your favorite journals to see what special features pose opportunities for your topic. You can find this information by reviewing a journal's table of contents, the articles themselves, or author guidelines. This information can usually be found on a journal's website.

For example, the *Oncology Nursing Forum* offers several options that vary in purpose and length: full-length articles focused on administration, clinical practice, education, or research

Table 8-1. Types of Manuscripts Included in Peer-Reviewed Journals

Type of Manuscript	Examples
Research	Curran, M.K. (2014). Examination of the teaching styles of nursing professional development specialists, part II: Correlational study on teaching styles and use of adult learning theory. *Journal of Continuing Education in Nursing, 45,* 353–359. Hunt, C.W., Sanderson, B.K., & Ellison, K.J. (2014). Support for diabetes using technology: A pilot study to improve self-management. *MEDSURG Nursing, 23,* 231–237.
Quality improvement/ evidence-based projects	Huffines, M., Johnson, K., Naranjo, L.L., Lissauer, M.E., Fishel, M., Howes, S.M., … Smith, R. (2014). Improving family satisfaction and participation in decision making in an intensive care unit. *Critical Care Nurse, 33*(5), 56–69. Palos, G.R., Zandstra, F., Gilmore, K., Russell, L., Flores, J., & Rodriquez, M.A. (2014). Transforming cancer survivorship care through quality improvement initiatives. *Clinical Journal of Oncology Nursing, 18,* 468–472.
Clinical	Nelson, W.K., Moore, J., Grasso, J.A., Barbarotta, L., & Fischer, D.S. (2014). Development of a policy and procedure for accidental chemotherapy overdose. *Clinical Journal of Oncology Nursing, 18,* 414–420. Mullholand, K.D., & Riley, R.M. (2013). Transesophageal echocardiography: Getting a clearer view. *American Nurse Today, 8*(9), 8–11.
Education	Lucas, A.N. (2014). Promoting continuing competence and confidence in nurses through high-fidelity simulation-based learning. *Journal of Continuing Education in Nursing, 45,* 360–365. Mathew, B. (2014). Using a social networking tool for blended learning in staff training: Sharing experience from practice. *Journal of Neonatal Nursing, 20,* 90–94.
Management	Harris, D., & Cohn, T. (2014). Designing and opening a new hospital with a culture and foundation of Magnet®: An exemplar in transformational leadership. *Nurse Leader, 12*(4), 62–77. Kallas, K.D. (2014). Profile of an excellent nurse manager: Identifying and developing health care team leaders. *Nursing Administration Quarterly, 38,* 261–268.
Theoretical	Petersen, C.L. (2014). Spiritual care of the child with cancer at the end of life: A concept analysis. *Journal of Advanced Nursing, 70,* 1243–1253. Park, M., & Jones, C.B. (2010). A retention strategy for newly graduated nurses: An integrative review of orientation programs. *Journal for Nurses in Staff Development, 26,* 142–151.
Continuing education (CE), including continuing nursing education (CNE)	[CNE Article] McAfee, N., Seidel, K., Watkins, S., & Flynn, J.T. (2010). A continuous quality improvement project to decrease hemodialysis catheter infections in pediatric patients: Use of a closed luer-lock access cap. *Nephrology Nursing Journal, 37,* 541–544. [CE] Narayan, M.C. (2013). Using SBAR communications in efforts to prevent patient rehospitalizations. *Home Healthcare Nurse, 31,* 504–517. Park, M., & Jones, C.B. (2010). A retention strategy for newly graduated nurses: An integrative review of orientation programs. *Journal for Nurses in Staff Development, 26,* 142–151.

(Continued on next page)

Table 8-1. Types of Manuscripts Included in Peer-Reviewed Journals *(Continued)*

Type of Manuscript	Examples
Special features	[Highlights From the Hill] Luther, A.P. (2014). A mid-year status report on issues of interest to nurses. *ORL–Head and Neck Nursing, 32*(3), 10–12. [Research Corner] Riesenberg, L.A., & Justice, E.M. (2014). Conducting a successful systematic review of the literature, part 1. *Nursing2014, 44*(4), 13–17.

topics; clinical challenges; genetics and genomics; methods and meaning; oncology updates on various topics; and leadership and professional development. The *Journal of Continuing Education in Nursing* offers many education-focused features, such as administrative angles, clinical updates, leadership and development, teaching tips, and CE articles that nurses can complete to obtain contact hour certificates.

Decide on Authorship

As you reflect on your topic and type of manuscript, decide if you will author the manuscript by yourself or if you will write it with a colleague or group of colleagues. If you plan on authoring with others, discuss authorship issues beforehand. First, decide the authors of the paper and discuss expectations of authorship. To be considered an author, an individual should have made a significant contribution to the manuscript (International Committee of Medical Journal Editors [ICMJE], n.d.).

According to ICMJE (n.d., para. 3), individuals who want to be considered for authorship need to meet four criteria:

- Substantial contributions to the conception or design of the work; or the acquisition, analysis, or interpretation of data for the work
- Drafting the work or revising it critically for important intellectual content
- Final approval of the version to be published
- Agreement to be accountable for all aspects of the work in ensuring that questions related to the accuracy or integrity of any part of the work are appropriately investigated and resolved.

Some journals request that authors confirm, in writing, the specific roles that they played in manuscript preparation. If individuals helped you with a manuscript but did not meet all of the criteria for authorship, recognize them in the article with an acknowledgment. A journal's author guidelines or editorial staff can specify how this information can be added.

After deciding on the authors, have a preliminary discussion regarding the order they will be listed. The first author listed is the person who assumes most of the work related to the manuscript process, such as the preparation, submission, and follow-up (Oermann & Hays, 2016). The first author is usually the contact person, the individual the editor corresponds with throughout the publishing process. Determine the order of the remaining authors using a cooperative approach. Arrive at an understanding about authorship prior to submitting your manuscript to avoid misunderstandings (Oermann & Hays, 2016).

Step 2: Research the Past

After identifying an idea for your manuscript, confirm and clarify your topic by researching it in published literature, limiting your search to the past five years (unless your topic warrants otherwise). Conduct a systematic search using reputable health-related databases, such as CINAHL (Cumulative Index to Nursing and Allied Health Literature), Medline, or PubMed. Ask your hospital's librarian for assistance with this search to ensure a comprehensive review on your topic. As you retrieve relevant articles, note the journals that published them, as this information may help you target a journal for your manuscript. Be sure to review the reference list at the end of each article to identify additional resources. If you discover that your idea has already been published, consider using a different perspective on the same topic, building upon that publication, or targeting a different audience. Suppose, for example, that you wanted to publish a clinical article about the postoperative care of patients with head and neck cancer following a total laryngectomy. Unfortunately, your review revealed that a considerable number of recent papers have already been published on the topic. Rather than abandoning your idea, you should explore creative and different perspectives on the topic. Write about a patient's post-laryngectomy homecare needs after discharge from the hospital, detail successful teaching strategies that helped promote patient self-care after surgery, or discuss how you managed a difficult clinical situation. You also could invite colleagues who work in the operating and recovery rooms of your organization to join you in coauthoring a paper about the perioperative phase of patient recovery. Step back and focus on ways that nurses promote health practices that individuals can use to prevent laryngeal cancer.

Step 3: Define Your Readers

After you have confirmed your idea, searched the literature, and determined coauthors, the next step is to identify and define your readers. Similar to previous steps, this task also can help refine the purpose of your manuscript and determine the journals you may want to target.

Journals identify their target readers and make this information publicly available on their websites. For example, the target readers of the *Journal of Continuing Education in Nursing* are "continuing education and staff development professionals, nurse administrators, and nurse educators in all healthcare settings" (Healio, n.d., para. 1), while the *Clinical Journal of Oncology Nursing* is aimed at the "practicing nurse specializing in the care of patients with an actual or potential diagnosis of cancer" (Oncology Nursing Society, n.d., para. 1).

If your target audience includes clinical nurses, you may want to focus on a specific specialty, such as medical-surgical, critical care, or oncology nursing. If you are targeting nurses who are generalists, determine their work setting, such as ambulatory, acute, home, or long-term care. If educators are included in your target audience, decide if they are patient educators, academic educators (faculty) in schools of nursing, NPDSs, or other clinical educators employed in community-based wellness centers. Use a similar approach when targeting nurse managers or researchers. The more specific you are, the easier it will be for you to develop your manuscript and identify journals. Also consider consumers, family caregivers, and other healthcare workers (e.g., assistive personnel, student nurses, physical therapists, occupational therapists, physicians) as possible audiences.

Step 4: Target a Specific Journal

Now that you have defined your readers, target two or three journals that fit your topic, audience, purpose, manuscript, and other factors important to you. Focus on journals you like or ones that are familiar to you. You can access a comprehensive list of nursing journals using the links in the Helpful Websites section at the end of this chapter. For example, a directory of nursing journals developed by the International Academy of Nursing Editors (INANE) and *Nurse Author & Editor* is available at http://nursingeditors.com/journals-directory. This directory provides an alphabetical listing of journals with descriptions and links to editors' email addresses and author guidelines. The Biosemantics Group also has a useful feature called Jane (Journal/Author Name Estimator), which includes a search function, ranking information about each journal, and sample articles (http://jane.biosemantics.org).

Submit your manuscript to only one journal at a time (Oermann & Hays, 2016). This point is crucial, as lack of compliance may be considered a violation of copyright laws. Because the journal's reviewers and editor invest a significant amount of time reviewing your manuscript after it is submitted, it is understandable to allow them time to provide you with their suggestions and decision. However, if you decide to withdraw your manuscript at any time or submit it to a second journal, it is important to immediately notify the first journal's editor.

Begin the submission process by retrieving a copy of the author guidelines from each journal's website. Although these guidelines may vary among your selected journals, they usually provide the journal's mission or purpose statements, target readers, requirements for manuscript preparation, and review processes. Figure 8-2 illustrates several characteristics that you may want to investigate when deciding on a journal. Use this form to record your findings and rank your top journals. Gain as much information about the journals as you can to help make your decision.

Peer Reviewed/Refereed

When selecting your top journals, make sure that they are peer reviewed or refereed. Being a refereed journal means that your manuscript will be reviewed by nurses across the country who are experts on publishing and your topic (Polit & Beck, 2012). These nurses are volunteers accepted by an editor to serve as a reviewer for a specific journal, read your manuscript, and offer their expert feedback using journal guidelines. The nurses who conduct a critical review of your manuscript and subsequently provide an editor with their suggestions regarding publication are known as *peer reviewers* (Polit & Beck, 2012). A journal's editor considers these recommendations and makes the final decision regarding manuscript publication. Most journals use a double-blind review process in which authors and peer reviewers do not have access to any identifying information about each other during the review process (Oermann & Hays, 2016). Having your manuscript withstand the scrutiny of expert nurses in your field adds prestige and value to the article. Christenbery (2011) emphasized the importance of the peer-review process as a means of ensuring the quality of both nursing knowledge and patient outcomes. The author also provided a detailed history and overview of the peer-review process and a template that can be followed by advanced practice nurses when preparing a manuscript.

Mission/Purpose

Review the mission or purpose of your targeted journals stated in their author guidelines or websites. Determine if the each journal is associated with a national professional nursing organization or a publishing company. Membership in a professional nursing organization usually includes access to its print or online journals. For example, the *Oncology Nursing Forum* and the *Clinical Journal of Oncology Nursing* are two journals both associated with the Oncology Nursing Society. Similarly, *MEDSURG Nursing* is affiliated with the Academy of Medical-Surgical Nurses, and the *Journal for Nurses in Professional Development* is associated with the Association for Nursing Professional Development. Conversely, the *Journal of Continuing Education in Nursing* and the *Nurse Educator* are not directly affiliated with a professional nursing organization and are managed by independent publishers. Find out if the journal you choose is an established publication or a newly created journal that may not yet have a significant backlog of manuscripts.

| Figure 8-2. Factors to Consider When Selecting a Journal for Publication ||
Journal Characteristics	Notes
Peer-reviewed/refereed journal	
Mission/purpose	
Target readers	
Types of articles published, special departments, or features (page limits)	
Acceptance and rejection rates	
Journal metrics/ranking	
Independent publisher or associated with a professional nursing organization	
Number of issues published each year; number of pages in each issue	
Manuscript preparation and submission process (style, electronic or hard copy)	
Preprint/early online viewing available	
New or established journal	
Journal prestige and reputation	
Editorial board members	
Use of images and photographs in articles	
Journal circulation	
Availability of print, online, and prepublication	
Supplements or themed issues	
Predatory publisher list	

Target Readers

As stated previously, a journal's author guidelines should contain information regarding the target audience. This readership may be as broad as professional nurses or as specific as perioperative nurses. Nursing education journals also may target academic educators (i.e., school of nursing faculty), NPD educators, or both. It is important to understand a journal's readership and use language appropriate for that group. Polit and Northam (2010) advocated that nurses should also explore publishing options in non-nursing journals. The authors identified 64 journals that would be appropriate publishing outlets for nursing information.

Journal Reputation

Explore the reputation of your journal candidates by doing homework on your own and asking colleagues and mentors about each journal. First, learn about the professional reputations of journal editors and editorial board members and determine if you, as a potential author, can directly communicate with each journal's editors (INANE Predatory Publishing Practices Collaborative, 2014). Next, ensure that each journal uses a quality peer-review process for submitted manuscripts and that each follows "sound business and publishing practices" (INANE Predatory Publishing Practice Collaborative, 2014, p. 4). Then, be sure that the journals are listed in the INANE/*Nurse Author & Editor* Directory of Nursing Journals, reports a valid impact factor, and explicitly communicates any author processing charges (INANE Predatory Publishing Practices Collaborative, 2014). Finally, investigate whether the journals hold membership in the Committee on Publication Ethics (n.d.), an international organization that provides editors and publishers an environment where they can discuss issues related to ethics and misconduct in both research and publishing.

As you investigate journal reputations, be aware of predatory publishers who use social media to solicit potential authors to publish in their open-access journals (Beall, 2013) that either do not exist or lack quality peer-review standards (Beall, 2012b). These publishers typically offer an extremely fast peer-review process (INANE Predatory Publishing Practices Collaborative, 2014), lack apparent contact information (Beall, 2012b), and charge authors a varied and often hidden processing fee (Beall, 2012b). If you have any concerns about a journal or its publisher, access Beall's *Scholarly Open Access* blog and List of Predatory Publishers (http://scholarlyoa.com/publishers) (Beall, 2012a).

In our recommendations to nurse educators to recognize and contend with predatory publishers, Nolfi, Myers, and I emphasized the importance of consulting with your hospital or school librarian to determine if a journal is predatory (Nolfi, Lockhart, & Myers, 2015). We also shared several resources to target reputable journals and ways to inform colleagues and newly graduated nurse researchers about the risks of predatory publishers.

Journal Metrics and Data

Discover all you can about your target journals by using statistics and metrics. If available, note each journal's ranking or impact factor. An impact factor is the "annual measure of citation frequency for an average article in a given journal . . . the ratio between citations and citable items published in the journal in a specified period" (Polit & Beck, 2012, p. 730). In basic terms, a journal's impact factor is how often articles from a journal have been cited in other journals during a specific two- or five-year period (Oermann & Shaw-Kokot, 2013). Impact factor scores may be posted on a journal's website or accessed from Thomson Reuters' Journal Citation Reports (http://thomsonreuters.com/journal-citation-reports). Journals must be indexed for two to three years before an impact factor is calculated. Impact factors for most nursing journals range from 0.027 to 2.926, with higher numbers found in research-based journals (Oermann & Shaw-Kokot, 2013, p. 483).

Review a journal's acceptance and rejection rates if this information is available. This information can help you estimate your chances of getting published in a specific journal.

Also, note the average time it takes for your manuscript to be reviewed and published once it has been accepted. More specifically, you should note the time it takes from manuscript submission to a decision such as a revision, rejection, or acceptance; from acceptance to publication via online early preview; and from acceptance to publication in print form. Knowing that it may take a year or longer to see your submitted manuscript in print form should put this process in proper perspective.

You may decide to submit your manuscript to a specific journal because, if published, it will be exposed to a large readership. One way to determine the size of a journal's readership is to check its circulation rate.

You may also want to consider the number and type of articles published in each journal issue and the number of issues published each year. For example, some authors choose journals that publish monthly issues or issues with a large volume of articles, assuming this approach may increase the odds of having their manuscript published in a timely manner. The number of issues published by journals each year varies, with some journals publishing monthly and others publishing as few as four or six issues each year.

Types of Articles Published and Journal Features

Review the types of articles that journals publish and their various features. Pay attention to whether a journal publishes primarily clinical articles, data-based (research) reports, theoretical papers, or other particular types. Some journals publish articles in print, while others publish online, allowing readers quick and easy access via a web-based, password-protected system. Some journals publish issues or supplements based on themes (e.g., palliative care). Themed issues are usually announced in advance to give authors time to adjust and prepare. Also, note if a journal allows figures, images, or photographs and if these appear in black and white or color. Some journals provide subscribers helpful information about articles using social media (e.g., Facebook, Twitter, LinkedIn), email blasts, and meeting exhibits.

Some journals publish articles using an open-access format, allowing readers to review, download, or print these articles from the Internet (Broome, 2014). Authors are charged a fee to publish in an open-access journal, and copyright status varies on a case-by-case basis. A listing of open-access journals can be found at https://doaj.org (Broome, 2014). While the number of nursing journals published using the open-access method is small compared to those in other disciplines, the format is rising in popularity. Later in this chapter, you will learn how to assess the quality of open-access journals.

Manuscript Preparation Logistics

Depending on the type of article you plan on publishing (e.g., feature, brief), review a journal's requirements on page/word limits, required sections, and designated lengths. Some journals include references, tables, figures, or images in their page/word limits, whereas others count only the body text. Note the formatting style required to prepare the paper, such as American Psychological Association (APA) or American Medical Association (AMA). Understand the process and timeline for the review process. Most journals use web-based electronic systems for journal submission, the peer-review process, and required documentation.

Step 5: Refine Your Paper With a Purpose and Outline

After a thorough search, determine the top journal choice for your manuscript submission. You must now adjust and refine your manuscript with a purpose and initial outline based on sample articles you retrieved from this journal. Start this process by developing a one-sentence statement that best describes the purpose of your manuscript. This task is often a challenge for new authors, as it forces them to refine the primary focus of their papers. A purpose statement should be included in the final manuscript so readers can understand its intended direction. For example, an article I published with colleagues concerning oncology content in prelicensure RN programs included this sentence as its purpose: "This article describes the findings of a national survey of accredited prelicensure RN (diploma, ADN, and BSN) academic programs" (Lockhart et al., 2013, p. 384). Similarly, Sobecki-Ryniak and Krouse (2013) shared the purpose of their literature review using this statement: "The purpose of this literature review is to explore the historical progression of treatment and its impact on care requisites in patients with head and neck cancer" (p. 660).

After identifying your purpose statement, draft an outline for your manuscript using a sample article as a model. Pay attention to each heading and subheading of this sample, using this style to draft your outline. Remember that you can change your outline as you further develop your manuscript's content; however, the more specific you are now, the easier it will be to prepare your final manuscript. Expect to spend a significant amount of time on this step.

Several reporting guidelines already exist for authors preparing certain types of manuscripts. For example, the traditional introduction, methods, results, and discussion (IMRAD) model is suggested when authors are preparing a research document (Oermann & Hays, 2016; Polit & Beck, 2012). For nonresearch articles, consider using the nursing process steps to organize your paper: assessment, plan, diagnosis, outcomes/planning, implementation, and evaluation (ANA, 2014). If you plan on preparing an article as a CE feature, follow an example of a CE article from your chosen journal. In addition, investigate who develops the post-test questions that readers need to complete to receive CE credits.

Several reporting guidelines for research, quality improvement, and integrative and meta-analyses are available at websites such as the EQUATOR Network (www.equator-network.org) and the Cochrane Collaboration (www.cochrane.org). These guidelines offer a standardized approach for reporting initiatives so that interpretations can be made across reports. Many of these guidelines include checklists, examples, and templates that authors can use in publications. Table 8-2 lists publication reporting guidelines that authors can use to prepare manuscripts.

As you draft the purpose statement and outline for your manuscript, think of a creative title for your paper. The style and length of the title should be consistent with titles of other articles published in your chosen journal. It should include your paper's key concepts and takeaway message while maintaining professionalism and uniqueness to capture readers' interest. One way to create a title is to write down several key words that are essential elements of your manuscript. Others may use key words of your title when they conduct computer searches on the

Table 8-2. Sampling of Reporting Guidelines Used in Publishing

Guideline	Guideline Focus	Website
SQUIRE (Standards for Quality Improvement Reporting Excellence)	Quality improvement projects	www.squire-statement.org
STROBE (Strengthening the Reporting of Observational Studies in Epidemiology)	Observational studies in epidemiology (cohort, case-control studies, and cross-sectional studies)	www.strobe-statement.org
CONSORT (Consolidated Standards of Reporting Trials)	Clinical trials	www.consort-statement.org
PRISMA (Preferred Reporting Items for Systematic Reviews and Meta-Analyses)	Systematic reviews and meta-analyses	www.prisma-statement.org
COREQ (Consolidated Criteria for Reporting Qualitative Research)	Qualitative research (interviews and focus groups)	http://intqhc.oxfordjournals.org/content/19/6/349.long

topic. Your working title may change as you develop your manuscript or as your paper undergoes the review process.

Step 6: Contact the Editor

Now that you have a clear purpose and outline for your paper, contact the editor of your chosen journal to determine the journal's interest in your manuscript. According to Oermann and Hays (2016), it is acceptable practice to submit a query letter to more than one journal editor at a time. Some journal editors prefer inquiries from prospective authors, whereas others request that you submit your manuscript directly. You can often find this information in a journal's author guidelines. You also can inquire about interest in your manuscript by discussing your plans in person with editors at conferences sponsored by professional nursing organizations.

Some authors prepare their manuscripts prior to contacting an editor, whereas others wait for an editor's response before finalizing it. Over time, you will develop your own preferences and styles. If it is your first attempt at publishing, you may want to have something prepared in writing ahead of time. Developing a manuscript in advance permits you to make minor changes in a timely fashion. A drawback to this approach is that you may need to make major changes if you have to switch your journal choice to one with different features.

Figure 8-3 contains a sample email query to a journal editor. An editor's name and contact information can be found on a journal's website or on the front cover of a journal's print copy. Be sure that you have the name of the journal's current editor. The query communication (via email) usually consists of three sections: the opening, body, and closing.

In the opening portion of your query communication, be precise with the spelling and format of the editor's name, credentials, and title. These elements should look exactly as they appear in the journal's current issue, author guidelines, or website. When in doubt, contact the journal directly to obtain this information.

The body is the most crucial part of the query. It is where you explain why you think your manuscript is exactly what the journal needs. In presenting your case, answer the following questions:

- What?—Provide the title of the proposed manuscript as well as a brief overview of its content. An attached outline of your manuscript will help clarify your point.
- Why not?—Convince the editor of the importance of your topic. Stress how innovative it is and how it may influence nursing practice and patient outcomes.
- Why you?—Describe your expertise and why you are qualified to write this article.
- Why now?—Emphasize the timeliness of your topic and how it fits into what is happening in health care now and in the near future.
- Why them?—Explain how your idea matches the journal's focus and how it will appeal to its target readers. It is a good idea to mention the journal's name in the letter.
- When?—Inform the editor when you foresee your manuscript being ready for submission. Keep your timeline realistic and marketable.

Finish the communication with a formal closing. Be sure to include your name, credentials (e.g., RN, BSN), and certifications. Because a query communication is often your first contact with an editor, make sure that it looks professional. Use correct spelling, grammar, and sentence structure. Provide your current contact information in the closing.

Remember, a promising response from an editor to your query only means that your idea may be publishable. It is not a guarantee that your manuscript will be accepted once it is received. Your manuscript still needs to undergo the peer-review process that was described

---

Figure 8-3. Sample Query Communication With Journal Editor

From: Joan Lockhart (lockhartj@dsd.com)

To: Dr. Eileen Carter

Subject: Manuscript Query: Being Alert After Routine Procedures (Joan Lockhart)

Date: January 8, 2015

Dear Dr. Carter:

As an experienced medical-surgical staff nurse at City Hospital, I recently encountered a clinical emergency that would be appropriate for your *Emergency!* feature column.

An elderly man diagnosed with cholangiocarcinoma returned to his room following a percutaneous transhepatic cholangiogram (PTC). This radiological procedure, used to visualize the biliary structures, is frequently performed as both a diagnostic test and a therapeutic intervention.

Unfortunately, the patient developed one of the common risks associated with a PTC: bleeding at the injection site. His preexisting liver failure and associated deficiency of clotting factors only complicated the situation. A nurse's assessment of early changes in the patient's mental and hemodynamic status and prompt treatment saved his life.

I hope that you will find this manuscript appealing to your readers, because nurses play a pivotal role in detecting early complications in patients following routine invasive procedures. I would be able to have this manuscript available to you for review within the next month.

Your consideration of my request will be greatly appreciated. Please feel free to contact me at my email address (lockhartj@dsd.com) or by telephone (xxx-xxx-xxxx) anytime between 8:30 am and 5 pm E.T.

Sincerely,

Joan Such Lockhart, BSN, RN
Clinical Staff Nurse II, City Hospital
Pittsburgh, PA 26667
Email: lockhartj@dsd.com

---

earlier in this chapter. Timely submission of your manuscript may make a positive difference in its final outcome.

Step 7: Plan and Prioritize

Now it is time to prepare your manuscript using the author guidelines and sample articles of your chosen journal. Revise your outline if suggestions were made by the editor after your query. Positively visualize what your final paper will look like in print. Draft a preliminary layout of your article, considering the use of supplements, such as figures, tables, graphics, or photographs. Imagine what elements are needed and where they may be located within your paper. Confirm that other articles published in the journal include such visuals. Consider using bullets, boxed material, or bold print to highlight important points, if appropriate. Some journals refrain from using photographs, whereas others may limit their use to only black-and-white images. Remember to reflect upon the mental image you had of your article when you first started. When in doubt, contact the editor to clarify the addition of graphics. Prepare a timeline to complete this final step based on the target date you provided to the editor.

Getting Your Ideas on Paper

Focus on writing one section of your manuscript at a time. It is important to get your thoughts on paper first, paying little attention to editing, spelling, and grammar. You will fine-tune the features of your manuscript in step 8. Refer to the information you retrieved from your literature search throughout this process.

Some authors find it helpful to start with a section of their manuscript that they feel most comfortable writing before moving to more challenging ones. For example, if you are writing about a research study or a quality improvement project, you may find it easier to begin with the "Methods" section, as it is often more concrete and logical. Or, you may elect to draft tables or figures that will capture the essence of your results or intervention.

After you draft your tables, focus on the narrative portion of their accompanying sections, sharing only highlights of the graphics without major duplication. If graphics are challenging for you to prepare, seek someone with skills in developing tables and figures. Make sure that these items are prepared according to the journal's required style guidelines (e.g., APA, AMA). Tables and figures are vital parts of a manuscript, as they provide readers with meaningful and concise summaries.

Continue this process until you have drafted your entire manuscript. After completing the rough draft, review your manuscript and focus on its organization, flow, and writing logistics (e.g., sentence structure, grammar, spelling). Most journals specify a maximum page length and minimum font and margin sizes for manuscripts. Arrange the parts of your manuscript as specified. These parts usually consist of a title page, abstract (limited to a specified number of words), narrative text, reference list, and appendices (e.g., tables, charts, figures, photographs). Use primary references as much as possible and properly cite them throughout the manuscript and in the final reference list. Check that all references in the paper match those listed in the reference list. Review author guidelines regarding the use of reference management software (e.g., EndNote, Zotero, RefWorks) when writing your manuscript.

Importance of the Abstract

Because an abstract conveys key information about your manuscript, pay close attention to its content. An abstract should be completed after the initial draft of your manuscript. Follow the journal's guidelines in preparing your abstract, paying attention to required headings and word count. Model your abstract after a sample article and make each sentence meaningful and substantial. The abstract introduces readers to your paper, so make it inviting and capture the readers' interest (Fowler, 2011a).

Step 8: Prepare to Submit Your Manuscript

At this point, you should be finalizing your manuscript and exploring your choice journal's required documents and submission process. To begin this process, conduct a final check to make sure that your manuscript is organized according to the journal's author guidelines and sample articles. Pay attention to the amount of space designated for each section of your manuscript and determine if it aligns with the sample article. You may have a reason to deviate from the sample article's spacing. Check that you adhered to the journal's page limitations and word count limit for an abstract. Double-check that the paper's format, headings, subheadings, citations, references, tables, figures, and pagination adhere to the journal's required style. Make sure that you referred readers to each graphic within the body of the paper and that the graphics are in sequential order.

Next, review the narrative portion of your manuscript, including the abstract. Make sure it flows logically and that its tone, language, and style match those of the journal. Knatterud (2008) highlighted seven "patient-unfriendly" and seven "reader-unfriendly" terms that authors should exclude from their clinical papers. For example, patient-unfriendly terms included using the word *case* in place of *patient*. Similarly, beginning sentences with the words *there* or *it* is considered reader-unfriendly (Knatterud, 2008).

In addition to checking the tone, language, and style of your work, be sure to double-check the accuracy of the data included in tables and figures. Some authors find that reading their paper aloud helps them determine the rhythm of their writing and recognize any problem areas. As you finalize your paper, try to think like a reviewer. If you have access to reviewer guidelines for the journal, use them to conduct your final edit. Take this opportunity to finalize the title of your paper and confirm that it best reflects your final product. Ask colleagues, both nurses and non-nurses, to provide you with an objective critique of the manuscript.

The Ethics of Writing

As an author, you are responsible for ensuring that all of the information in your manuscript is accurate and true. Pay close attention to references, data, and other citations. Double-check your final manuscript for errors and ask a colleague to provide a second review.

Be alert to issues related to plagiarism, self-plagiarism, fabrication, and falsification. Plagiarism occurs when you submit someone else's work as your own (APA, 2010). Avoid plagiarism by carefully citing sources and quotations within your manuscript according to the specific guidelines outlined in official publication manuals, such as the *Publication Manual of the American Psychological Association* (APA, 2010). Detection of plagiarism will result in rejection and may prevent you from publishing in a journal in the future. Self-plagiarism is similar to plagiarism and occurs when you, as the author, paraphrase or use verbatim quotes from your previously published work and present them as new scholarship (APA, 2010). Review any exceptions using your publication manual guidelines. Fabrication occurs when the author reverts to "making up data or study results" (Polit & Beck, 2012, p. 169). Falsification differs in that it implies actions by the authors such as "manipulating research materials, equipment, or processes" or "changing or omitting data, or distorting results such that the research is not accurately represented in reports" (Polit & Beck, 2012, p. 169).

If you have coauthors for your manuscript, make sure they have met the criteria addressed in step 1. Some journals require authors to confirm coauthorship and designate the specific roles played in manuscript development. Make sure that all authors agree upon the final version of the entire manuscript before it is submitted to the journal.

Confirm that you have obtained written permission for images used in your manuscript, even if these photographs are of your students, colleagues, or family. Most institutions have prepared permission forms available for such situations. Check with author guidelines to determine other preferences regarding the use of images. Instructions describing how to obtain copyright permission should be available on the website of the journal in which an article and its image appeared. Copyright holders may charge a fee to use or adapt an image. Scan the visual and note the exact source and its page numbers, and include your emailed copyright request with your manuscript submission. Obtaining permission may take several weeks, so allow yourself sufficient time. Once copyright permission is granted, follow the journal's formatting style to determine the credit that should be noted with the image.

The Submission Process and Additional Documents

Most nursing journals use Internet-based commercial software systems for manuscript submission and review processes. Plan time to familiarize yourself with this software. Learn the various documents that you will need to upload, the required file formats, and how to upload them. Although you prepared your manuscript according to the journal's author guidelines, you may be asked to upload your manuscript as separate files with additional documents, such as a cover letter to the editor; a signed author statement regarding conflict of potential interest, authors' specific contributions to the manuscript, and copyright transfer to the publisher; and any copyright permissions you have secured. If your manuscript was coauthored, each author will need to complete and sign author forms. Although journals use different software systems, tracking your manuscript's progress during the review process and receiving reviewers' comments should be common features. You will use the same system to upload revisions, as needed.

If your journal does not use a software program for submission, simply follow the guidelines of the journal. Unless otherwise specified, the required documents can be attached in an email to the editor.

Be sure to keep copies of all the materials you used and submitted during the preparation of your manuscript, including the return receipt or email acknowledging receipt of your manuscript. Because this process may take more than a year, these come in handy if questions arise or if clarification is needed. For example, you may be asked to respond to a letter written to the editor in reference to your article. References may be useful when you prepare your next article. These documents also may be helpful to use as examples as you mentor other nurses in publishing.

Step 9: Deal With the Outcome

Waiting for a final response from a journal editor can be an exciting yet stressful time for authors. After the editor receives your paper, it is forwarded to two or more reviewers with expertise on the topic. Reviewers are usually given three or more weeks to submit their review using journal-specific guidelines. The editor needs time to consolidate the reviews and forward the final outcome of your manuscript to you. If at any time you feel that the review process has taken longer than expected, contact the editorial office of that journal for clarification.

In most situations, you can expect one of three possible decisions regarding your manuscript: acceptance, with or without minor revisions; major revisions needed and resubmit for second review; or rejection.

Acceptance

Congratulations! Your manuscript was accepted. Consider yourself very fortunate if you have no revisions to make. It is common to make minor revisions suggested by an editor and manuscript reviewers. Read these suggestions very carefully as you incorporate them into your draft, and resubmit your manuscript in a timely fashion per the journal's request. Be sure to contact the editor if you have any questions about reviewer comments or if you disagree with some suggestions.

The editor probably will ask you to complete some documents at this time. You will need to sign an author's agreement form that describes your role in the publishing process, such as copyright and ownership issues (Oermann & Hays, 2016). This means that the journal will be the legal owner of your work and that you cannot submit or publish it in any other journal. Be sure to clarify any questions with the editor before signing these forms.

The editor may ask you to revise your manuscript slightly and resubmit a revised version for review. You also may be asked if you are interested in purchasing reprints of your article once it is published. Most journals provide each author with a complimentary copy of the journal in which the article appears.

You will be given a tentative date of publication at this time, which varies depending on the journal. This time may be as long as a year or more from the date your manuscript was accepted. Although this date may change, it will give you an estimate of when to expect requested edits and a layout of your manuscript, called a *galley proof*, to review. You may be expected to review the galley in a very short turnaround time; be prepared to make this task a priority. Check the galley for accuracy against your original manuscript. Do not be surprised if the galley looks very different from the manuscript you submitted. Maintain a copy of the galley file and keep it with your manuscript documents.

Once your manuscript is accepted for publication, the editor may ask each author to complete a brief biographical form that includes questions about their expertise and educational background. You may be asked to sign a document to declare any conflict of interest and to transfer copyright to the journal. Return these forms promptly to avoid delays in processing your manuscript.

Revision

Some journals ask authors to make major revisions to their manuscript and resubmit it for a second review. Most often, the second review is conducted by the same reviewers who completed the first. Although this response is not an acceptance, neither is it a rejection. It may be best to consider this a second chance. Depending on reviewer comments, go back to the steps described previously in this chapter and repeat them, as needed. Follow the same author guidelines as you did when you first submitted your manuscript.

When developing your revised manuscript, carefully review the comments made by the editor and reviewers, responding to each comment appropriately (Happell, 2011; Wachs, Williamson, Moore, Roy, & Childre, 2010; Yoder-Wise, 2012). Unless the editor specifies differently, address the reviewers' comments in a cover letter attached to your revised manuscript. Yoder-Wise (2012) suggested creating a changes log, a five-column table labeled with a reviewer number, reviewer comment, author response, actions taken (by the author), and location in the manuscript. Contact the editor if you are unclear about a particular comment or if you feel a comment does not warrant a change. Be open to suggestions when discussing these issues and thank the reviewers for their time and helpful comments. In a study reported by Moos and Hawkins (2009), 14 editors identified the barriers that they perceived nurse authors faced during revision requests: author disagreement, reviewer disagreement, clarity, resources, and research methodology.

However, you may choose not to revise your manuscript. Instead, you might want to start from the beginning and submit your manuscript to your second journal choice. Take some time and reflect if this is the best option for you. If so, inform the editor of the first journal of your decision.

Rejection

No one likes rejection. It is important to remember that the editor rejected your manuscript, not you. According to a survey of 63 nursing journal editors, the most common reasons for the rejection of manuscripts included poorly written content, a topic not appropriate for the journal, or methodology issues (Northam, Yarbrough, Haas, & Duke, 2010).

After you have had some time to react and reflect, read the comments of the reviewers and editors closely and try to understand them from their perspective. Remember that learning to write for publication is similar to perfecting clinical skills; they both take practice and time. Be sure to ask the editor for specific suggestions regarding how to improve your manuscript and where to submit your manuscript in the future.

Many things may have occurred as the result of your manuscript being rejected. Perhaps you reacted emotionally with anger or despair, or maybe you concluded that you were a failure and vowed to never write again. It is all right to feel that way. Just set your manuscript aside for a few days until your negative emotions clear. Then, take a closer look at your manuscript and try to be objective. Rather than giving up and thinking that your work is not up to standards after a rejection, it is important to persevere (Illman, 2011). Learn something positive from the rejection of your manuscript, and keep the situation within the proper perspective. How important is this one experience in the total scheme of things? You did not lose anything. You only experienced a delay in meeting your goal. Start incorporating changes into your manuscript, targeting your second-choice journal. Be sure to reflect upon the tips for successful writing listed in Figure 8-4.

Figure 8-4. Tips for Becoming a Successful Author

Think positive.
Repeat to yourself, "I know I can do it!" Visualize yourself as an author. Imagine what your article will look like once it is published.

Be creative.
Think of a creative way to meet the objectives of your paper. How would you, as a learner, best understand the content?

Do your homework.
Conduct a self-assessment as an author. List your strengths and weaknesses and develop a plan to strengthen areas. Enroll in a writing course or attend a presentation on writing for publication. Seek out an experienced mentor or a self-help book.

Use proper English.
Time to review your old English notes. Proper grammar and sentence structure are a must.

Follow the rules.
A journal sets specific guidelines to follow for a reason. Do not jeopardize your chances for successful publication by not complying with details. If this is not your strength, ask a friend strong in this area for help.

Follow your plan.
Follow the strategic approach described above. Do not get discouraged if you need to use all your targeted journals. Learning to write is a process that often takes time.

Think like an editor or reviewer.
Imagine you are a reviewer who just received your manuscript. What impression does it make?

Practice, practice, and more practice.
Attempt to gain all the writing experience you can. Volunteer to write for your nursing organization's newsletter. Write a letter to the editor in your local newspaper or nursing journal.

Celebrate successes.
Celebrate your article with your peers and encourage them to publish.

Never give up!
Be persistent, keep trying, and learn from feedback.

Step 10: Celebrate!

If your manuscript is accepted, congratulate yourself on your success! Share this success and your article with colleagues in your organization's newsletter or in a poster or presentation at a professional conference. Also, consider using social media to share your accomplishment. Maintain a copy of your manuscript in your secure professional files and in your professional portfolio (see Chapter 10). Send a copy of the article to your manager for your work record. If you are enrolled in school, share a copy with a faculty mentor. Submit your article for display during the National Nurses Week celebration at your organization. Maintain a copy your journal article along with the information you collected in preparing the manuscript. Most publishing companies provide you with a few free physical copies of the journal that contains your article. You should also receive an electronic version, usually as a PDF. This will allow you to retrieve this information for future articles or in the event that a reader poses a question about your article. Now it is time to get started on your next manuscript and to help other nurses get involved in publishing. You are now an experienced author!

If you were not successful with your submission and your paper was rejected, still take pride in navigating the publishing process and learn from the feedback. Then, use the feedback for your next submission.

Summary

Writing for publication benefits the nursing profession, patients, and employers and offers both personal and professional rewards for authors. Nurses should consider creative strategies to overcome possible barriers to publishing, such as a lack of time and incentives; fear of failing; and limited resources, ideas, and publishing skills. The 10-Step Approach to Publishing (Lockhart, 2000) provides nurse authors with a practical guide to preparing a manuscript for publication in a nursing journal. This guide begins with identifying a publishable topic and ends with dealing with the final outcome and celebrating successes. NPDSs and unit-based educators can apply these steps with their own publishing goals and with clinical staff nurses in the writing for publication process.

Helpful Websites

- Biosemantics Group—Jane: Journal/Author Name Estimator: http://jane.biosemantics.org
- Committee on Publication Ethics—Promoting Integrity in Research Publication: http://publicationethics.org
- Elsevier Publishing Campus: www.publishingcampus.elsevier.com
- International Academy of Nursing Editors and *Nurse Author & Editor*—Directory of Nursing Journals: http://nursingeditors.com/journals-directory
- International Committee of Medical Journal Editors—Defining the Role of Authors and Contributors: www.icmje.org/recommendations/browse/roles-and-responsibilities/defining-the-role-of-authors-and-contributors.html
- Johns Hopkins University Press—Project MUSE: http://muse.jhu.edu/browse/titles/all?browse_view_type=list&limit_content_type=journal

- Lippincott Nursing Center—Nursing Articles and Publications: www.nursingcenter.com/articles-publications
- Publish, Not Perish: The Art and Craft of Publishing in Scholarly Journals: www.publishnotperish.org
- Purdue Online Writing Lab (OWL): https://owl.english.purdue.edu
- University of Toledo, Ramon Mulford Library—Instructions to Authors in the Health Sciences: http://mulford.utoledo.edu/instr

References

Alspach, G. (2010). Converting presentations into journal articles: A guide for nurses. *Critical Care Nurse, 30*(2), 8–15. doi:10.4037/ccn2010788

American Nurses Association. (n.d.). The nursing process. Retrieved from http://nursingworld.org/especiallyforyou/what-is-nursing/tools-you-need/thenursingprocess.html

American Nurses Association & National Nursing Staff Development Organization. (2010). *Nursing professional development: Scope and standards of practice.* Silver Spring, MD: American Nurses Association.

American Nurses Credentialing Center. (n.d.). Magnet Recognition Program® overview. Retrieved from http://www.nursecredentialing.org/Magnet/ProgramOverview

American Psychological Association. (2010). *Publication manual of the American Psychological Association* (6th ed.). Washington, DC: Author.

Ashton, K.S. (2012). Nurse educators and the future of nursing. *Journal of Continuing Education in Nursing, 43*, 113–116. doi:10.3928/00220124-20120116-02

Bandura, A. (1977). Self-efficacy: Toward a unifying theory of behavioral change. *Psychological Review, 84*, 191–215. doi:10.1037/0033-295X.84.2.191

Beall, J. (2012a). Beall's list of predatory publishers 2013. Scholarly Open Access. Retrieved from http://scholarlyoa.com/2012/12/06/bealls-list-of-predatory-publishers-2013

Beall, J. (2012b). Predatory publishers are corrupting open-access. *Nature, 489,* 179. doi:10.1038/489179a

Beall, J. (2013). Predatory publishing is just one of the consequences of gold open-access. *Learned Publishing, 26,* 79–83. doi:10.1087/20130203

Benton, M.J. (2014). Dissemination of evidence: Writing research manuscripts for successful publication. *Clinical Nurse Specialist, 28*(3), 138–140. doi:10.1097/NUR.0000000000000040.

Berkey, B., & Moore, S. (2012). Preparing research manuscripts for publication: A guide for authors. *Oncology Nursing Forum, 39,* 433–435. doi:10.1188/12.ONF.433-435

Broome, M.E. (2014). Open-access publishing: A disruptive innovation. *Nursing Outlook, 62,* 69–71. doi:10.1016/j.outlook.2014.02.004

Carlson, D.S., Masters., C., & Pfadt, E. (2008). Guiding the clinical nurse through research publication development. *Journal for Nurses in Staff Development, 24,* 222–225. doi:10.1097/01.NND.0000320679.73448.bf

Christenbery, T.L. (2011). Manuscript peer review: A guide for advanced practice nurses. *Journal of the American Academy of Nurse Practitioners, 23,* 15–22. doi:10.1111/j.1745-7599.2010.00572.x

Committee on Publication Ethics. (n.d.). About COPE. Retrieved from http://publicationethics.org/about

Driscoll, J., & Aquilina, R. (2011). Writing for publication: A practice six step approach. *International Journal of Orthopaedic and Trauma Nursing, 15,* 41–48. doi:10.1016/j.ijotn.2010.05.001

Fowler, J. (2010a). Writing for professional publication. Part 1. Motivation. *British Journal of Nursing, 19,* 1062. doi:10.12968/bjon.2010.19.16.78336

Fowler, J. (2011a). Writing for professional publication. Part 6: Writing the abstract. *British Journal of Nursing, 20,* 120. doi:10.12968/bjon.2011.20.2.120

Fowler, J. (2011b). Writing for professional publication. Part 9: Using client case studies. *British Journal of Nursing, 20,* 330. doi:10.12968/bjon.2011.20.5.330

Fowler, J. (2011c). Writing for professional publication. Part 10: Publishing a project report. *British Journal of Nursing, 20,* 371. doi:10.12968/bjon.2011.20.6.371

Gately, R. (2011). What's your story? *Nursing Spectrum, 21*(8), 31.

Gennaro, S. (2014). Writing: Ensuring the stars align [Editorial]. *Journal of Nursing Scholarship, 46,* 217. doi:10.1111/jnu.12098

Happell, B. (2008). From conference presentation to journal publication: A guide. *Nurse Researcher, 15*(2), 40–48. doi:10.7748/nr2008.01.15.2.40.c6328

Happell, B. (2011). Responding to reviewers' comments as part of writing for publication. *Nurse Researcher, 18*(4), 23–27. doi:10.7748/nr2011.07.18.4.23.c8632

Happell, B. (2012). Writing and publishing clinical articles: A practical guide. *Emergency Nurse, 20*(1), 33–38. doi:10.7748/en2012.04.20.1.33.c9042

Harrison, E. (2012). How to develop well-written case studies: The essential elements. *Nurse Educator, 37,* 67–70. doi:10.1097/NNE.0b013e3182461ba2

Healio. (n.d.). *Journal of Continuing Education in Nursing.* Retrieved from http://www.healio.com/nursing/journals/jcen

Heinrich, K.T., Tafas, C., & Jackson, C. (2011). Write a clinical narrative that clinches your advancement. *American Nurse Today, 6*(9), 24–25.

Holzmueller, C.G., & Pronovost, P.J. (2013). Organising a manuscript reporting quality improvement or patient safety research. *BMJ Quality and Safety, 22,* 777–785. doi:10.1136/bmjqs-2012-001603

Horstman, P., & Theeke, L. (2012). Using a professional writing retreat to enhance professional publications, presentations, and research development with staff nurses. *Journal for Nurses in Staff Development, 28,* 66–68. doi:10.1097/NND.0b013e31824b417a

Illman, J.C. (2011). If at first you don't succeed. *Nursing Standard, 25*(27), 62–63.

INANE Predatory Publishing Practices Collaborative. (2014, September). Predatory publishing: What editors need to know. *Nurse Author & Editor, 24*(3), 1–4. Retrieved from http://www.nurseauthoreditor.com/article.asp?id=261

International Academy of Nursing Editors & *Nurse Author & Editor.* (n.d.). Directory of nursing journals. Retrieved from http://nursingeditors.com/journals-directory

International Committee of Medical Journal Editors. (n.d.). Defining the role of authors and contributors. Retrieved from http://www.icmje.org/recommendations/browse/roles-and-responsibilities/defining-the-role-of-authors-and-contributors.html

Jackson, D. (2009). Mentored residential writing retreats: A leadership strategy to develop skills and generate outcomes in writing for publication. *Nurse Education Today, 29,* 9–15. doi:10.1016/j.nedt.2008.05.018

Kable, A.K., Pich, J., & Maslin-Prothero, S.E. (2012). A structured approach to documenting a search strategy for publication: A 12 step guideline for authors. *Nurse Education Today, 32,* 878–886. doi:10.1016/j.nedt.2012.02.022

Knatterud, M.E. (2008). With respect to patients and readers: Deadly terms to excise. *AMWA Journal, 23,* 113–117. Retrieved from http://www.amwa.org/files/Journal/2008v23n3.pdf

Knievel, J.E. (2008). Instruction to faculty and graduate students: A tutorial to teach publication strategies. *Portal: Libraries and the Academy, 8,* 175–186. doi:10.1353/pla.2008.0020

Lockhart, J.S. (2000). Writing for health care publications: A partnership between service and education. *Nurse Educator, 25,* 195–199. doi:10.1097/00006223-200007000-00016

Lockhart, J.S., Galioto, M., Oberleitner, M.G., Fulton, J.S., McMahon, D., George, K., … Mayer, D.K. (2013). A national survey of oncology content in prelicensure registered nurse programs. *Journal of Nursing Education, 52,* 383–390. doi:10.3928/01484834-20130529-01

Moos, D.D. (2009). *Barriers to the publication of scientific literature by academic certified registered nurse anesthetists* (Doctoral dissertation, College of Saint Mary). Retrieved from http://www.csm.edu/sites/default/files/Moos.pdf

Moos, D.D., & Hawkins, P. (2009). Barriers and strategies to the revision process from an editor's perspective. *Nursing Forum, 44*(2), 79–92.

Morgan, N.P. (2014). Writing for good health: Expressive writing can be a coping tool for nurses. *American Nurse Today, 9*(7), 22–23.

Morton, P.G. (2013a). Publishing in professional journals, Part I: Getting started. *AACN Advanced Critical Care, 24,* 162–168. doi:10.1097/NCI.0b013e318285db7c

Morton, P.G. (2013b). Publishing in professional journals, Part II: Writing the manuscript. *AACN Advanced Critical Care, 24,* 370–374. doi:10.1097/NCI.0b013e3182a92670

Nolfi, D.A., Lockhart, J.S., & Myers, C.R. (2015). Predatory publishing: What you don't know can hurt you. *Nurse Educator, 40,* 217–219.

Northam, S., Yarbrough, S., Haas, B., & Duke, G. (2010). Journal editor survey: Information to help authors publish. *Nurse Educator, 35,* 29–36. doi:10.1097/NNE.0b013e3181c42149

Oermann, M.H., & Hays, J.C. (2016). *Writing for publication in nursing* (3rd ed.). New York, NY: Springer.

Oermann, M.H., & Shaw-Kokot, J. (2013). Impact factor of nursing journals: What nurses need to know. *Journal of Continuing Education in Nursing, 44,* 293–299. doi:10.3928/00220124-20130501-14

Oncology Nursing Society. (n.d.). About *CJON*. Retrieved from https://cjon.ons.org/content/about-cjon

Polit, D.F., & Beck, C.T. (2012). *Nursing research: Generating and assessing evidence for nursing practice* (9th ed.). Philadelphia, PA: Wolters Kluwer Health/Lippincott Williams & Wilkins.

Polit, D.F., & Northam, S. (2010). Publication opportunities in nonnursing journals. *Nurse Educator, 35,* 237–242. doi:10.1097/NNE.0b013e3181f7f1ea

Price, B. (2008). Designing continuing professional development articles. *Nursing Management, 15*(8), 26–32. doi:10.7748/nm2008.12.15.8.26.c6879

Price, B. (2010). Disseminating best practice through publication in journals. *Nursing Standard, 24*(26), 35–41. doi:10.7748/ns2010.03.24.26.35.c7568

Price, B. (2014). Writing a journal article: Guidance for novice authors. *Nursing Standard, 28*(35), 40–47. doi:10.7748/ns2014.04.28.35.40.e8582

Price, B. (2015). Writing up research for publication. *Nursing Standard, 29*(19), 52–59. doi:10.7748/ns.29.19.52.e8764.

Richardson, A., & Carrick-Sen, D. (2011). Writing for publication made easy for nurses: An evaluation. *British Journal of Nursing, 20,* 756–759. doi:10.12968/bjon.2011.20.12.756

Smith, L.S. (2010). Good news about writing for your local newspaper. *Nursing Management, 41*(5), 43–45. doi:10.1097/01.NUMA.0000372033.52605.a6

Sobecki-Ryniak, D., & Krouse, H.L. (2013). Head and neck cancer: Historical evolution of treatment and patient self-care requirements. *Clinical Journal of Oncology Nursing, 17,* 659–663. doi:10.1188/13.CJON.659-663

Stone, T., Levett-Jones, T., Harris, M., & Sinclair, P.M. (2010). The genesis of 'the Neophytes': A writing support group for clinical nurses. *Nurse Education Today, 30,* 657–661. doi:10.1016/j.nedt.2009.12.020

Wachs, J.E., Williamson, G., Moore, P.V., Roy, D., & Childre, F. (2010). You're a published author! *AAOHN Journal, 58,* 233–236. Retrieved from http://whs.sagepub.com/content/58/6/233.abstract

Yoder-Wise, P. (2012). Responding to feedback: Making clear the changes made. *Nurse Author & Editor, 22*(1), 3.

CHAPTER 9

Sharing Your Expertise Through Abstracts, Oral Presentations, and Posters

I MAGINE that you have been asked to present a paper at a national conference for a professional nursing organization—or maybe you are interested in preparing a poster for a local clinical nursing workshop. Most of your colleagues have given presentations such as these, and their successes in these endeavors have made you eager to contribute your own expertise as well. Where do you start? What topic could you possibly present?

If you are like most nurses, you will have mixed emotions when presenting to other nurses or healthcare professionals. Part of you is thrilled that you were asked to share your nursing expertise, but another part is scared to death, wondering why you ever agreed to present in the first place.

Do not be alarmed, as you already have what it takes to create an excellent project. As a nurse, you have encountered many complex, stressful experiences, especially in the clinical setting. You came through most of these experiences with increased skills and confidence in dealing with similar clinical situations.

The approach you need to take to be effective at presentations is very similar to that of learning new clinical skills in nursing practice. You need to carefully assess the situation, develop a strategic plan, do your homework, and practice, practice, practice. Try to rely on the leadership and interpersonal skills that you developed in nursing school. Remember to always visualize a positive outcome. You can do it!

According to *Nursing Professional Development: Scope and Standards of Practice*, NPDSs are expected to report the outcomes of their continuing education (CE) efforts with others (American Nurses Association [ANA] & National Nursing Staff Development Organization, 2010; Dickerson, 2013). NPD standards related to research and leadership support this expectation and can be fulfilled through professional abstracts, posters, podium presentations, and publications (Dickerson, 2013). NPDSs also are expected to be role models in professional development activities, sharing their expertise and mentoring clinical nurses. As a unit-based educator, it is important that you demonstrate these professional behaviors in your own role and when helping staff nurses on your clinical unit.

As an NPDS, it is important to design practical, creative strategies that will help clinical nurses develop professionally with very few barriers. For example, Durkin (2011) promoted the professional development of staff nurses within a hospital by helping them create posters that were shared annually at an in-house event during National Nurses Week. Staff development specialists provided two to three hours of assistance per poster. The posters were categorized as Research, Education, Project, or Quality Improvement. Durkin reported an increase in the number and quality of posters over time, while nurses reported a greater level of comfort in poster development. Expenses related to this event were assumed by the hospital and determined as being more cost-effective than budgeting travel funds for individual nurses (Durkin, 2011).

Types of Presentations

Presentations can be viewed as being either formal or informal. A formal presentation often includes speaking in front of an audience, either at a podium or in a less formal environment. This oral or paper presentation, as it is sometimes called, is accompanied by audiovisuals, such as a PowerPoint® presentation, video, or other media. At some conferences, several speakers may present on related topics during a special session called a *symposium*.

Informal presentations can include roundtable sessions, panel discussions, and poster presentations. During a roundtable session, presenters informally share their projects with others and may use audiovisual supports such as flipcharts or whiteboards. Panel discussions consist of a group of experts who present contributions related to a particular topic. Each panel member may briefly present and respond to questions posed by an audience. A poster presentation is a visual representation of your project using a poster format. In this scenario, presenters stand next to their poster during a scheduled session and answer questions for viewers. Some conference personnel ask poster presenters to provide a brief oral summary of their poster for participants during a formal part of a conference.

Both formal and informal presentations are effective and efficient methods of sharing clinical projects with peers and publications (see Chapter 8). Although both types of presentations involve some preparation, each relies on different presenter skills. Some conferences require you to present exclusively using one of these formats. If it is your first time presenting, choose the option you feel most secure with and have the resources to complete. Table 9-1 outlines some advantages and disadvantages of both oral and poster presentations.

Pursuing Opportunities to Share Your Expertise

Let us assume that you are interested in sharing your expertise with colleagues either inside or outside your organization but are unsure how to find these opportunities. You can start by searching the websites of professional nursing organizations that you belong to or that pique your interest (see Chapter 7). You may have even already received an email inviting you to submit an abstract for a national or regional conference from one of your affiliated organizations. Most organizations advertise their calls for abstracts as far as six months prior to the conference date (Hedges, 2010).

If you are an NPDS and want to present on a topic related to your role, consider accessing the Association for Nursing Professional Development website (www.anpd.org) for information about its annual convention and other educational events. After finding an interesting program at this site, note the opening and closing dates of the abstract submission period. If you already missed the deadline, make a personal reminder to visit the site earlier next year. If the site contains a call for abstracts, carefully review the guidelines and save them in a file (hard copy or electronic) for your records and future retrieval.

Similarly, if you are mentoring clinical nurses interested in sharing their expertise in an oncology specialty, search oncology organizations such as the Oncology Nursing Society (ONS) (www.ons.org).

Table 9-1. Advantages and Disadvantages of Oral and Poster Presentation Types

Presentation Type	Advantages	Disadvantages
Oral	• By some sources, it is viewed as more prestigious than posters. • Content is portable and conducive to travel. • Presenter has more time to convey message than poster presenter. • Audiovisuals can be used in other projects. • Creativity can be used to influence content.	• Audiovisual production may be costly and time consuming. • Oral presentation may be overwhelming or cause anxiety. • It requires the presenter to convey information to learners using good oral presentation skills.
Poster	• Most of the preparation work is completed prior to the conference. • It allows individual interaction between viewer and presenter. • It permits informal sharing and networking with viewers. • Process may be less intimidating than an oral presentation. • Primary focus is on questions posed by the viewer. • Mutual learning on shared interests may occur between viewer and presenter. • Learning may occur without the presence of a presenter.	• Presentation may be viewed as less prestigious by some sources. • It may be time consuming to prepare by yourself. • If commercially prepared, costs are likely to increase significantly. • Creation requires artistic talent or resources. • Size may pose barriers related to portability. • Format limits time and space to convey message. • Materials require assembly, dismantling, and storage space. • It is difficult to reuse pieces in future projects.

More details on how to choose a topic and prepare an abstract for submission to a conference will be discussed in the next section. In addition, the Helpful Websites list at the end of this chapter provides resources that can help you develop professional presentations and posters.

Choosing a Topic to Present

If you do not have a topic in mind for your abstract, think about your role and responsibilities as an NPDS or unit-based educator. Consider your accomplishments in clinical practice, leadership, research, quality improvement, teaching, or education. You may also include topics related to one of the throughputs of the NPDS practice model (see Chapter 2). For example, you could share a successful leadership development program you implemented for nurse managers at your organization, the outcomes of a mentoring program you developed for newly hired nurses, or your use of simulation to help nurses become preceptors (see Chapter 5). Dickerson (2013) recommended that NPDSs share the outcomes of their CE programs through podium and poster presentations.

If you are mentoring staff nurses who work on a surgical oncology unit, have them reflect on their role expectations or criteria included in their organization's clinical advancement program (see Chapter 10). For example, they can share a unique case presentation illustrating a difficult patient situation that they managed, a quality improvement project on their clinical unit that helped reduce patient falls, or a mentoring project completed by a local chapter for student nurses interested in oncology.

Topics derived from either professional issues or life experiences also can provide ideas for presentations. Many of these approaches are similar to those used to generate topics for publication purposes (see Chapter 8). A poster, for example, can be an effective way to update peers at your workplace about new clinical policies or procedures.

Once you have an idea for a topic, match it with the theme and objectives of the conference, or use the conference theme to brainstorm ideas. Find out who the learners (audience) will be at the conference and what their expectations or learning needs may be regarding your topic.

If you already have a topic in mind but are having trouble ironing out its details, consider rethinking the perspective or angle you will take when presenting it. For example, a presentation that describes the steps involved when performing an advanced neurologic assessment is appropriate for a clinical nursing conference attended by RNs who provide direct care for patients at risk for neurologic impairments. In this case, the focus of your presentation is on the content of the assessment. On the other hand, if the conference is geared toward nurse educators, you may want to describe a simulation that you used in an online CE program aimed at helping nurses learn how to conduct a neurologic assessment. Using this approach, the perspective of the topic is on the teaching strategy rather than the content.

Preparing and Submitting an Abstract

Now that you have a topic, prepare your abstract according to your chosen conference's guidelines. If others also "own" the topic, be sure to invite them to provide input early in the preparation phase. Review the abstract guidelines again and develop a timeline. Begin with the due date for the abstract and work backward, allowing sufficient time to obtain input from your colleagues or a mentor. Determine and assign specific responsibilities with due dates.

The process for developing your abstract is very similar to the process described for drafting a manuscript (see Chapter 8). Develop a template (outline) using the headings stated in the abstract guidelines and prepare a rough draft. Abstract headings often differ depending on the conference and the type of abstract. Linder (2012) identified six common types of abstracts: research-related, theoretical, systematic reviews of the literature, clinical practice projects, education projects, and quality improvement projects. A few examples of abstract formats required by professional nursing conferences are presented in Table 9-2. If available, retrieve examples of abstracts used in the previous year's conference as models for your own abstract. If guidelines include the criteria that will be used by reviewers in judging the abstract, make sure that you address each criterion.

During this phase, focus on capturing the key points of your project, paying little attention to details such as grammar, spelling, word count, or sentence structure. Although word limits for abstracts can vary from 150 to 500 words (Linder, 2012), address this restriction after you have established the abstract's content. Gradually revise each section until your abstract is complete and resembles your model. Pay attention to the amount of information provided under each section. The "Results" and "Discussion" sections will garner the most interest from readers and should have more content than other sections. Some nurses find it beneficial to first work on less challenging sections of the abstract before moving on to more challenging ones.

Table 9-2. A Sampling of Abstract Headings

Headings	Source	Purpose
Purpose and Goals Background Methods Results	Robert Wood Johnson Foundation New Careers in Nursing, 2014 Annual Summit www.newcareersinnursing.org	General project
Problem Statement and Aims Methods Results Implications for Nursing	2014 Oncology Nursing Conference, Cleveland Clinic www.clevelandclinicmeded.com/live/courses/oncologynursing/default.asp	Oncology topics
Purpose Problem Significance Intervention Evaluation and Summary	41st Annual National Conference on Professional Nursing Education and Development, Professional Nurse Educators Group http://pneg.org/2014-conference	Nursing education
(Quantitative) Purpose Background Theoretical Framework (if applicable) Methods (Design, Sample, Setting, Measures, Analysis) Results Conclusions and Implications	ENRS 27th Annual Scientific Sessions, Eastern Nursing Research Society (ENRS) www.enrs-go.org/html/2015-conference.html	Research
(Qualitative) Purpose Background Methods (Design, Participants, Setting, Data Collection, Analytic Approach) Results Conclusions and Implications		

Create an informative title for your abstract that not only aligns with the conference's theme but also captures the attention of your readers. Your title needs to be professional and reflect the key message of your presentation. If developing a research abstract, include words that convey key aspects of your study, such as its variables, target population, and design (Russell & Ponferrada, 2012). Check whether abstract guidelines state any word limits for the title.

According to Ickes and Gambescia (2011), outstanding abstracts possess four qualities, referred to as the four Cs: complete, concise, clear, and cohesive. At this point, focus on these qualities as you review your abstract, now paying close attention to grammar, spelling, word count, and sentence structure. Each sentence of the abstract should be substantial, add value, and have meaning. Word count can often be managed by eliminating repetition, deleting words not vital to a sentence, and rephrasing sentences. Adhere to guidelines regarding the use of margins, font, style, size, capitalization, and other elements. Read your abstract aloud to confirm its flow. Ask colleagues and mentors to review your abstract and provide you with constructive feedback. You also may consider inviting reviewers unfamiliar with your project to take part in this evaluation (Linder, 2012).

Submit your abstract using the process outlined by the conference guidelines, saving a copy of these files for your records. If asked, indicate if you would accept presenting a podium presentation, a poster presentation, or both. Note the date of when decisions will be made, and follow up with a conference contact person if notification is not received by that date.

Anticipating Resources in Advance

Once your abstract has been accepted for a presentation, you will need to begin anticipating what resources you will need. Before you begin developing your presentation, review the instructions provided by the conference leaders regarding the specifications for your presentation and the due dates of key documents, such as objectives, audiovisual requests, speaker biographies, and conflict of interest forms. Carefully determine the resources (e.g., money, expert advice, special services) you will need to finish and present your project. Be sure to match your specific needs with resources available at your workplace. The resources available to you also will determine how you need to ultimately structure and present your topic. Check whether your workplace has a media center or instructional designer who can help you create audiovisuals for your presentation, such as PowerPoint slides, videos, photographs, images, or illustrations. Make an appointment with the center to discuss questions related to cost, format, and time that may be pertinent to your project. After you have researched the need for additional resources and other supplies, develop a tentative budget for your project. Include anticipated costs, such as typing, conducting literature searches, creating PowerPoint presentations or videos, duplicating handouts, and making poster materials. Do not forget the other costs associated with the conference, such as travel, lodging, meals, and registration. Some organizations offer either a reduced or waived registration fee for speakers. Also, check with your supervisor or adviser to see if your employer or school can share in any related costs. If not, seek opportunities that may have been advertised by conference planners. Next, think about other supplies or services you may need for your presentation. This may include typing text for your project, duplicating handouts, or even constructing your poster. Enter the cost of these items in your projected figures for your presentation.

Once you see the financial figures on paper, you will need to make decisions that keep your project within a range reasonable for your budget. For example, if your total costs exceed your budget allotment, you may choose to make your poster yourself rather than paying a media center.

Finally, develop a timeline for completing tasks related to your presentation, working backward from the day of the presentation to the time your topic was accepted. Allow sufficient time to prepare your presentation and meet the deadlines included in your conference acceptance letter. Although individuals require different timelines, give yourself several weeks to prepare, organize, and think through your project. Allow time for unexpected events, such as family and work crises, mistakes, or retyping, as well as time for obtaining colleagues' reviews and securing supplies. Figure 9-1 illustrates essential steps when developing your timeline.

Figure 9-1. Essential Steps Included in a Timeline for a Presentation
• Identify a topic.
• Target learners.
• Investigate time allotted.
• Consider the location.
• Specify and clarify objectives/outcomes.
• Outline essential content.
• Prepare a draft.
• Design visuals.
• Purchase materials (posters).
• Organize presentation.
• Create handouts.
• Perform a mock presentation.
• Practice, practice, practice.

Developing the Content

In developing content for your presentation, use an approach similar to those previously discussed in creating content for an in-service program (see Chapter 6) and preparing a manuscript (see Chapter 8). If you plan on presenting a research project (see Chapter 12), consider relying on the major headings used for most research proposals, such as the IMRAD (introduction, methods, results, and discussion) template (see Chapter 8) (Polit & Beck, 2012).

If you are presenting at a conference, ask a session coordinator or a conference contact if any specifications exist for your presentation. Perhaps your topic came about as the result of a needs assessment conducted by the conference planning committee. If this is the case, the contact person may have some additional information that may help you develop your project. If no background information is available about your topic, think your project through logically, as though you were a member of the audience.

As you develop your content, adhere to appropriate reference manuals for including citations to support your statements. Some conference organizers recommend that presenters integrate current evidence throughout their presentations. An example of evidence-based education guidelines for presenters developed by ONS can be found at https://onsopcontent.ons.org/SpeakerUpload/Guidelines/FAQ.aspx.

Identifying Target Learners

It is vital that you know who your learners are as you prepare your presentation. You need to tailor your presentation's content level according to the learners' existing knowledge or skill levels. If your learners possess a beginning level of understanding on your topic, establish a baseline. If your audience consists of learners with a more advanced knowledge of the topic, customize your presentation at a higher, more complex level. You may need to quickly review the basics on your topic before you start your presentation at a more involved level. Regardless, you want to be in sync with your learners to maintain their interest. Attempt to create a balance of content that will not leave them either bored or overwhelmed.

Longo and Tierney (2012) advised presenters to carefully review the principles of adult learning theory and tailor this information to their audience of learners. After identifying who your learners are and their respective work settings, seek more information about their proficiency levels, performance gaps, and expected outcomes of your presentation (Longo & Tierney, 2012). As a presenter, it is important to design an evaluation tool to help recognize whether your presentation was perceived by the audience as successful in meeting their learning needs.

Investigating Time Allotted

Find out how much time is allotted for your presentation and practice staying within this time frame. If you have 20 minutes, be sure to subtract some time for introductions, questions, and other procedures. It often is advantageous to end a presentation a little earlier than scheduled rather than to extend it or take some of the next speaker's time. It is also helpful to investigate what presentations learners will most likely attend before and after yours. If they will experience several formal lectures before they arrive at your presentation, you may prefer to change yours to a discussion format with more audience participation.

If you are presenting a poster, you will be told when and where to set it up and when to dismantle it. Some conferences have a scheduled time when poster presenters provide a brief summary of their projects. Be sure you are available during these times by scheduling accordingly.

Hedges (2010) recommended that presenters prepare their "elevator speech" in advance of a poster viewing event. This speech is intended to serve as a takeaway message or a brief summary of the main points and key outcomes of your project. Avoid sharing too many details while conversing with viewers, allowing time for them to pose questions.

Specifying and Clarifying Objectives and Purpose

Similar to the process for manuscript preparation (see Chapter 8), think about the overall purpose of your presentation and try to state it succinctly to yourself in one sentence. As you do this, keep the knowledge level of your learners in mind. An example might be: *The purpose of this presentation is to enable the learner to describe the development of a unit-based education program for RNs assigned to a specialty unit.*

Outline specific objectives or outcomes that you hope learners will be able to demonstrate following your presentation. This will help you focus the direction of your content. Remember that objectives must be learner centered and should not be too simple nor extremely complex. Develop these objectives using a process similar to the one described for in-service programs (see Chapter 6). The number of objectives you develop may be influenced by a variety of factors, including the content and length of your presentation. Experts in CE programs recommend having one or two objectives per hour of presentation (Pennsylvania State Nurses Association, 2013). If you are preparing a poster, design it so that viewers will be able to quickly capture its essence.

Outlining Essential Content

Systematically research information related to your topic, seeking assistance from a local librarian or the Internet, as needed. Be sure to talk with various experts on your topic, and supplement your content with materials prepared by community agencies, if appropriate.

Once you have carefully organized your materials, draft a detailed outline of the presentation. Be sure to follow the directions established by your objectives, as the content should help learners in meeting these objectives. If your presentation is a description of a research project, use the main headings of your proposal as a guide.

Preparing a Draft

Prepare a draft of your presentation that is based on your outline. The amount of detail needed for your draft will depend on whether you plan to read your presentation verbatim or closely follow primary points. Although some presenters prefer preparing a script ahead of time, others record only general thoughts and use slides as cues. If it is your first presentation, it may be best to have your speech written verbatim on paper, as you can rely on it if other options fail. Although the decision is yours, be sure to practice your approach before you decide on a method.

One of the most convenient ways to prepare your script is to type it on a computer, allowing the ability to change font size and double-space text to facilitate reading in dim lighting. The use of upper- and lowercase letters is more readable than using all capital letters. Try to use the fewest number of pages possible during your talk, minimizing the chance that shuffling papers will distract participants. If you record your speech on small note cards, be sure to write sufficient information.

If you are developing your presentation using PowerPoint, you can use its various features to develop your script, such as the "Notes" feature that allows you to add text below each slide that only you can view. You can also choose to use the "Handout" option that records keynotes next to your slide images. Regardless of what option you choose, be sure the strategy is comfortable for you.

Planning and Developing Audiovisuals

Once you are fairly satisfied with the overall outline and draft of your presentation, plan to enhance it with some type of visuals. You need to use audiovisuals that are appropriate for your presentation and match both your resources and your budget. Conference planners will ask you in advance what equipment you will need for your presentation.

One approach to visuals is to divide your presentation into major sections of content and identify at least one image or slide for each section. You can use slides that contain words or illustrations that reflect each section of your presentation. Creating a grid or storyboard that contains categories based on your purpose may help you visualize an overall picture.

Start with an image, such as a logo or photograph, that depicts your workplace, school, or the agency that is sponsoring you to attend the conference. Obtain the appropriate permissions to use this image, asking public affairs representatives for assistance. Pay close attention to authorship issues (see Chapter 8) and give appropriate acknowledgment for content used.

Federal copyright laws protect the work of an individual or company that owns a copyright (Catalano, 2014). Some use of works falls within a category as an educational exception. Such exceptions allow you to use the work if your presentation is of an educational nature, is offered in a classroom, and will not be recorded for learners to access after the presentation (Catalano, 2014). Your use also needs to comply with standards of brevity (use only a limited portion of the work), spontaneity (use the image only once), and cumulative effect (use only one source by the author) (Catalano, 2014). If you own the work, you are permitted to use it as you choose. You can obtain copyright permission to use the work of others by contacting the owner of the copyright and crediting the owner, as advised by the owner or writing style manual.

You can access images and videos that are free of most copyright limitations at the Creative Commons website (http://creativecommons.org/about) (Catalano, 2014). The Helpful Websites section at the end of this chapter provides a list of additional sources where you can obtain visuals for your presentation.

Images and Slides

PowerPoint assists you in designing slides that contain text or graphics, such as charts or pictures, with color options that can either be chosen by the user or selected from software templates. Explore using sound and slide transition features to add extra punch to your presentation. PowerPoint is fairly easy to master, but seeking expert help the first time you create a presentation is advised.

If you decide to use PowerPoint for your presentation, acquire and set up the equipment needed for this program ahead of time. You will need to use an LCD projector to project your PowerPoint presentation from your laptop to a large screen. LCD projectors vary in size, weight, brightness, resolution, and cost, but are compatible with most laptop platforms. Check with your conference contact person in advance to determine if this equipment is available.

Investigate if a laptop computer is provided or if you will need to bring your own. Also, clarify access to anything else that you requested upon acceptance of your presentation, including a speaker podium, light, microphone (portable or stationary), and Internet access.

Some centers have the ability to copy pictures or graphics from books or journals using software programs or a scanner. If you are talented in this area, capture images with a digital camera and obtain permissions for use, as appropriate. Be sure to factor in some extra time for retakes. If you need to capture a very close shot outside the focal range of your camera, you may need to rely on expert help. Regardless of your resources, prepare to hold the interest of your audience with slides that contain both text and graphics.

Do not forget to address issues with font size, text and background color, and the number of words per line. Consider using the prepared templates with ideal color combinations of text, background, and style.

Once you create your slides, make sure that they are arranged in order based on their appearance in the presentation. Using the Slide Sorter view option in PowerPoint makes this step easier. Keep a copy of your presentation with you as you travel, and avoid placing it in checked luggage.

Videos

If you plan on using videos or accessing the Internet during your presentation, start by obtaining written permission from the proper authorities. Practice using the video or accessing the Internet with your presentation in advance. Be alert to details such as accurate timing of video and sound. View the seating arrangement of the conference room to make sure the audience can both see and hear the video adequately. If an audiovisual expert is not available at the conference, arrange for someone with experience to operate this equipment and troubleshoot problems if they arise.

Handouts

Supplement key points of your presentation with printed or electronic handouts. These allow learners to spend time listening to your presentation rather than focusing on note-taking. A few good handouts can also add additional content to your topic, especially if you have limited time to present. To save time, avoid including images that need copyright permissions in these handouts.

Handouts are also a useful supplement to a poster presentation. If your poster is research based, a printed abstract of your project, reference list, or details on data analysis can enhance its content. Sharing your mailing address, telephone number, or email address on a handout is a common way to develop a network with others interested in your topic.

Investigate if the software you used to prepare your presentation also has the ability to generate a smaller version of your presentation that can be used as a handout, as is the case with PowerPoint. Talk with the conference planning committee to decide who is responsible for duplicating handouts and to clarify how participants will access your presentation. If it is your responsibility to provide handouts, ask conference planners for the anticipated number of participants attending your presentation. Prepare a few more handouts in case unexpected participants arrive. Be sure to monitor the cost of duplicating large numbers of handouts, especially when printed in color.

Considering Location

Find out as much as you can about the location of the conference and what is planned for your presentation. As soon as you have the opportunity, visit your assigned presentation space and confirm available resources. Doing this well in advance of your presentation will afford you some time to make any last-minute changes.

If you are scheduled to give an oral presentation, visit the room in which you will present. It is a good idea to do this when no one is in the room, such as during breaks or when the conference has finished for the day. Simulate your presentation and make sure all its components (e.g., audiovisuals, PowerPoint, Internet) are working properly. Sometimes, speaker-ready rooms are offered as an alternative practice setting for presenters. The location of these practice rooms is often listed in the conference materials. If not, ask staff at the conference registration desk. If using your own laptop, save your presentation file on your desktop and practice advancing slides with the conference room's remote control. Use a laser pointer if it will help with your presentation.

Be sure to dim the lights in the conference room appropriately, checking if lighting is sufficient for learners to view the slides and for you to see your notes. Practice using the room's microphone, and make sure you have water available to sip during your presentation.

Look at the seating arrangements of the room and plan where you will sit prior to your presentation. It is often helpful to sit close to the front so that you will not take too much time getting to the stage prior to your talk. If possible, listen to several speakers present their topics in the same room before you present. Carefully observe what works for them.

If you are giving a poster presentation, visit the location where the posters will be exhibited ahead of time.

Using Posters to Share Clinical Expertise

Poster presentations can be a creative and effective way to communicate your clinical and research expertise with others. Although some nurses may view posters as being less esteemed than oral presentations, Bindon and Davenport (2013) viewed both forms of scholarship as being equal to each other, asserting the value of posters in promoting collaboration, communicating valuable outcomes, and highlighting accomplishments.

Poster presentations also provide an opportunity to share ideas with colleagues in a more relaxed, informal environment than an oral presentation (Bindon & Davenport, 2013). The poster arrangement allows you, as a presenter, to interact on a one-on-one basis with conference participants and network with professionals with similar interests.

Spend some time consulting with other nurses (e.g., NPDSs, clinical nurse specialists, faculty from affiliated schools of nursing) who have recently prepared posters for presentation. These nurses can provide helpful information and insight into the process (Linder, 2012).

Posters can be created in a number of ways depending on conference specifications and presenter resources. Advances in technology have enabled authors to create posters using software templates in PowerPoint, PosterGenius®, Adobe InDesign, and Adobe Illustrator (Bindon & Davenport, 2013; McCulloch, 2010). Some conferences may provide you with a template (or poster shell), allowing you to easily create your poster. Templates provide a general structure for your poster and allow you to add your own headings, content, and images. Some authors create a low-budget poster using individual PowerPoint slides printed in color and logically arranged. A more professional-looking, expensive poster can be printed from your template as a one-piece, photographic document by a media department or local paper supply store. Examples of templates and hints on developing a poster can be found in the Helpful Websites section at the end of this chapter.

Posters can also be displayed a number of ways depending on the conference and type of poster. At large conferences, posters often are mounted on a freestanding bulletin board, freestanding trifold cardboard, or a lightweight foam poster board displayed on a tabletop (Bindon & Davenport, 2013). The location for your poster is often preassigned by conference staff. Posters can be attached to boards using thumbtacks or long metal pushpins, or to a trifold using double-sided tape, pins, or adhesive fabric. Some conferences allow presenters to display posters on a laptop. Figure 9-2 illustrates samples of posters on various topics and displayed using different methods.

In addition to printed displays, posters also may be showcased electronically, referred to as *e-posters* (Shin, 2012). E-posters can be presented in various formats. Similar to printed posters, conference organizers will indicate the specifications for e-posters. Some e-posters are presented on display monitors where viewers can zoom in on a particular slide or section of the poster for additional information (Szalinski, 2013). E-posters can be created in PowerPoint, Adobe Acrobat Professional, or Prezi (https://prezi.com) (Szalinski, 2013).

E-posters have been evaluated as a method for providing nurses CE contact hours. A virtual poster session was developed by ANA's Center for Continuing Education and Professional Development to offer additional CE prior to face-to-face conferences (Sloan, 2012). Posters were accompanied by a brief voice recording made by each author. This innovative strategy enabled the American Nurses Credentialing Center to calculate contact hours for the session, obtain funding, validate the integrity of the approach, and manage the processes used for submission and content.

Figure 9-2. Examples of Different Poster Displays

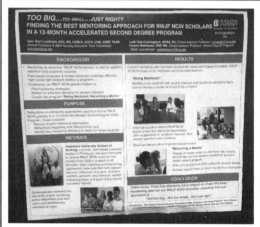

Hanging Poster

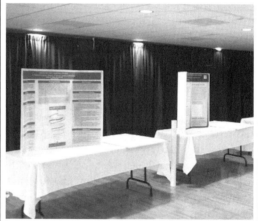

Trifold Poster

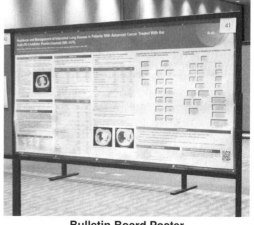

Bulletin Board Poster

Depending on your budget, you can create the poster yourself or use the assistance of a professional media service or office supply service at your workplace or in your community. Regardless of your choice, it is important that you focus on the message that your poster conveys.

Designing a Mock Outline and Layout

Before you start creating your poster, design a mock outline to map essential content. Sherman (2010) advised that less is more when designing your poster. Use your poster to convey a short story to viewers about your project rather than to simply duplicate your abstract (Sherman, 2010). Decide on the main content areas and headings that you want to include. These major categories can be adapted from the outline you previously developed. Do not forget to include the title of the poster, along with the names of authors and places of employment, as needed. Acknowledge any sources of funding for your project, such as grant monies, and include references either on the poster or as a handout.

After outlining the sections of your poster, consider creating individual slides for each section in black and white with no background. You can use these slides to manage your mock layout. Add the background, color, and font features later.

Find out what the display specifications (sizes) are for your poster, as required by conference leaders. These specifications will tell you whether you should design your poster to be freestanding, on a tripod, or attached directly to a large display board provided at the conference. The committee also should provide you with the outside dimensions of the bulletin board or table upon which you will place your poster.

Once you know the maximum outside dimensions for your poster, develop a mock layout. This step will help you plan the content of your poster and make it aesthetically pleasing. One helpful strategy is to create an outline of your poster with masking tape marking the outside dimensions. Use a flat surface, such as a large tabletop or the floor. After you have typed a draft of each content area, trim the paper to size. Then, organize these pieces within the marked outline. Be sure to leave plenty of space for content such as photographs or other graphics to add interest and balance your poster. Adjust the size of each content area as needed.

Be aware of both the content and physical appearance of your poster. Your poster must create a good first impression to gain audience interest. Remember to keep your poster simple and professional. It should look appealing, yet contain essential content. One way to accomplish this professional look is to replace the details of tables and other data using color visuals, such as pie charts, bar graphs, or photographs. Because viewers have limited time to spend at each poster, adding graphics such as arrows or lines will help guide them through the essential points of your poster.

Choosing Color

Color can be used either in the text or the background of your poster. Be sure it is readable and appealing. Incorporate color combinations that complement each other when deciding on the poster background and borders for each content area. Test these color combinations both at a distance and in the lighting anticipated at the poster session. McCulloch (2010) suggested limiting your poster to two or three colors with white and pale colors used for the background. If appropriate, use color combinations that reflect your workplace, school, conference theme, or project topic. Prepare a draft of the color scheme before you finalize your plans.

Factors to Consider With Text

If possible, rely on computer software for your text decisions. Allow space around the edges of your poster for a sufficient border surrounding the text. Choose a print style that is attractive, simple, and readable. Fancy fonts, such as gothic, may interfere with your poster's legibility. McCulloch (2010) suggested limiting your fonts to two types: sans serif (such as Arial) for the poster title and serif (such as Times New Roman) for the poster body. Titles should be one-inch tall (100 point), subheadings one-half inch (50 point), and the body about a quarter of an inch (24 point) (McCulloch, 2010). Make sure your print is large enough that viewers can read it at a reasonable distance of five feet (Hedges, 2010). Print the text for your poster using a quality printer and enlarge images using a quality copier.

Enhancing Your Poster

Photographs can be used to enhance the appearance of a poster presentation, especially in illustrating overall themes or concepts. Photographs should be enlarged so viewers can see them at a reasonable distance. As with manuscripts, be sure to obtain permission to use photographs from their owners.

Create a poster that is pleasing to the viewer's eye. One way is to offer a balance between text and graphics. Once you have developed your draft, stand a distance from your poster and judge its overall appearance. McCulloch (2010) suggested placing the most vital portions of your poster at eye level.

In addition to using computer software, you can enhance your poster in various other ways with the use of special features. Consider the use of an enlarged poster title or institution logo above the main body of your poster. Borders can add zest to simple text. Be sure to include a holder for your business card, abstract, and handouts. Attempt to use creative, professional approaches for your poster presentation and title. Remember that you need to get your message across to viewers in a very brief time. If appropriate, consider a novel approach, such as a faded background that conveys the topic.

Selecting Materials

It is important to decide how your poster should look at the conference, as it needs to be professional looking and comparable with other posters at the event. If you are composing your poster by hand rather than using a software program, think about its creation in two sections: the backboard and the content areas. A backboard can be constructed using a variety of available materials, such as the cardboard or foam trifold panels previously described. In fact, some stores sell freestanding poster displays that contain three connected cardboard panels coated with a white or black finish and require no additional preparation. As mentioned earlier, large bulletin boards often are provided as backboards at some conferences. These boards are usually left natural (white or cork) or covered with colored paper or cloth.

Depending on the backboard, the smaller content sections of the poster can be made using similar materials, such as foam board, poster board, or paper. These sections can be created with rubber cement or spray adhesive and adhered to the backboard with small pieces of adhesive hook and loop tape. This permits easy removal and storage of the content areas. If you plan on using the display or bulletin board as a backboard, affix content sections of your poster with attractive thumbtacks. Staples may be used in some cases. Long metal pushpins often are required to penetrate the depth created by several layers of poster or foam board.

Considering Assembly and Portability

In designing your poster, plan for ease of its assembly, portability to the conference site, and storage. This is especially true if you need to carry your poster a distance when traveling. You want to design a poster that requires minimal time to assemble and dismantle.

Depending on your needs, you may decide to check a large poster as baggage using a commercial cardboard box or carry it as dismantled pieces in a garment bag or suitcase. If your poster is flexible, it can be rolled and carried in a protective cardboard cylinder for travel. You can also mail your poster using an overnight option (Sherman, 2010). Be sure to contact the conference site to confirm the mailing address and procedure to ensure your poster is safely delivered in a timely manner.

Capturing the Final Product

Now that your poster is finished, take a picture of it. You can use this photograph to supplement your portfolio (see Chapter 10), share in your hospital's newsletter, or develop future posters. Use this opportunity to evaluate the content and overall appearance of your poster. Look at the photograph objectively to determine if it contains the qualities of good posters mentioned previously. Judge whether the overall message of your project is conveyed.

Finally, when you arrive at the conference, compare the quality of your poster with others. Take notes about features of other posters you particularly enjoyed. If permitted by the authors, photograph posters that were especially well done. Review these images when it is time to develop your next poster presentation.

Overcoming Presentation Jitters

Most presenters have experienced their share of jitters prior to presenting either posters or oral podium sessions. In fact, even the most experienced presenters report some degree of anxiety associated with this activity.

Although you cannot control all aspects of a situation when presenting, you can use several strategies to help decrease your anxiety. Just as in writing for publication, presentations involve a great deal of homework and practice.

Knowing Your Topic

Knowing your topic thoroughly can reduce some anxiety associated with a presentation. This involves not only memorizing your presentation but also truly understanding the topic.

You should be able to describe your project to someone without notes. Prior research that you conducted on your topic will help you accomplish this task.

Refining Your Presentation Skills

Once you understand your topic, refine your presentation skills through practice. Discover what approach is most comfortable for you to use. Although some presenters read verbatim from their notes, others let their slides and a few notes guide their presentation.

One helpful way to gradually perfect your presentation skills is to practice them at local meetings or conferences. These settings may pose a lesser threat to you and may enable you to perform better at larger national conferences.

Take the opportunity to closely observe experienced presenters as they share their work in front of others. Watch how they organize their content and how they present themselves. Decide what impressed you and what these presenters could have improved upon in their performance. You may decide to model some of these successful behaviors in your own presentations.

If you have the opportunity to listen to some of the speakers before it is your turn to present, be alert to content that is related to your topic. Then, during your presentation, try to address these issues and incorporate them into your talk, if appropriate. This adds to the overall continuity of the program.

Knowing Your Equipment

Be certain that you are comfortable with the equipment you plan to use for your presentation. As mentioned earlier in this chapter, practice with your equipment both at home and at the conference, making sure any technical difficulties are discovered well in advance. Many large conferences have speaker-ready rooms where presenters can review their audiovisuals prior to their presentations.

Dressing the Part

It is important that you create a good impression as a presenter. Start by dressing appropriately for the conference and your presentation. Most often, a conservative business ensemble is suitable. Dress in an outfit that is comfortable yet professional. Feeling good about your appearance often creates a positive self-image in your mind. This can boost your confidence and help you perform well. Have faith in yourself.

Do not forget that your presentation needs to be just as professional as your physical appearance. It is not impressive for the audience to see you carrying various unorganized pieces of paper to the podium. Place your speech or notes in a nice, plain folder. Because no one will see your notes, you can mark them as needed.

Performing a Mock Presentation

Conduct several mock presentations well in advance of your scheduled talk. Try capturing your practice sessions on audiotape or video, unless this increases your anxiety. As you review your mock session, try to be objective. Be sure to maintain good posture and eye contact (Hayne & McDaniel, 2013). Watch for distracting gestures, such as hand or head movements, when you speak. Be alert to errors with pronunciation and the use of extraneous words, such as "uh" or "OK?" Be sure that you are speaking at a proper speed, as nervous speakers often talk too fast. Focus on reducing these problems in future tapings. Imagine yourself as an admired speaker, and always remember to smile.

Preparing for the Worst Scenario

Even with the most experienced presenters, an unexpected situation can arise. One way to lessen your anxiety is to anticipate and prepare for the worst. The following are situations that may occur when giving both formal and informal presentations. After each problem situation, a solution is provided.

Situation #1: You become short of breath and nervous during your presentation.

Solution: Remember that a difference exists between your nervous feeling and others being aware that you are nervous. Most often, you may feel more nervous than others perceive you to be. If you find yourself a little breathless during your presentation, stop for a few seconds, take several deep breaths, and then start again. The time period may seem like forever, but in reality, it is only a brief moment. Some speakers just acknowledge their nervousness and continue with their presentations.

If your presentation is more informal, this is a good time to pose a few questions to the audience and to talk with others. Do not assume the audience is focused on you. Most likely, their attention is focused on your audiovisuals or handouts.

Regardless, slow down, make eye contact, and smile. Some presenters relax if they mingle with participants before their presentation. Do not forget that the lights will be low. Try wearing a turtleneck or scarf if this makes you feel more at ease while presenting.

Situation #2: Your mind goes blank during your presentation. You lose your place within your talk.

Solution: No problem. You have prepared some backup notes clearly marked with the headings of your content. Take a few seconds to regroup your thoughts.

Situation #3: Your talk does not match the audiovisual on the screen. Your slides will not advance.

Solution: Perhaps you got a little ahead of yourself with your slides. Excuse yourself to the audience and advance or reverse to the appropriate slide. Because you have marked your script with the appropriate slide number or image that accompanies it, you can easily relocate your place. If your slides do not advance, ask for assistance. While this is happening, proceed with your presentation to keep the program on schedule. Once your slide projector is working, briefly run through the key slides, if appropriate and as time permits.

Situation #4: You are running behind schedule or have less time to present than previously thought.

Solution: Quickly regroup your thoughts. You may need to advance ahead to the essential portions of your presentation. Maybe you can use the question and answer time of the program to finish explaining these key points. You can agree to meet with participants during a break to answer their questions. Practice and careful timing of your presentation should minimize the risk of this scenario happening. Again, it may be useful to prepare a shorter version of your talk in the event that you have less time than anticipated.

Situation #5: You do not know the answers to questions posed by the audience. Some participants become rude and challenge your patience.

Solution: Remember that no one expects you to know the answers to every question. However, your prior research on the topic should enable you to know most of them. Do not hesitate to say that you do not know the answer to a question. Ask the audience for assistance. You may offer to investigate the question later and get back to the participant via email. You should be courteous and professional to participants, even the most annoying ones. Do not be intimidated. Remember, you are the one giving the presentation because of your expertise.

Situation #6: You lose your presentation.

Solution: No problem, because you have kept duplicate copies of your talk in your carry-on and checked baggage. Prevent this from happening by keeping your slides and presentation with you at all times prior to the conference. Do not check your only copy. It is also a good idea to have an extra copy of your presentation at home so it can be sent to you in the event of an emergency. Another strategy is to email yourself a copy of the presentation and notes as attachments or save a copy in a cloud-based storage service, such as Dropbox.

Evaluating the Results

Now that your presentation is over, be objective and personally evaluate the strengths and weaknesses of your performance. If you recorded your speech, you can play it back to critique your efforts. Give yourself credit for your strong points, and decide to work harder on the areas that were not as strong.

Hayne and McDaniel (2013) published a valuable rubric for nurses to assess their professional presentations using 10 key attributes: "appearance, organization, knowledge of subject, graphics, mechanics, eye contact, engagement, elocution, posture, and movement" (p. 290). This rubric was developed using evidence extracted from sources on public speaking. Each attribute is scored using a scale labeled from 0 to 6 points, with 0 being "most negative" and 6 being "most positive." Some attributes have more than one subsection that is scored. A total score is calculated by summing the scores across all 10 attributes (Hayne & McDaniel, 2013). Results provide focused and constructive feedback that can be used to strengthen future presentations.

A different approach to evaluate your presentation uses Kirkpatrick's Four Levels of Evaluation (Kirkpatrick, 1998; Longo & Tierney, 2012). The four levels include the audience's reaction, the level of learning that occurred, changes in learners' behavior as a result of the presentation, and the measurement of results as they relate to return on investment (Kirkpatrick, 1998). Kirkpatrick provided measures for the four levels and methods that can be used to capture components of your presentation.

Most conferences request their audience participants to evaluate each presentation with particular attention to the designated objectives, quality of the speaker, and teaching strategies used. Conference organizers often send presenters a summary of these scores. If not, ask the conference planners for them.

Reflect back to the primary purpose of your presentation and its predetermined outcomes or objectives. Determine whether the learners actually gained information. Capture the general consensus of the audience from your evaluation summary. Presenters have the habit of focusing on the negative comments rather than the overall feedback. You cannot please everyone. Remember that some individuals have not learned how to offer criticism in a polite and constructive manner.

While the topic is still fresh in your mind, think about making the most of your efforts by using your presentation as a stepping stone for publication. Learning about your presentation from the perspectives of colleagues at a conference can help you transform your project into a publishable manuscript (Sherman, 2010). You can begin this process by recording and transcribing your presentation or by purchasing a recording of your presentation. If you created a poster, use your abstract as an outline to draft your manuscript (see Chapter 8) (Davis, 2012).

Before you convert your oral podium (or poster) presentation into a journal article, you will need to determine whether it is feasible. Alspach (2010) advised potential authors to consider if their topic is publishable and appropriate for a manuscript by comparing a journal's target readership with the audience that attended their presentations. Receiving feedback from an audience during and after your presentation allows you to evaluate the quality of your presentation and revise it into a manuscript for a journal (Alspach, 2010).

Before you disassemble your presentation, be sure to share it with your coworkers. Think about presenting it at a unit-based in-service program (see Chapter 6).

Summary

Both NPDSs and clinical nurses need to share their professional nursing expertise both formally and informally through abstracts, oral presentations, and posters. When preparing your presentation, pay attention to choosing a topic and purpose, developing content and audiovisuals tailored to your expected audience, practicing and perfecting your presentation skills, and evaluating its outcomes. In addition, plan for anticipated resources and prepare for unexpected challenges. It is important that NPDSs engage in sharing their successes through presentations and in mentoring clinical nurses within their work setting.

Helpful Websites

- AllNurses—Effective PowerPoint Presentations: http://allnurses.com/nursing-educators -faculty/effective-powerpoint-presentations-406620.html
- Creative Commons—About: https://creativecommons.org/about
- Microsoft Office—Posters: https://store.office.live.com/templates/Posters?ui=en-US&rs= en-US&ad=US
- Microsoft Office—Tips for Creating and Delivering an Effective Presentation: https://support .office.com/en-US/article/Tips-for-creating-and-delivering-an-effective-presentation -F43156B0-20D2-4C51-8345-0C337CEFB88B
- NN/LM National Network of Libraries of Medicine—Nursing on the Net: Health Care Resources You Can Use: http://nnlm.gov/training/nursing/sampler.html
- Oncology Nursing Society—Speaker Upload: Frequently Asked Questions: https://ons opcontent.ons.org/SpeakerUpload/Guidelines/FAQ.aspx
- Presentation-Pointers.com—Presentation Tips: www.presentation-pointers.com
- Slideworld: www.slideworld.org/slidestag.aspx/COMMUNITY-HEALTH-NURSING
- University of Virginia Health System, Claude Moore Health Sciences Library—How Do I Create a Poster Using Microsoft PowerPoint? www.hsl.virginia.edu/services/howdoi/how -do-i-create-poster-using-powerpoint

- United States Copyright Office—Copyright Law of the United States: www.copyright.gov/title17
- Vanderbilt University Nursing Research Department—Step by Step: Scientific Poster Making Using Microsoft PowerPoint 2010: www.mc.vanderbilt.edu/documents/evidencebasedpractice/files/Step%20by%20Step-Poster%20making%20tips.pdf

References

Alspach, G. (2010). Converting presentations into journal articles: A guide for nurses. *Critical Care Nurse, 30*(2), 8–15. doi:10.4037/ccn2010788

American Nurses Association & National Nursing Staff Development Organization. (2010). *Nursing professional development: Scope and standards of practice.* Silver Spring, MD: American Nurses Association.

Bindon, S.L., & Davenport, J.M. (2013). Developing a professional poster: Four "Ps" for advanced practice nurses to consider. *AACN Advanced Critical Care, 24,* 169–176. doi:10.1097/NCI.0b013e318287a3fb

Catalano, L.A. (2014). Avoiding copyright violations in educational presentations. *American Nurse Today, 9*(5), 53–54.

Davis, L. (2012). Developing your poster presentation into a manuscript. *Journal of the Association for Vascular Access, 17,* 174. doi:10.1016/j.java.2012.10.008

Dickerson, P.S. (2013). Making your voice heard: Sharing outcomes of continuing nursing education. *Journal of Continuing Education in Nursing, 44,* 101–102. doi:10.3928/00220124-20130222-02

Durkin, G. (2011). Promoting professional development through poster presentations. *Journal for Nurses in Staff Development, 27*(3), E1–E3. doi:10.1097/NND.0b013e318217b437

Hayne, A.N., & McDaniel, G.S. (2013). Presentation rubric: Improving faculty professional presentations. *Nursing Forum, 48,* 289–294.

Hedges, C. (2010). Poster presentations: A primer for critical care nurses. *AACN Advanced Critical Care, 21,* 318–321. doi:10.1097/NCI.0b013e3181e138da

Ickes, M.J., & Gambescia, S.F. (2011). Abstract art: How to write competitive conference and journal abstracts. *Health Promotion Practice, 12,* 493–496. doi:10.1177/1524839911413128

Kirkpatrick, D.L. (1998). *Another look at evaluating training programs.* Alexandria, VA: American Society for Training and Development.

Linder, L. (2012). Disseminating research and scholarly projects: Developing a successful abstract. *Journal of Pediatric Oncology Nursing, 29,* 362–366. doi:10.1177/1043454212456087

Longo, A., & Tierney, C. (2012). Presentation skills for the nurse educator. *Journal for Nurses in Staff Development, 29,* 16–23. doi:10.1097/NND.0b013e318240a699

McCulloch, B. (2010). Don't ignore that call for posters! *Journal of Continuing Education in Nursing, 41,* 392–393. doi:10.3928/00220124-20100825-04

Pennsylvania State Nurses Association. (2013). *Continuing education approval manual* (R-2013 ed.). Harrisburg, PA: Author.

Polit, D.F., & Beck, C.T. (2012). *Nursing research: Generating and assessing evidence for nursing practice* (9th ed.). Philadelphia, PA: Wolters Kluwer Health/Lippincott Williams & Wilkins.

Russell, C.L., & Ponferrada, L. (2012). How to develop an outstanding conference research abstract. *Nephrology Nursing Journal, 39,* 307–311, 342.

Sherman, R.O. (2010). How to create an effective poster presentation. *American Nurse Today, 5*(9), 13–15.

Shin, S.J. (2012). Evaluation of electronic versus traditional format poster presentation. *Medical Education, 46,* 519–520. doi:10.1111/j.1365-2923.2012.04253.x

Sloan, R. (2012). Poster presentations in the virtual world. *Journal of Continuing Education in Nursing, 43,* 485–486.

Szalinski, C. (2013, September 17). What on earth is an ePoster and how do I make one? *ASCB Post.* Retrieved from http://www.ascb.org/what-on-earth-is-an-eposter-and-how-do-i-make-one

CHAPTER 10

Recording Your Professional Nursing Achievements in a Portfolio

AS a professional nurse, you realize the important role that meticulous documentation plays in validating and tracking key components of patient care. On a more personal note, documentation of your professional nursing accomplishments serves a similar purpose with respect to your career goals. Whether you are a recent graduate or an experienced RN, maintaining a systematic and accurate record of your professional life is an essential activity that serves a variety of purposes.

After you have collected and organized your professional accomplishments, place them in a document commonly referred to as a professional nursing portfolio (American Nurses Association [ANA], 2000). A portfolio not only provides a way for you, as a staff educator, to record your professional development, but also serves as a method to record your "career planning, demonstration of learning, and maintenance of continuing professional competence" (ANA, 2000, p. 25).

As an NPDS, you are responsible for maintaining your own career development, as well as facilitating the career development of clinical nurses in your practice setting (ANA & National Nursing Staff Development Organization [NNSDO], 2010). This responsibility may include not only creating your own professional portfolio but also coaching clinical nurses in this same endeavor. When planning your portfolio coaching sessions, include creative strategies with nurses that will minimize barriers and result in an evidence-based professional portfolio tailored to the needs and purpose of your organization.

Barriers to portfolio development were addressed by Pellico and Violano (2010), who designed and implemented a successful portfolio development class for nurses employed at Yale–New Haven Hospital in Connecticut, a university-affiliated medical center. The authors created the class after recognizing an organizational need to encourage more nurses to apply to a clinical advancement program. Therefore, they provided qualified nurses with the knowledge and protected time to create a portfolio for this purpose. The program included providing qualified nurses with a dedicated computer room where they received instruction and hands-on experience in creating portfolio elements required for the clinical advancement program application, such as a letter of intent, clinical narratives or exemplars, curriculum vitae (CV), self-evaluation, and clinical practice goals (Pellico & Violano, 2010).

Although templates were used to guide nurses in developing their letters and CVs, the authors paid particular attention to increasing the nurses' comfort levels in sharing personal stories that illustrated their clinical expertise in the form of clinical narratives and exemplars. Nurses also needed support in conducting a self-evaluation of their performance.

In this program, nurses learned how to engage in future goal setting for clinical practice by using personal goal-setting examples. This portfolio development approach provided the nurses with a foundation for lifelong learning and ongoing professional development.

Validating Reasons for Portfolios

Why should you spend time collecting and organizing evidence that reflects your professional nursing achievements? A variety of reasons exist, some of which are global in nature and others that are more specific and personal. Only you can determine what is essential at this point in your career. While some portfolios provide a mechanism to document your progress toward career goals, others will help you manage clinical advancement and job opportunities or provide evidence of your expertise and competencies.

Assessing Progress Toward Career Goals

Assembling, organizing, and documenting your professional accomplishments in a portfolio will help you stay focused and evaluate your progress in reaching career goals (Oermann, 2002). A portfolio is a way to take responsibility for your own learning. Although developing a professional career plan will be discussed in more detail in Chapter 14, the following examples may help clarify this purpose.

Suppose you are currently a nurse on a surgical oncology unit and are interested in pursuing a career as an oncology nurse in home care. Collecting, organizing, and reviewing your professional records using a portfolio format can help you reflect on your accomplishments and assess your ongoing progress toward this goal. The evidence contained in your portfolio will enable you to make informed decisions on participating in new professional opportunities. In the future, you can rely on your professional portfolio to evaluate opportunities based on their alignment with your short- and long-term career goals.

Cangelosi (2008) reported on an initiative focused on career transition. In this assignment, graduate nursing education program students extended their learning profiles to include reflection on their future roles as nurse educators. In their final capstone course, students were asked to reflect on their past learning and clinical expertise and visualize their future teaching roles. Key components of this portfolio included a revised CV, an experiential learning reflection paper, a sample course syllabus, and a critique of a published nursing education research study. This expanded portfolio assignment received positive feedback from learners and course faculty in preparing students for new specialty roles.

Seeking Job Opportunities, Promotions, and Advancements

When submitting a résumé or CV for a new position or job advancement, consider the positive impression a professional portfolio gives to your potential employers or reviewers. Your portfolio provides them with focused evidence that supports your professional achievements.

For example, portfolios were used by graduates of a recent clinical nurse leader (CNL) program for job interviews related to their new roles (Norris, Webb, McKeon, Jacob, & Herrin-Griffith, 2012). The portfolios served as vehicles for CNLs to showcase evidence of competencies highly valued by employers of healthcare organizations, such as "quality improvement, patient safety, error prevention, and teamwork" (Norris et al., 2012, p. 47). The portfolios were organized using CNL role competencies, as outlined by the American Association of Colleges of Nursing (AACN, 2007) at that time, and were accompanied by various clinical examples of their work.

Keeping a record of your professional outcomes in a portfolio can also help you prepare for a performance review meeting. Consider using criteria listed in your position description as a guide to document essential outcomes if no template is available for this purpose.

Capan et al. (2013) demonstrated the value of portfolios for validation of professional development during the annual performance review process at Children's Hospital of Pittsburgh of UPMC, a pediatric urban academic medical center in Pennsylvania. Both staff nurses and their unit directors viewed electronic portfolios as a valuable source of evidence to validate specific areas of the nurses' professional development during performance reviews. Specific areas of professional development addressed in the portfolios included professional certifications, specialty training, honors/awards/recognitions, attendance at conferences, presentations, participation on committees or councils, and community service (Capan et al., 2013). Surveys completed by directors and nurses prior to and after using portfolios during annual reviews revealed that this new approach gave added attention to the nurses' professional accomplishments compared to the traditional performance review process. While staff nurses felt that portfolios enabled them to be recognized for their professional certifications, honors, awards, and recognitions, directors cited the nurses' conference attendance and community service efforts as gaining more recognition (Capan et al., 2013).

Maintaining a professional record can give you an edge in promotions or clinical advancements within your organization or open you to opportunities outside your workplace. Use documented criteria, such as those identified in your organization's clinical advancement or career ladder guidelines, to direct you.

At Maine Medical Center, Owens and Cleaves (2012) used portfolios in their revised clinical nurse advancement program that aimed to acknowledge and reward bedside nurses for their commitment to clinical expertise, the nursing profession, and the organization. Eligible applicants submitted portfolios that contained the required evidence, including a statement of purpose, the nursing director's endorsement letter, résumé, two clinical exemplars, two peer support letters, educational/activity record, and goals related to their professional practice (Owens & Cleaves, 2012). A nurse-led review committee evaluated the portfolios according to predetermined criteria and decided the final outcome. Nurses who were promoted in the clinical ladder continued to use their portfolios in annual performance reviews.

Similarly, professional portfolios were used to document outstanding clinical performance and leadership in advanced practice RNs (APRNs) employed at Akron General Hospital (Hespenheide, Cottingham, & Mueller, 2011). Key elements for the APRN model were derived from the Standards of Professional Performance in APRN (ANA, 1996), Relationship-Based Care (Koloroutis, 2004; Koloroutis, Felgen, Person, & Wessel, 2007), and the Forces of Magnetism (American Nurses Credentialing Center [ANCC], n.d.). Portfolios included evidence on the following topics: introduction, quality of care, self-evaluation, education, research, leadership, ethics, interdisciplinary process, and future goals (Hespenheide et al., 2011). Stakeholders evaluated the approach as being a significant way to recognize excellence in clinical practice and promote ongoing professional development in APRNs.

Validating Prior Learning, Expertise, and Competencies

It is helpful to have an organized record of your professional accomplishments when applying for awards, such as scholarships, grants, or other types of professional recognitions. For example, perhaps you need evidence of teaching cardiopulmonary resuscitation (CPR) classes to maintain your volunteer position as a CPR instructor.

Similarly, validation of items such as clinical practice hours, continuing education (CE) programs attended, and contact hours earned often can help you when verifying specialty nursing certification requirements. For example, Byrne, Schroeter, Carter, and Mower (2009) designed, implemented, and evaluated the use of evidence-based portfolios to document continuing competence when applying for recertification or reactivation as a perioperative nurse. Required documentation in the portfolio reflected domains related to the practice of perioperative nursing. Applicants had to provide documentation that supported 4 of 12 predetermined professional activities. Procedures to evaluate the portfolio applications were developed along with a scoring system and an evaluation tool.

An organized collection of documents that reflect your clinical competency in a particular area can be used when pursuing formal education in nursing. Because they focus on assessing learning outcomes, some schools accept portfolios as verification of one's past professional achievements, accomplishments, and other personal learning experiences. Following careful evaluation of this portfolio, faculty determine a learner's individual strengths and weaknesses and use this information to develop an individualized plan that builds upon existing competencies. In some instances, a school also may grant advanced standing credits or some type of recognition for these prior learning experiences.

Certification Application or Renewal

Many nursing specialty certifications require new applicants to successfully pass a valid and reliable examination to obtain certification status. Nurses seeking recertification often have the opportunity to renew through either retesting or a portfolio application. ANCC (2014) has developed a handbook for nurses seeking certification using a portfolio option. This handbook instructs applicants to submit evidence in four major categories: evaluations and certifications, practice hours and licensure, professional development record, and employment and career information (ANCC, 2014). Applicants also submit résumé information using a template as well as an exemplar or clinical narrative (ANCC, 2014). Although designed for certification purposes, the ANCC portfolio handbook can serve as a helpful resource in preparing your portfolio for other purposes, such as those described in this chapter.

Preparing for Organization Mergers and Restructuring

Healthcare systems in the United States have undergone various mergers and restructures related to changes in healthcare reimbursement, such as the 2010 Patient Protection and Affordable Care Act. Nurses may find themselves in the midst of unexpected career changes within their own practice settings. One proactive strategy to prepare for possible organizational changes or career moves is to develop a professional portfolio to confirm your level of nursing knowledge and clinical skills and to help you prepare for unexpected events. This approach forces you to organize your professional achievements while you are actively employed rather than while you are experiencing emotional stress. This strategy may provide you with a sense of control over your future, especially during a time of uncertainty and change in the workplace (see Chapter 1).

Creating a Professional Portfolio

Before you create your professional portfolio, you will need to consider and include several important elements of the portfolio creation process. The following section provides such elements and explains their importance.

Clarifying Its Purpose

One of the first things you should do is determine the purpose of your portfolio and in what context it will be used. Clarify how the portfolio is defined by the individual or group that requested it. Some of the situations in which portfolios are used include serving as a source of evidence for clinical advancement programs, renewal for specialty certifications, annual performance reviews, or job interviews. Determine if your portfolio content is intended to represent your recent accomplishments within a short time frame or if it should provide evidence of your ongoing professional development over the span of your nursing career. If you are an NPDS or unit-based educator and plan on creating a portfolio for your own personal development, consider including evidence related to your job description, competencies outlined in *Nursing Professional Development: Scope and Standards of Practice* (ANA & NNSDO, 2010), or your long-term career goals (see Chapter 14) to guide the content of your portfolio.

Gathering Information About the Process

After confirming the purpose of your portfolio, outline the portfolio creation process from initial submission to the final outcome. For example, say that you just had your annual performance review. Your manager told you that NPDSs and clinical staff nurses will be required to submit a portfolio for review prior to their next evaluation sessions. Carefully review and maintain any documentation that describes this new endeavor and keep it in a folder or electronic file. Pay particular attention to the portfolio submission process and the due date. Develop a realistic timeline to manage this project, working backward from the due date. Recognize that this date will most likely occur well in advance of next year's annual review session. If creating a portfolio is a new activity for you, be generous with the amount of time that you allot to this project. Also, clarify to whom you will initially submit your portfolio, who will review and evaluate the portfolio after its submission, and how the reviewer's decisions will be weighted in terms of the final decision and outcome. In this example, you obtain the new policy regarding portfolios and file it electronically in your computer. You also file a printed copy in a labeled folder stored among your professional documents. You recognize that your portfolio is due one month prior to your annual review next year. Only your manager will be reviewing your portfolio and making the final decision regarding whether the evidence included supports effective and excellent performance.

Focusing on Criteria and Required Evidence

After you understand the portfolio's purpose and review process, pay close attention to the evaluative criteria and recommended documents. Review the expected levels of competency at each rank (i.e., intended outcomes to be measured) to understand what evidence you will need to provide. For example, what does "excellence" look like? The sources of evidence should illustrate these evaluative criteria and will be used by reviewers to determine excellence and effectiveness. If the criteria are based on a guiding framework, reading more about these criteria may help you frame or word your document more appropriately. Take advantage of any professional development sessions that are offered, such as the program by Pellico and Violano (2010), to learn more about portfolio development. Investigate any samples of portfolios created by others and consult other nurses who may be willing to help mentor you during this process. Remember to seek any supplies, such as folders, notebooks, access to websites or computer software, or software training programs, well in advance of your due date.

As an example, suppose you, as an NPDS, realize that your portfolio needs to address the key components of your job description framed by core competencies outlined in *Nursing Professional Development: Scope and Standards of Practice* (ANA & NNSDO, 2010). Knowing this, you obtain this document from your hospital library and familiarize yourself with its content as you plan your portfolio. Because you will be helping clinical staff nurses develop their portfolios, your manager sends you to a CE program on portfolio development. Through networking at the program, you connect with an NPDS with experience in portfolio development who agrees to serve as your mentor. At the conference, you pay special attention to the creative teaching-learning strategies and samples used by the speakers as you think about designing future portfolio sessions for nurses at your organization. Given the information that you have learned so far, you are able to draft a realistic timeline to produce your portfolio.

Understanding the Reviewer's Perspective

After reviewing the purpose, criteria, and documents required for your portfolio, be sure to obtain information regarding how the reviewer (or reviewers) will be evaluating your materials. It may be helpful to understand the instructions provided for the review process and the evaluation tools that will be used. As mentioned before, it is helpful to know who will be reviewing your documents so that you can tailor your writing accordingly.

Picturing the Final Product

Based on your guidelines, imagine what your final portfolio will look like. Picture your portfolio as a three-ring binder with dividers or as an electronic version. Keeping a mental image of your portfolio can confirm your timeline and resources. As with other new projects, it is important to break your portfolio's creation into manageable, smaller steps and to think positively.

Putting It All Together

Be creative when developing your portfolio and tailor it to meet your specific needs. Unless otherwise specified by guidelines, you can develop a portfolio using a variety of practical approaches. For example, create a portfolio incorporating a file folder with two or more pockets. Try making one with a three-ring binder to organize data. Or, perhaps you will develop your portfolio electronically using software designed for portfolios. You also may consider organizing your portfolio according to categories and ordered by dates. Whatever method you use to compile it, be sure that your portfolio is more than just a collection of documents; it needs to tell a story about your ongoing development and growth as a professional nurse.

The portfolio development process can be viewed as an exercise, whereas the portfolio itself can be viewed as a tool or worksheet to help plan and evaluate your career development. By using both the process and the outcome (product), you can assess your professional accomplishments and reflect upon your strengths and weaknesses. These data enable you to develop a plan based on your career goals that includes specific interventions or strategies to meet these goals. You can then evaluate your success in meeting your goals.

Organizing and filing your professional achievements also provides you with a mechanism to develop and update your résumé (see Chapter 11) and other professional documents. Because most of the data and vital documents you will need fall into one of several major content categories used in both résumés and portfolios, this makes creating and updating them much easier.

As an NPDS, suppose you discover that your organization's first attempt at portfolios will be done in printed form using a notebook. Plans for next year include electronic portfolios, allowing time for software purchases and staff training. You are optimistic about this new opportunity and are excited about seeing your professional accomplishments organized into one place. Your organization's guidelines include the reviewer evaluation tool that will be used by your manager. Be sure to familiarize yourself with this tool and the NPDS documents.

Developing a Painless Record-Keeping System

What is the best way to start collecting and organizing your professional documents? Keeping track of all these details can be a nightmare unless you develop an organized record-keeping system. This system should be sophisticated enough to accomplish the outcome yet easy to use. This way, you are more likely to use it and make it work for you. Your system can consist of hard copies maintained in a series of folders labeled by content or an electronic set of folders using scanned or filed documents on your computer. The organization that requested your portfolio also may provide you with a template to store your portfolio while it is in progress. Regardless of your approach, maintain a backup copy of your portfolio's content.

Establishing a Time Frame for Your Records

Choose a time span that matches your needs. For some nurses, this may be a calendar year that starts in January and ends in December. For others, it may comprise a fiscal year, such as one that begins July 1 and ends June 30 of the following year. Or, maybe you choose to organize your record-keeping system in accordance with your date of hire or annual performance appraisal. Whatever timeline you choose, match it with your needs.

Creating a System to Collect and Organize Data

Once you have established a time frame, develop a system to collect and organize your professional data. Use your smartphone or personal calendar to record important events and other occurrences, such as clinical successes. This strategy will help you create an overall picture for the year and order events chronologically.

Now that you have an idea about what to record, how do you begin the process? One simple approach involves assembling several file folders in an expandable, accordion-like file pocket.

Use colored file folders for easy identification and label each with the headings you will need in your portfolio. You can also recreate the same system using electronic file folders on your computer if this is more comfortable for you. For example, Hespenheide et al. (2011) described a portfolio that used the headings of Introduction, Quality of Care, Self-Evaluation, Education, Research, Leadership, Ethics, Interdisciplinary Process, and Future Goals.

If you do not have any specific heading system to follow, try using the ones provided in Figure 10-1. Then, go through your documents and place each in the appropriate folder based on the topic. Develop a three-ring notebook with dividers labeled according to your categories, if that is the required format.

> **Figure 10-1. Suggested Headings for Folders**
>
> - Educational experiences
> - Professional work experiences and exemplars
> - Licensure, certifications, and certificates
> - Awards, honors, and special recognitions
> - Professional memberships
> - Publications
> - Research and quality improvement participation
> - Consulting
> - Presentations
> - Community volunteer activities
> - Attendance at continuing education programs
> - Letters of support, endorsement, and recommendation
> - Cover letter
> - Résumé
> - Self-evaluation statement
> - Future career goals

A similar approach can be taken using computer software. Consider creating a table, such as the one illustrated in Table 10-1, using word processing software. This figure provides you with a map of the main categories (labels) of either your portfolio or record-keeping system, the file name of each document, and a section for notes or descriptions of items. Save a hard copy as well as an electronic version on a jump drive for your files. Combine the two approaches using folders or binders for storage and a computer for recording and organizing data. Regardless of the approach you use, it needs to be manageable for you to view, add, compile, and retrieve information. Repeat the process with new folders for each year that follows.

Identifying Documents to Collect, Organize, and Record

Your portfolio guidelines should dictate the documents you will need to collect, organize, and record. You may want to focus your efforts on a variety of essential materials. As you review your professional materials, sort them accordingly. Be sure to place valuable original documents, such as official school transcripts, diplomas, licenses, and certifications, in a safe place, and use copies of these documents, if acceptable, for the purposes of your portfolio. Avoid sharing professional documents that contain personal data, such as your Social Security number or clinical exemplars that contain patient identification data.

The following components are intended to provide you with a start as you collect and organize your professional data throughout the year. You will need to decide which of these components belong in your portfolio based on guidelines. Most likely, you will need to include an updated résumé (see Chapter 11) and a cover letter. Be sure to frame your cover letter and organize your résumé according to the purpose of your portfolio and determine if templates are provided to guide you in their development.

Educational Experiences

Organize documents that deal with your formal education, such as programs or courses that you completed (Hespenheide et al., 2011). Include materials such as copies of your school

Table 10-1. Map of Record-Keeping System

Category (Folder Label)	Document (File Names)	Description (Notes)
Educational Experiences	Pitt_BSN Transcript Pitt_BSN_ProgramofStudies	BSN courses with grades BSN program outcomes, program of studies, and course descriptions
Professional Work Experience	Staff Nurse 1_Job Description_ General Hospital 2014Evaluation _General Hospital Shared Governance Committee – Professional Development Preceptor_FeedbackfromFaculty Preceptor_FeedbackfromStudent	First job description Year 1 performance appraisal Description of professional development projects Preceptor evaluation from nursing student and faculty
Clinical Exemplars	DischargeTeaching_General Hospital Pain Management_ General Hospital StaffInservice_Pain Management_ GeneralHospital	Samples of clinical exemplars from General Hospital
Licensure, Certifications, and Certificates	RN License	Copy of license
Awards, Honors, and Special Recognitions	RecognitionAward2014_General Hospital	General Hospital Award Certificate 2014
Professional Memberships	Oncology Nursing Society	Evidence of Oncology Nursing Society (ONS) membership
Publications	PainManagement_General Hospital-Newsletter2013	Short paper in pain management published in hospital newsletter
Research and Quality Improvement	QIPainProject_Description_General_ Hospital QI PainProject_FinalReport_General-Hospital	Materials used for pain management project implemented on the unit
Consulting	ICU_Inservice	Notes about in-service with intensive care unit nurses about head-neck patient transfer
Presentations	Cancer Basics_Invitation Cancer Basics_LessonPlan Cancer Basics_Slides CancerBasics_Evaluation	Information about the cancer basics lecture for juniors at Duquesne University
Community Service	Volunteer_Hospice	Description of volunteer activities at hospice
Continuing Education Programs	Certificate_EvidenceBasedPractice Certificate_Pain_Management	Refer to separate file for listing of continuing education programs by dates
Letters of Support	ManagerLetter_2013 ManagerLetter_2014 SSmithPeerLetter_2013	Support letters from manager and peer

(Continued on next page)

Table 10-1. Map of Record-Keeping System *(Continued)*		
Category (Folder Label)	**Document (File Names)**	**Description (Notes)**
Cover Letter	CoverLetter_Draft	Cover letter draft
Résumé	Résumé_July2013	Latest résumé
Self-Evaluation	Self-Evaluation_Draft	Self-evaluation draft
Future Career Goals	CareerGoals2014_Draft	Career goals draft

transcripts, diplomas, and the results of required admission tests. Be sure to keep a copy of a school catalog or web page that illustrates the program outcomes and the curriculum that you completed, including the program of studies and course descriptions with objectives. You also may want to keep some key correspondence that describes your progress, such as admission, advanced standing, program completion, evaluations, and financial agreements. Samples of outstanding papers or projects you completed during school can be useful in documenting your creativity and writing skills.

Professional Work Experiences and Clinical Successes

Similar to how you organized your educational experiences, collect and organize evidence related to your clinical performance. Start by focusing on your present job and then reflecting on previous ones. Keep a copy of your position or job descriptions along with samples of any evaluations received from your supervisors and peers. Retain not only the positive evaluations but also the not-so-good ones as a means to document your progress in certain areas. Remember to include any interdisciplinary (interprofessional) initiatives that you have been involved in or any ethical narratives that you have encountered and managed appropriately (Hespenheide et al., 2011).

File copies of any other correspondence, such as thank-you letters received from patients or families, peers, and supervisors or letters of appreciation from faculty regarding your experiences in precepting or mentoring nursing students. Include your roles and accomplishments while participating on committees, such as those related to professional development or the quality council in your institution's shared governance structure.

In addition to these obvious documents, keep a daily record of your clinical successes, specifically those that set you apart from colleagues, often referred to as *clinical exemplars* (Owens & Cleaves, 2012) or *clinical narratives* (Heinrich, Tafas, & Jackson, 2011). Focus on the scenario, including assessment, planning, implementation of interventions or solutions, and evaluation of outcomes. Reflect on what outcomes resulted because of your expertise. Possible scenarios include development of an individualized plan of care for a patient, completion of a quality improvement project, creation of a patient care standard, or introduction to a new piece of equipment, procedure, or documentation system on the unit. Share information about your leadership role with the unit-based in-service programs you have presented for your coworkers. Try to recall a specific clinical situation or critical incident in which your nursing skills and behaviors positively influenced the outcome.

Whether it is participation in committees or unit-based projects, be sure to save some documentation of the project along with any evaluation comments or feedback received. Remember to document your success on an annual clinical competency test.

Licensure, Certifications, and Certificates

Maintain a copy of your nursing license along with any certifications or certificates you have obtained. You also may choose to keep any correspondence related to these items, such as test scores or certification results.

Awards, Honors, and Special Recognitions

Copy documents that reflect awards or honors you have received, such as membership in Sigma Theta Tau International Honor Society of Nursing, outstanding work accomplished, recognition received from professional or community work, or inclusion on a dean's list at school. Include how you met criteria for each award you received.

Professional Memberships

Document your membership in professional nursing organizations, such as ANA or the Oncology Nursing Society. Keep copies of membership cards and correspondence that describe your involvement on committees or as an elected official. Be sure to note any evaluative comments you have received regarding your work in these organizations. Similar to examples of clinical accomplishments, include examples of the influence that you had on outcomes of the committee or position.

Publications

Keep the original and hard or electronic copies or reprints of any of your published works, including journal articles, editorials, topical journal issues, book chapters, or books (see Chapter 8). Be sure to mention experience as a manuscript or book reviewer. Clinical publications of a more informal nature include patient teaching guides, clinical or critical pathways, policies and procedures, discharge guides, staff education materials, newsletters, and charting samples (e.g., patient assessment forms, discharge instructions). Be aware of confidentiality standards when recording these documents.

Research and Quality Improvement Participation

Keep a copy of your participation or leadership roles in research or quality improvement activities (Hespenheide et al., 2011). This documentation can range from a letter written by a principal investigator or project manager thanking you for helping with data collection or a literature review to the actual publication of results in a journal. Or, perhaps you organized and led a unit-based journal club in which staff nurses read and discussed clinical research articles. Do not forget to file a copy of any research grants or quality improvements submitted or any other accompanying correspondence. Maintain a copy of the abstract and executive summary that describes the completed project.

Consulting

Include any experience you may have as a consultant, for example, serving as an expert witness or sharing your expertise with staff at an affiliated agency. Mention more informal consulting activities as well, such as helping intensive care nurses understand the care of a head and neck surgical oncology patient who has been transferred to the intensive care unit. Explain what happened as a result of you sharing your expertise.

Presentations

Include a copy of any professional presentations you have completed. Also include photographs or images of posters you have developed both inside and outside of your organization. Try to keep original conference fliers that list you as a participant. Be sure to include any evaluations or copies of correspondence that address the quality of your efforts.

Community Volunteer and Service Activities

Just as with presentations, be sure to document any of your volunteer activities, especially those that relate to your expertise as a professional nurse. Enclose any feedback received about the outcomes of your involvement.

Attendance at Continuing Education Programs

Keep an ongoing record of CE programs that you have attended, along with evidence of contact hours earned or certificates of completion granted. Be sure to include any independent learning or home study modules you have completed at work or through nursing journals (see Chapter 13). Maintain a record of your attendance at conferences and include the titles, dates, locations, and providers and approvers, and any contact hours earned. Keep your certificates of attendance in a secure file for easy retrieval. Table 10-2 illustrates one way of recording and organizing your attendance at such conferences. Consider tracking these programs according to your specialty certification requirements, especially if you have more than one certification.

Letters of Support, Endorsement, and Recommendation

Save any letters of recommendation you received during your professional career. Also, include documents such as thank-you notes that reflect your professional performance. If letters of support or endorsement are required from your managers or peers, inquire if templates are available. Be sure to give these individuals sufficient time and information regarding the purpose and focus of the letter. Consider drafting highlights about your accomplishments for those who will submit letters. Be sure to follow up with a thank-you note.

Self-Evaluation Statement

You most likely will need to include a self-evaluation or reflection related to the criteria and components of your portfolio (Fowler, 2012; Hespenheide et al., 2011). This statement should be a clear and succinct description of your accomplishments supported by documents related to the purpose of your portfolio (e.g., performance evaluation, clinical advancement program). Organize your self-evaluation statement in a logical manner, make sure it reflects the mission and philosophy of your workplace and nursing department, and frame it to your reviewers.

Table 10-2. Example of Documenting Attendance at Professional Conferences

Date	Title	Location	Provider	Approver	Contact Hours
5/13/2014	2014 UPMC Skin Health Conference	UPMC, Pittsburgh, PA	UPMC	ANCC	5.5
4/17/2014	Safe Handling of Hazardous Drugs	Webinar	ONS	ANCC	1
2/16/2014	Postoperative Pulmonary Complications	UPMC, Pittsburgh, PA	UPMC	ANCC	1.5
2/5/2014	Cancer Genetics	Webinar	ONS	ANCC	2

ANCC—American Nurses Credentialing Center; ONS—Oncology Nursing Society; UPMC—University of Pittsburgh Medical Center

Future Professional Goals

Many portfolios include a section where you address your short- and long-term career goals (Hespenheide et al., 2011). Think carefully when writing this section, and reflect on where you are now in your professional career and where you hope to be in two to five years (see Chapter 14). Maybe you have a definitive plan, or perhaps you need to conduct further career exploration.

Other Helpful Materials

Remember to include personal reflections of experiences that illustrate your professional knowledge, skills, and attitudes in nursing. Include introspective evidence that reflects the qualities that make you a unique, competent, and exceptional professional nurse.

It is a good idea to obtain several copies of a small professional photograph of yourself. A black-and-white or color wallet-sized photo saved as an electronic JPG or GIF file usually works best. Ask the media center at your workplace or a copy center in your community for details. Photographs come in handy when you are asked for one in a hurry, such as for the newsletter at your workplace or for a local professional organization. Sometimes editors request a photograph to accompany manuscripts for publication.

Keep your old calendars or appointment books until you have had a chance to transcribe their content. Recording professional events and personal accounts on your calendar provides a helpful means of making sense and organizing your yearly professional activities.

Consider sharing some of your documents using a professional, web-based network where they can be viewed by other professionals with similar interests. Such sites include LinkedIn (www.linkedin.com), Zerply (https://zerply.com), and Meetup (www.meetup .com). It is important to choose these websites carefully, ensuring their authenticity and professionalism.

Learning From the Outcome

Regardless of the final decision regarding your portfolio, learn from the feedback you receive from reviewers. Record this feedback and make notes to strengthen weak areas before you create your next portfolio. Set aside time to update your portfolio during the following year. In fact, Fowler (2012) suggested dedicating about a half-day every two months to accomplish this task. Celebrate your successes and share your expertise with other nurses new to the portfolio process.

Summary

Recording your professional achievements in a portfolio will help you track your progress toward career goals and support new job opportunities, promotions and professional advancements like clinical ladders. Portfolios also can help you validate your prior learning, professional expertise, and competencies. When creating a portfolio, be sure to clarify the type of portfolio that you will need and pay attention to required criteria and supporting evidence. Develop a practical record-keeping system and a realistic time frame that allows you to easily record your accomplishments and store key documents as supporting evidence. Whether you create your portfolio using a traditional print or electronic format, assemble its contents in a systematic and organized manner. Learn from the feedback you receive about your portfolio and revise it accordingly. Share your expertise with colleagues who may be new to portfolios.

Helpful Websites

- AllNurses—A Nursing Exemplar; One New Nurse's Experience: http://allnurses.com/general -nursing-discussion/a-nursing-exemplar-546481.html
- American Association of Critical-Care Nurses—2013 Award-Winning Exemplars: www .aacn.org/wd/memberships/content/2013-coe-chapter-exemplars.pcms

References

American Association of Colleges of Nursing. (2007). *White paper on the education and role of the clinical nurse leader.* Retrieved from http://www.aacn.nche.edu/aacn-publications/white-papers/cnl-white-paper

American Nurses Association. (1996). *Scope and standards of advanced practice registered nursing.* Washington, DC: Author.

American Nurses Association. (2000). *Scope and standards of practice for nursing professional development.* Washington, DC: Author.

American Nurses Association & National Nursing Staff Development Organization. (2010). *Nursing professional development: Scope and standards of practice.* Silver Spring, MD: American Nurses Association.

American Nurses Credentialing Center. (n.d.). Forces of Magnetism. Retrieved from http://www.nursecredentialing .org/ForcesofMagnetism.aspx

American Nurses Credentialing Center. (2014). *Certification through portfolio application requirements.* Retrieved from http://www.nursecredentialing.org/CertificationPortfolioRequirements

Byrne, M., Schroeter, K., Carter, S., & Mower, J. (2009). The professional portfolio: An evidence-based assessment method. *Journal of Continuing Education in Nursing, 40,* 545–552. doi:10.3928/00220124-20091119-07

Cangelosi, P.R. (2008). Learning portfolios: Giving meaning to practice. *Nurse Educator, 33,* 125–127.

Capan, M.L., Ambrose, H.L., Burkett, M., Evangelista, T.R., Flook, D.M., & Straka, K.L. (2013). Nursing portfolio study: The use in annual performance reviews. *Journal for Nurses in Staff Development, 29,* 182–185. doi:10.1097/ nnd.0b013e31829aec0f

Fowler, J. (2012). Professional development: From staff nurse to nurse consultant. Part 7: Polishing your portfolio. *British Journal of Nursing, 21,* 367. doi:10.12968/bjon.2012.21.6.367

Heinrich, K.T., Tafas, C., & Jackson, C. (2011). Write a clinical narrative that clinches your advancement. *American Nurse Today, 6*(9), 24–25.

Hespenheide, M., Cottingham, T., & Mueller, G. (2011). Portfolio use as a tool to demonstrate professional development in advanced nursing practice. *Clinical Nurse Specialist, 25,* 312–320. doi:10.1097/NUR.0b013e318233ea90

Koloroutis, M. (Ed.). (2004). *Relationship-based care: A model for transforming practice.* Minneapolis, MN: Creative Health Care Management.

Koloroutis, M., Felgen, J.A., Person, C., & Wessel, S. (Eds.). (2007). *Relationship-based care field guide: Visions, strategies, tools and exemplars for transforming practice.* Minneapolis, MN: Creative Health Care Management.

Norris, T.L., Webb, S.S., McKeon, L.M., Jacob, S.R., & Herrin-Griffith, D. (2012). Using portfolios to introduce the clinical nurse leader to the job market. *Journal of Nursing Administration, 42,* 47–51.

Oermann, M.H. (2002). Developing a professional portfolio in nursing. *Orthopaedic Nursing, 21,* 73–78. doi:10.1097/00006416-200203000-00013

Owens, A.L., & Cleaves, J. (2012). Then and now: Updating clinical nurse advancement programs. *Nursing2012, 42*(10), 15–17. doi:10.1097/01.NURSE.0000419437.60674.45

Pellico, L.H., & Violano, P. (2010). Creating a room of our own. *Journal for Nurses in Staff Development, 26,* 104–107. doi:10.1097/NND.0b013e318199387d

CHAPTER 11

Preparing Your Résumé or Curriculum Vitae and Cover Letter

Y OU are faced with a quandary. You need to prepare a résumé for a new position that is available in a local community center but are not quite sure where to begin. You also are not sure what information should be included in a résumé.

Merriam-Webster describes a *résumé* as "a short document describing your education, work history, etc., that you give an employer when you are applying for a job" ("Resume", n.d.). Although nurses frequently associate preparing a résumé with the job-searching process, they may develop a résumé for a variety of other professional reasons.

A résumé should be more than just a summary of your past experiences. Experts have recently emphasized the importance of tailoring your résumé according to the needs of the receiver—in most instances, a prospective employer (Haseltine, 2013; Welton, 2013). In fact, some individuals perceive a résumé as a visual representation of one's professional image or self-image. Your résumé needs to show who you are as a professional nurse. It should reveal your identity and be framed within your experiences, accomplishments, and progress in self-development activities. An effective résumé can send a message that tells others how motivated you are as a professional and how you stand apart from other nurses.

You may have also heard of the term *curriculum vitae* (CV) but are unsure how it differs from a résumé. Merriam-Webster defines a *curriculum vitae* as "a short account of one's career and qualifications prepared typically by an applicant for a position" ("Curriculum Vitae", n.d.). Although some sources use the terms *résumé* and *curriculum vitae* interchangeably, in reality, a CV is a more extensive and detailed account of an individual's career history, including information about educational preparation, training, prior and current employment, teaching experience, presentations, awards, and service to the profession. A CV especially focuses on scholarly publications (Haseltine, 2013). A CV is usually required of faculty who work in schools of nursing within university or college settings. Because of the CV's lean toward education, Haseltine (2013) suggested that a résumé may be a stronger, more diverse document to use to market your skills to a prospective employer.

Regardless of your choice to create a résumé or a CV, the process described in this chapter can be helpful in designing either one; however, a résumé will be used as a primary example. Be sure to adhere to specific guidelines provided by prospective employers when you submit your résumé or CV. For example, if a newspaper ad for a nurse educator position requests that applicants submit a one-page résumé, then adhere to that request.

Reasons for Preparing a Résumé

Most nurses will agree that it is an expected practice to submit a résumé when you are applying for a new position or when you are changing work settings. However, developing a résumé for other professional situations can create a first impression that may help you with many of your career goals. A professional résumé can set you apart from other nurses competing for the same opportunity. Keeping an updated résumé available can allow you to respond quickly to opportunities, such as advancements in your workplace, new job opportunities, and awards, as soon as they are advertised. You will need to modify your résumé in these instances, but having a draft on hand allows you more time to prepare a new version.

Although a formal résumé is not required in all professional situations, nurses often are asked to provide content that is similar to that contained in a résumé on various applications. For example, application forms needed for admission into a school of nursing may ask about prior education and work experience. If your résumé is updated and readily available, using it as a reference will save you a great deal of time and aggravation.

Developing your résumé is very similar to conducting a professional self-assessment. In fact, the process of developing a résumé can help you realize your strengths or accomplishments, as well as your weaknesses or areas that need to be developed. Because a résumé traditionally contains several categories related to your professional development, it can be used as a focal point for a career plan (see Chapter 14).

Perhaps, while drafting your résumé, you discovered that you have nothing to enter under certain categories, such as professional organizations, continuing education (CE) programs attended, community involvement, or publications. Rather than fretting about not having these activities, view this discovery within its proper perspective and as a learning opportunity. By preparing your résumé, you discover potential areas in which you can focus your career goals. Plan to explore the professional activities that are missing in your résumé, such as writing a journal article or volunteering at a local nurse-managed wellness center, and incorporate them into your career plan. In this instance, include publishing an article in a nursing journal among one of your short-term goals. Pay special attention to the criteria required to advance in a clinical ladder system within your healthcare organization.

As an NPDS, developing your résumé can help you mentor staff nurses in creating their own in the future, as you will already be familiar with the process and the content that needs to be included. Rely on available resources, experts, and team-building strategies when helping staff nurses on your clinical unit develop their résumés. For example, consider inviting the nurse recruiter from your organization or faculty members from a local school of nursing to share their expertise on developing a strong résumé. Or, navigate through one of the free professional résumé websites available on the Internet. One example is Developing Your Résumé, a 75–90-minute workshop designed for students and offered by the Purdue University Online Writing Lab (n.d.). This source consists of a series of PowerPoint® slides organized into modules. Dialogue in the "Notes" section of each slide assists users in creating their own résumés. A YouTube version of this presentation can be found at www.youtube.com/watch?v=bdhs0VRJODo. You can locate other helpful resources for résumé writing at career services departments or the websites of educational institutions.

Job Application

As mentioned earlier, résumés are commonly used when applying for a job. Whether you are looking for your first nursing position or are changing jobs, your résumé should accurately and honestly match your expertise with the employer's mission and philosophy and the job qualifications advertised (Green, 2010; Welton, 2013). Be honest in describing your professional expertise, as you will need to provide evidence to support your claims.

A résumé often is used to supplement the information required on an organization's job application. A well-prepared, professional, and attractive résumé can set you apart from others who are applying for the same position. As mentioned in Chapter 10, your résumé should be part of your professional portfolio.

Promotion or Clinical Advancement

In addition to securing new positions, résumés can be tailored by more seasoned professionals to demonstrate evidence of their experience in a particular clinical specialty (Mathieu, 2010). Depending on your workplace, résumés may be required or preferred as part of the promotion process, especially in clinical advancement programs. Résumés are an effective means of summarizing your overall accomplishments and demonstrating progress within your career plan. Be sure that your résumé accurately and honestly reflects the stated expectations of a promotion or advancement.

Admission to School

A résumé can be included when applying for admission to a school of nursing. Depending on the web-based software program that a school uses, you may be asked to enter individual sections of your résumé or CV into an application template. Your document sends the message to an admissions committee that you recognize key activities of professional nursing practice. A résumé also can reflect the consistency of your contributions in clinical practice, nursing scholarship, and community service.

Scholarships, Awards, and Recognition

Include your résumé when applying for scholarships and awards, grants, or other forms of recognition. The next time you ask a former employer or teacher for a letter of recommendation, attach an updated résumé with your request. Your résumé can help these individuals organize the content of their letter so that it accurately reflects your accomplishments.

Conference Speaker

A résumé or a biographical sketch (a document that resembles a résumé) is requested of nurses who present papers or posters at professional nursing programs that award contact hours for attendance. Organizations that sponsor these programs often serve as approved providers of CE activities (American Nurses Credentialing Center [ANCC], 2012). As such, these organizations need to prepare several documents for review by their accredited approver (e.g., state nurses association), who must ensure the organization followed criteria for CEs established by ANCC (2012).

Once you are confirmed as a speaker, the conference planning committee will send you several forms to complete a few weeks prior to the conference. Even if a formal résumé is not required, information available from your résumé can simplify this process. Résumés also are used by conference planners to introduce you to participants immediately prior to your presentation.

Manuscript or Educational Program Reviewer

If you are interested in serving as a manuscript reviewer for a nursing journal, a résumé can provide an editor with an overall impression of your professional qualifications. Once you have become a manuscript reviewer for a journal, be sure to add this accomplishment to your résumé as a professional service activity. Similarly, your service as a pilot or field reviewer for a CE program should be added to your résumé to reflect this expertise.

Consultant

Maybe you possess expertise in a particular area of nursing, such as establishing an early discharge program for new mothers or providing nursing care for patients diagnosed with head and neck cancer. Perhaps you have the expertise to serve as a legal nurse consultant on cases where professional judgment of nursing care is required. Regardless of the type of consulting you provide, a résumé can inform others of your qualifications.

Certifications

Although applications for obtaining or renewing specialty certifications do not typically require submission of a résumé, the information included in a résumé is often needed. For example, certification renewals may ask for clinical practice positions and hours, professional presentations and publications, preceptor experience, completed academic coursework, and attendance at CE programs. Having this information readily available on your résumé can make the application process easier to complete.

What to Include in a Résumé

Although minor variations exist, most résumés contain common categories or content areas. Some of these common categories can be found in Figure 11-1. Create a document listing the categories you will use. Be sure to leave sufficient space after each category so that you can fill in your specific information.

Do not worry about being neat right now, because this is your personal worksheet; only you need to understand it at this point in the process. As you enter information from your personal files into the résumé draft, try to be accurate and record detailed information. Pay less attention to style, format, and order of content at this point. Consider using a résumé template provided by professional networking sites such as Monster (www.monster.com) or LinkedIn (www.linkedin.com) (Mathieu, 2010).

Depending on your experience, you may need to search several sources to compile information for these categories, such as your personal calendar, certificates received from attending CE programs, school files, conference records, presentations, and performance evaluations. Ask the nurse educator in the staff development or nursing education department at your workplace for more details about the programs you have attended, if needed. You also may need to review your professional file at work to fill in some gaps. A brainstorming session with your peers can be a productive means of completing missing data, such as conference dates or college courses.

Figure 11-1. Main Categories Frequently Used in a Résumé

- Identification information
- Career objective (optional)
- Education
- Professional work experience
- Licensure, certifications, and certificates
- Awards, honors, and special recognition
- Professional activities
  - Membership in professional organizations
  - Publications
  - Research
  - Consulting
  - Presentations
- Community volunteer activities
- Attendance at continuing education programs (past five years)
- References (optional)

Identification Information

This section contains identification information and provides the heading for your résumé. Start with your full name followed by your credentials. Be sure to include any certifications you may have, such as RNC, OCN®, or CORLN. Your highest degree in nursing appears before the RN listing. Follow this information with your mailing address, phone number, and email address. Avoid using your work email if you are applying for a position at another healthcare organization. Make sure that your email address is professional in nature and does not include any nicknames (Welton, 2013).

Because this is contact information, it is important that it is both accurate and current. Omit personal or confidential information on your résumé, such as your Social Security number, age, marital status, or names of family members.

Career Objective

Next, include a career objective on your résumé, especially if you are applying for a job. This objective informs prospective employers of your goals. It also helps them determine a match between your goals and their needs. If your résumé is intended for a reason other than job placement or promotion, you may want to omit this category.

An example of a career objective might be, *To obtain a beginning staff nurse position in cardiovascular nursing*. Perhaps you are an experienced RN interested in obtaining a nursing management position. If so, your objective may look like this: *To obtain a first-level management position within a progressive university-affiliated medical center*. Tailor your career objective to the prospective employer. Keep it realistic, concise (one or two sentences), and within the limits of your qualifications.

Education

The next category is education, in which you will describe your educational background relevant to the overall purpose of your résumé. Include the names of educational institutions you have attended, such as your school of nursing and college or university. You can also include any college credits obtained at institutions where you did not complete a degree. If you are currently completing a degree, include your anticipated date of graduation. Be sure to add the locations of schools, years attended, your major and/or minor areas of study, and degree(s) awarded. Some nurses choose to supply their grade point average at each school attended, especially if it will support your application. In most instances, it is not necessary to list your high school education.

You might, for example, list a diploma in nursing, an associate degree in nursing, a bachelor's degree in nursing, or a master of science in nursing degree. Check your school transcript or official diploma if you are uncertain of the wording of your degree. Most likely, your major is in nursing, although you may have completed a minor in another discipline, such as psychology or a language. If nursing is your second degree, be sure to list your previous degree.

This information informs readers of your formal preparation in nursing and other fields. It also makes them aware of any advanced nursing preparation you have received.

Professional Work Experience

The next section affords the opportunity to describe your previous professional employment (paid) experiences. As mentioned before, include content that is essential to the purpose of your résumé. Start by listing your present and past job titles or positions, dates of employment, employers, and their locations. Provide a succinct review of your major responsibilities. Include activities such as serving as a clinical preceptor for nursing students or new employees on your unit. If you are applying for your first position as an RN, include your experience working as a nursing assistant or participating in student internships.

List each major responsibility as a separate, brief statement. Begin each statement with an action verb such as the ones listed in Figure 11-2. Unless you want to emphasize a particular point, provide more details about your most recent positions and less about your previous positions. You may choose to include your membership in various committees in this section.

If possible, organize your past positions so that they demonstrate progression or make some sort of sense. For example, if you have had several nursing positions within one organization, develop a creative way to illustrate how these positions are connected. Avoid making them appear simply as a listing of jobs. If you are applying for your first job as an RN, list previous jobs that represent your positive qualities, such as your ability to organize and lead groups, your independence and competence when completing assignments, and your effective communication skills.

Licensure, Certifications, and Certificates

List any current licensures that you hold, including the state in which you received each licensure and the expiration dates. In this category, include any specialty certifications you have attained (e.g., OCN®, CORLN), the sponsoring agencies providing each certification, and the effective dates of your certifications. Be sure to include special certificates you have obtained, such as cardiopulmonary resuscitation (CPR) or advanced cardiac life support. Specify if you are qualified as an instructor or instructor trainer in these areas.

Although proof of licensure as a professional nurse is a requirement when obtaining an RN position, certifications demonstrate that you voluntarily excelled above and beyond in a nursing specialty and have assumed a leadership role by choosing to prepare for and take the certification examination. These activities can set you apart from other RNs who possess similar work experience.

Figure 11-2. Examples of Action Words

Accomplishments

Achieved	Exceeded	Pioneered	Reversed	Surpassed
Benchmarked	Expanded	Reduced (losses)	Spearheaded	Transformed
Completed	Improved	Resolved (issues)	Succeeded	Won

Analytical and Research

Analyzed	Detected	Formulated	Investigated	Reviewed
Assessed	Determined	Gathered	Located	Searched
Calibrated	Diagnosed	Identified	Measured	Specified
Clarified	Evaluated	Inspected	Observed	Summarized
Collected	Examined	Interpreted	Organized	Surveyed
Compared	Experimented	Interviewed	Proved	Tested
Conducted	Explored	Invented	Researched	Validated
Critiqued	Extracted			

Communication and Persuasion

Addressed	Convinced	Elicited	Joined	Recruited
Advertised	Corresponded	Enlisted	Judged	Referred
Arbitrated	Debated	Established	Lectured	Reinforced
Arranged	Defined	Explained	Marketed	Reported
Articulated	Demonstrated	Expressed	Mediated	Resolved
Authored	Described	Formulated	Moderated	Responded
Clarified	Developed	Furnished	Modified	Solicited
Collaborated	Directed	Illustrated	Observed	Specified
Composed	Discussed	Influenced	Participated	Spoke
Condensed	Dissuaded	Informed	Persuaded	Suggested
Conferred	Documented	Interacted	Presented	Summarized
Consulted	Drafted	Interpreted	Promoted	Synthesized
Contacted	Edited	Interviewed	Proposed	Translated
Conveyed	Educated	Involved	Publicized	Wrote

Creative

Acted	Created	Drew	Instituted	Performed
Adapted	Customized	Entertained	Integrated	Photographed
Began	Designed	Established	Introduced	Planned
Combined	Developed	Fashioned	Invented	Revised
Composed	Devised	Formulated	Modeled	Revitalized
Conceptualized	Directed	Founded	Modified	Shaped
Condensed	Displayed	Illustrated	Originated	Solved

Financial and Data

Adjusted	Balanced	Determined	Prepared	Researched
Administered	Budgeted	Developed	Programmed	Retrieved
Allocated	Calculated	Estimated	Projected	Tabulated
Analyzed	Computed	Managed	Purchased	Tracked
Appraised	Conserved	Marketed	Quantified	Trimmed
Assessed	Cut	Measured	Reconciled	
Audited	Decreased	Planned	Reduced	

(Continued on next page)

Figure 11-2. Examples of Action Words *(Continued)*

Helping

Adapted	Cared for	Diagnosed	Helped	Rehabilitated
Advocated	Clarified	Educated	Insured	Represented
Aided	Coached	Encouraged	Intervened	Resolved
Answered	Contributed	Ensured	Motivated	Simplified
Arranged	Cooperated	Expedited	Prevented	Supplied
Assessed	Counseled	Facilitated	Provided	Supported
Assisted	Demonstrated	Guided	Referred	Volunteered

Interpersonal and Teamwork

Advised	Focused	Involved	Mentored	Partnered
Collaborated	Initiated	Listened	Moderated	Solved
Enabled	Interacted	Mediated	Negotiated	

Leadership and Management

Accomplished	Decided	Founded	Launched	Reorganized
Acted	Decreased	Generated	Led	Replaced
Administered	Delegated	Governed	Lowered	Represented
Advanced	Determined	Guided	Managed	Restored
Advised	Developed	Headed	Merged	Reviewed
Analyzed	Directed	Hired	Modified	Saved
Appointed	Dispatched	Hosted	Motivated	Scheduled
Approved	Disseminated	Improved	Organized	Secured
Assigned	Diversified	Incorporated	Originated	Selected
Attained	Eliminated	Increased	Overhauled	Shaped
Authorized	Emphasized	Influenced	Oversaw	Solidified
Chaired	Enforced	Initiated	Pioneered	Stimulated
Completed	Enhanced	Inspected	Planned	Streamlined
Considered	Enlisted	Inspired	Presided	Strengthened
Consolidated	Ensured	Instigated	Prioritized	Supervised
Contracted	Established	Instituted	Produced	Terminated
Controlled	Examined	Instructed	Proposed	Trimmed
Converted	Executed	Integrated	Recommended	Updated
Coordinated	Explained	Introduced	Recruited	Verified
Counseled				

Organization and Detail

Approved	Coordinated	Inspected	Processed	Scheduled
Arranged	Corrected	Logged	Provided	Screened
Catalogued	Corresponded	Maintained	Purchased	Set up
Categorized	Distributed	Monitored	Recorded	Standardized
Charted	Executive	Obtained	Registered	Submitted
Classified	Expedited	Operated	Reserved	Supplied
Coded	Filed	Ordered	Responded	Updated
Collected	Generated	Organized	Restructured	Used
Compiled	Implemented	Planned	Reviewed	Validated
Contained	Incorporated	Prepared	Routed	Verified

(Continued on next page)

Figure 11-2. Examples of Action Words (Continued)

Teaching and Training

Adapted	Coordinated	Evaluated	Informed	Simulated
Advised	Critiqued	Explained	Instilled	Taught
Appraised	Demonstrated	Facilitated	Instructed	Tested
Clarified	Developed	Focused	Motivated	Trained
Coached	Educated	Guided	Persuaded	Transmitted
Communicated	Enabled	Influenced	Set	Tutored
Conducted	Encouraged			

Technical

Adapted	Conserved	Fortified	Prevented	Retrieved
Advised	Constructed	Identified	Printed	Solved
Analyzed	Controlled	Implemented	Programmed	Specialized
Applied	Converted	Inspected	Proposed	Specified
Assembled	Debugged	Installed	Recorded	Standardized
Automated	Designed	Located	Rectified	Studied
Built	Determined	Maintained	Regulated	Supported
Calculated	Diagnosed	Monitored	Remodeled	Trained
Coded	Drafted	Networked	Repaired	Troubleshoot
Computed	Engineered	Operated	Replaced	Upgraded
Computerized	Fabricated	Overhauled	Restored	

Note. From "Action Verbs," by Duquesne University Career Services Center, n.d. Retrieved from http://www.duq.edu/Documents/career-services/_pdf/Action%20Verbs.pdf. Copyright by Duquesne University. Reprinted with permission.

Awards, Honors, Special Recognitions, and Scholarships

List any awards, honors, special recognitions, or scholarships you have received, especially those that have resulted from a review of your accomplishments by your peers. Include the names of the awards, their sponsoring agencies, and the dates they were acquired. Examples include attaining membership into Sigma Theta Tau International, achieving the dean's list at your school, receiving a professional nursing organization's literary award, or acquiring other service awards.

This information shows that you not only have experience in particular areas within the profession of nursing but also were recognized by colleagues or community members for your accomplishments.

Professional Activities

This section of a résumé contains an assortment of your professional experiences in nursing. These activities can either be grouped together or listed separately based on what experiences you have had in these areas. If you have very few activities to list, then you may choose to organize them together under the heading of "Professional Activities." On the other hand, if you have many experiences, list them separately under each subheading. Exclude any subheadings for which you have no experience. Avoid the practice of listing headings or subheadings followed by the explanation "none."

Membership in Professional Organizations

In this section, detail any professional organizations to which you are a paid or nonpaid member. These may include international, national, state, local, or private organizations (e.g., Oncology Nursing Society, Sigma Theta Tau International Honor Society of Nursing, ANA). Include memberships you hold within these organizations at the local chapter and state levels. Try clustering smaller state and chapter groups under their larger parent organizations to provide order to your listing.

Be sure to include the official name of the professional organizations (and acronyms), dates of membership, and your specific roles (e.g., member, committee chair, treasurer, president) within each organization.

This section demonstrates to people viewing your résumé that you are an involved professional who is concerned about what is happening within nursing and your specialty. Holding an office or committee chair position demonstrates your ability to lead or direct others related to a particular project. It also speaks of your communication skills. Because your peers voted for you to lead them, holding an elected office reflects that your skills are valued.

Publications

List any publications that you have authored or coauthored, if available. If you are listing an article, be sure to include the full names and first initials of all authors, year of publication, the title of the article, journal name, volume number, and inclusive pages. If you are citing a book, include the book title, the city and state of the publisher, and the publishing company. When noting a chapter, indicate the author(s) and title of the specific chapter you are citing. Unless a particular format is specified, use any format or publication manual style to document the details of your publication(s), and use this style consistently when citing your entries. You can obtain copies of these manuals through your library's reference section or see formatting guidelines online at the Purdue Online Writing Lab (https://owl.english.purdue.edu/owl). The sample résumé shown in Figure 11-3 illustrates a publication formatted according to American Psychological Association (2009) style, which is frequently used to cite references in nursing journals. Listing your publications provides evidence of your diversification as a professional nurse.

Research and Evidence-Based/Quality Improvement Projects

This section provides an opportunity to share your research activities. Research experience often varies among nurses and frequently depends on job type, opportunities available at school or work, and the guidance available. Research participation can be viewed as either formal or informal. Formal activities in research often involve assuming the role of an investigator or researcher. Informal participation may include helping a unit-based research team with various activities needed to carry out the research process, such as conducting a review of the literature, assisting with data collection on the clinical unit, or helping with data entry.

Be sure to include your participation in any quality improvement or evidence-based projects and note specific reports that were produced as a result.

If appropriate, describe the extent of your involvement in any research project. Be sure to include a list of investigators (specify who was the principal investigator or leader of the project), the title of the study, the agency that funded the study, the amount in dollars awarded (if applicable), and the year(s) the research was conducted. If the research is still in progress, clarify this point. If you are not listed as a formal investigator or worked on the project as a research assistant or student while in school, provide information that describes your specific role in the project.

This section demonstrates your involvement and initiative in nursing scholarship and related clinical problem-solving activities. It also illustrates many of the reasons for participating in research, as described in Chapter 12.

Consultant

Describe your involvement in consulting activities, such as serving as an expert witness for a law firm. Include your general area of consultation, such as labor and delivery or trauma nursing, along with the dates you were involved in this activity. To maintain confidential-

---

Figure 11-3. Sample Résumé

EMILLIE M. BROOKS, BSN, RN, OCN®
126 Oaktree Drive
Pittsburgh, PA 35871
(xxx) xxx-xxxx (Cell)
E-mail: brooksem@cmm.org

OBJECTIVE:
To obtain a staff nurse position in oncology home care.

PROFESSIONAL WORK EXPERIENCE:
University Medical Center, Pittsburgh, PA 15213
Clinical Nurse II, Medical Oncology Unit (2010 to present)
• Provided direct care to medical patients with cancer
• Supervised staff nurses and ancillary healthcare workers
• Functioned as charge nurse as needed
• Chaired the Patient Education Committee
• Coordinated a unit-based education program
• Served as a preceptor for staff nurses during cross-training

EDUCATION:
BSN, Nursing, 2010, Duquesne University School of Nursing, Pittsburgh, PA

LICENSURE AND CERTIFICATIONS:
PA RN License (2010 to present)
OCN®, Oncology Nursing Certification Corporation (2012 to present)
Basic Cardiac Life Support, American Heart Association (2010 to present)

AWARDS AND HONORS:
Sigma Theta Tau International Honor Society of Nursing, 2010
Graduated summa cum laude, Duquesne University, 2010

MEMBERSHIP IN PROFESSIONAL ORGANIZATIONS:
Oncology Nursing Society (2010 to present)
Sigma Theta Tau International Honor Society of Nursing, Epsilon Phi Chapter (2010 to present)

PUBLICATIONS:
Brooks, E.M. (2014). Teaching the medical oncology patient. *Nursing Journal, 1*(4), 123–125.

COMMUNITY ACTIVITIES:
Volunteer for Eastside Shelter, Pittsburgh, PA, 2009 to present

CONTINUING EDUCATION PROGRAMS ATTENDED:
Cancer Nursing Course, Oncology Programs Inc., March 3–7, 2014
Case Management, L. Jones, Townsend Conferences, June 5, 2013
Pain Management, J. Goodman, University Hospital, January 5, 2013

REFERENCES:
Available upon request

ity, avoid disclosing the names of the parties involved in the case. Use the same guidelines for other opportunities you have had as a consultant.

This section tells people viewing your résumé that your nursing expertise is recognized and valued by others. Your prior experience as a consultant may also show that you are qualified for particular job opportunities.

Presentations

List any presentations you have given at the local, regional, national, or international level. Be sure to include the title of your presentations, the conferences and organizations they were presented for, and their dates and locations (city and state).

The presence of presentations on your résumé informs people of your ability to disseminate professional information. It also reflects that you assumed a leadership role in communicating with groups, such as professional nursing organizations and lay communities.

Community Volunteer Activities

Use this section to identify any community activities in which you volunteer your expertise and time. For example, perhaps you serve lunch at a local homeless shelter and provide monthly educational programs on health promotion topics. Or, maybe you taught CPR to a neighborhood community group. Be sure to list the dates involved, the names of the volunteer organizations or groups, their locations, and a general statement about the specific services you provided.

This listing of community activities tells others that you share your nursing expertise voluntarily with the community. It demonstrates that you recognize the need to participate in community service as a healthcare professional.

Attendance at Continuing Education Programs

List any professional CE programs you have attended. Try to limit this list to the past three to five years, depending on the purpose of your résumé. Start with the most current program you have attended. Include the following with each entry: date attended, title of the presentation, speaker, sponsoring organization, and location (city and state). Indicate the contact hours you received, the provider, and the accrediting or approval organization. If your list is particularly long, prepare this section as an appendix or attachment to your résumé. You will need to maintain a file of CE program attendance for other purposes (see Chapter 13), such as when applying for or renewing a specialty certification or RN license.

Regular attendance at clinically relevant professional conferences tells others that you take personal responsibility to keep abreast of changes in your discipline.

References

If appropriate, supply the names, addresses, emails, and telephone numbers of individuals who are willing to serve as professional references for you. Choose two or three individuals whose expertise matches the goal of your résumé. References should include people who know you on a personal level, as well as colleagues who can speak on the quality of your professional work. In some instances, you may be asked to provide names of individuals as references who possess particular backgrounds or specifications, such as a former clinical instructor or supervisor.

Be sure to obtain permission from these individuals before you list them as references, as it is unprofessional to assume that they will grant permission without being asked first. You might want to call and ask them to serve as a reference for you. Follow the call with a note or letter that explains the details of your request. The sample cover letter described later in this chapter can be adapted for this purpose. Supply a copy of your résumé for their review. Because some agencies ask for references written on an official application form rather than in letter form, investigate the requirements prior to making arrangements. Be sure to follow up with a thank-you note to those who provided you with a reference.

Organizing the Content of Your Résumé

Once you have drafted the main content of your résumé, organize the data you compiled under each heading. Decide what content areas you plan on including, combining, or eliminating. Decide on the order of the headings, as was previously mentioned. Most résumé guides suggest a similar sequence of headings, but you can design yours to emphasize certain areas. Although you want to avoid "padding" or adding false information to your résumé, you have the freedom to fashion it so that it effectively communicates your strengths to the reader. This is particularly important because a résumé is often the first information a potential employer sees.

Try preparing two drafts of your résumé and asking your peers or a mentor to choose the one that is most appealing. You may decide to design several versions, depending on your intended goal or overall objective.

Choosing a Format

Résumés are commonly organized using either a chronological or functional format; however, most health-related employers prefer the chronological approach (Welton, 2013). If you choose the traditional chronological format for your résumé, arrange your information under each category in reverse chronological order. For example, organize your professional experience section by listing your most recent job and description first, followed by the jobs you held earlier. Your oldest job should be listed last.

Although nurses commonly use the chronological format, choose this approach only if it meets your particular professional needs. Some experts suggest a chronologically formatted résumé for graduate or novice nurses who are just beginning the job search process or for those who have been continually employed throughout their professional careers. Because information listed first within a category on your résumé is likely to receive the most attention by the reader, the chronological format also may be appropriate for nurses who are seeking positions at a level higher than their previous occupation.

Alternatively, a functional résumé centers on the applicant's particular skills or competencies (Welton, 2013), such as management skills or special technology skills developed from prior jobs or training. These strengths are stated at the beginning of the résumé and accompanied with examples from your various experiences. This focal section is followed by the usual information, such as job positions, dates, employers, and locations.

Because functional résumés focus more on achievements and less on dates, this approach may benefit nurses with less traditional work experiences. Although these résumés can help minimize gaps in employment or "job hopping" that occurred throughout your professional work history, they are not typically used in health care (Welton, 2013).

Relying on Resources

If you choose to prepare your own résumé, be sure that you have access to word-processing software and a quality printer. If your budget permits, rely on the graphical expertise of a professional résumé service. If you use a professional company to prepare your résumé, be sure to choose one with a good reputation and investigate the confidentiality policy related to any information you provide. Ask others who have used a company about the quality of its résumés and services. While some word-processing software include résumé templates in which you simply enter the content, these templates may limit your ability to modify sections (Welton, 2013). For example, you can access sample résumé template in Microsoft® Word® by clicking on the "File" tab at the top of the screen and choosing "New."

Regardless of the approach, you are the author of your résumé and need to provide accurate, complete, and current content. Once you have developed your résumé, update it regularly. Consider updating your résumé each year, for example, prior to your performance evaluation at work.

Preparing the Layout: Aesthetic Considerations

Now that you have planned and organized the content of your résumé, focus on its overall appearance. The first impression that your résumé makes to others is important. Try to think from the perspective of the viewer and develop a résumé that requires the least amount of effort to read. Because you are competing against other nurses with similar credentials, every element of your résumé is vital. Although you do not want to exaggerate your experiences, you also do not want to underestimate them.

If you are preparing a hard copy of your résumé, carefully choose the quality, color, and weight of paper you will use. If an employer prefers to receive your résumé electronically as an attachment in an email or as an uploaded file within the organization's online management system, consider changing your Microsoft Word document into a PDF to maintain its original format (Welton, 2013).

Mathieu (2010) suggested creating a résumé in three formats: a print version (hard copy with design features), a scannable version (without many design features), and a plain text version (to cut and paste into an online system). The Purdue University Online Writing Lab (n.d.) offers a workshop presentation that can help you create a scannable résumé document.

Although a variety of attractive colors and textures are available for a reasonable cost at most paper supply stores, be sure that the one you select captures a professional image. Neutral shades, such as white, off-white, beige, and ivory, are appropriate color selections (Feery & Tierney, 2002). Avoid the use of pastel-colored papers. Although these may be attractive, their unprofessional look may be the deciding factor in eliminating your résumé. Consider using quality, letter-sized bond paper with at least a 20-pound weight (Feery & Tierney, 2002).

Print and Special Effects

Similar to preparing a poster presentation, pay special attention to the size and type of print used in your résumé. Choose a font size (at least 11 point) and style that are both readable and professional (Haseltine, 2013). A résumé is not the place to experiment with extreme graphics. Use a quality printer to produce a crisp and attractive output. Use features such as boldface, capitals, underlining, and large type sizes selectively. Try outlining essential points, such as job responsibilities, with bullets (Haseltine, 2013). Avoid adding handwritten comments or corrections on your printed résumé.

Length

Limit your résumé to one or two pages, especially if you are a beginning professional. More experienced professionals might consider two to three additional pages to capture pertinent experience (Welton, 2013). Unless otherwise specified by the employer, allow essential information (not page restrictions) to guide the length of your résumé. If you have just one or two lines on a second page, reorganize your content to make your résumé fit on one sheet of paper. You can accomplish this by shortening earlier job experiences or combining two entries into one. Whatever your approach, review your résumé and exclude unnecessary information.

Grammar, Spelling, and Punctuation

Pay close attention to grammar, spelling, and punctuation when developing your résumé. These need to be perfect. Similar to the techniques described when refining a manuscript for publication (see Chapter 8), read your résumé aloud or ask colleagues to proofread it. Be consistent and concise when listing points, such as your major work responsibilities or accomplishments. For example, start each responsibility with an action verb and limit it to one or two lines. Figure 11-2 provides a list of action-oriented words that may be helpful for this part of your résumé.

Margins and Spacing

Pay close attention to the margins and spacing on your résumé. Allow at least a one-inch margin or more around the borders. Be sure to single-space within an entry and double-space between entries. You may need to be creative with this option if you are limited on space. Center your name and demographic information, or align it to the left side of the page.

Evaluating the Results

Once you have prepared the polished draft of your résumé, ask several colleagues and family members to critique it again for both appearance and content. Ask them about their first impression of your résumé. Was the layout attractive and professional? Did the print direct their attention to the essential points? Was the content relevant and action oriented? Did it reflect a valuable potential employee? Incorporate their suggestions into your résumé's final edit.

Pay attention to details. Insert the date at the end of your résumé to help you maintain its currency. Include your name and the page number on each page. Always use original copies of your résumé rather than photocopies. Keep a master version and copies of your résumé along with the file (plus a backup file) in a safe place, such as with your professional files or portfolio materials.

Creating a Cover Letter

Always prepare a cover letter to accompany your résumé, unless directed otherwise (Welton, 2013). Because the content of this letter will vary depending on your purpose or intention, tailor this letter carefully to the receiver. The basic guidelines are similar to the instructions given in preparing a query communication, as described in Chapter 8 on publishing. Figure 11-4 provides an example of a cover letter used for employment purposes.

A cover letter consists of three primary parts: the opening paragraph; the body, which describes your qualifications for the job (Welton, 2013); and the closing. Because this letter is commonly limited to one page, you need to carefully plan its content to capture your intended message.

The opening of your letter should contain the date and your mailing address, along with the exact name, title, and address of the recipient. Be sure to spell the name correctly and include appropriate credentials. Consider creating your own letterhead by centering your name, address, and contact information at the top of the page.

The body of the letter consists of several essential elements. Start with a brief statement regarding the purpose of the letter. For example, if you are applying for a nursing position, first state the title of the position and how you became aware of it, and briefly describe your interest. Next, introduce yourself and highlight your essential experiences. Focus on how they match the requirements for the position and why you want to work for this organization. For example, perhaps you had the opportunity to visit this organization during one of your clinical experiences as a student. When addressing your professional qualities, try using self-descriptive words, such as "motivated," "conscientious," and "energetic." A list of similar words can be found at www.uow.edu.au/careers/recycle-bin/applications/actionwords/index.html. Finally, explain how and when you can be contacted for an interview. For example, you may ask them to call you at work or at home during your available hours, instruct them to leave a message, or suggest that they email you, if appropriate. Close the letter with your name, credentials, and title (if appropriate). Be sure to sign your name in blue or black ink above the typed version.

Pay close attention to spacing, paper quality, and font size and style. Have your colleagues critique your cover letter and résumé, examining their layout and attractiveness. Be sure that the content is distributed over the entire paper. Often, nurses make the mistake of crowding the text at the top third of the paper. Pay close attention to the quality of the envelope and text if you intend to mail or personally deliver your résumé. Some organizations may simply request you to submit your résumé electronically via email or a web-based system.

Summary

Résumés and curricula vitae are important documents needed when applying for a new job, a promotion, clinical advancement, or admission to graduate studies. These documents also may be used when applying for scholarships and awards or when serving as a conference speaker, manuscript reviewer, or consultant. This chapter described the essential components of a résumé and a cover letter and offered suggestions for organizing and developing a résumé with or without a template. Careful use of action words to describe your accomplishments were also addressed. Attention to layout and aesthetics helps to make a good first impression.

Figure 11-4. Sample Cover Letter for a Job Application

EMILLIE M. BROOKS, BSN, RN, OCN®
126 Oaktree Drive
Pittsburgh, PA 35871
(617) 333-8979 (Work) (617) 987-4957 (Home)
Email: brooksem@cmm.org

September 15, 2015

Ms. Joan Kenneth, Personnel Director
Oncology Home Care, Gateway Center
Pittsburgh, PA 35871

Dear Ms. Kenneth:

This letter is in application for the position of Oncology Home Care Nurse that was advertised in the September 14 issue of the *Pittsburgh Post-Gazette*. You are seeking a BSN-prepared RN certified in oncology nursing to provide direct nursing care to medical oncology patients within the community in which I currently reside.

I am presently employed as a Clinical Nurse II on a medical oncology unit at University Medical Center. My career goal is to obtain a homecare position that utilizes both my professional experience and leadership abilities. As a nursing student, I had the pleasure of having my community practicum at your agency and admired the professionalism of your nursing staff.

Enclosed is my résumé, which details my professional background. Should you need any additional information, please feel free to contact me by email or telephone. I can be reached at work during the day or at home during the evening. My contact information is listed in the letterhead. Thank you for your time. I look forward to hearing from you.

Sincerely,

Emillie M. Brooks

Emillie M. Brooks, BSN, RN, OCN®

Helpful Websites

- Georgetown University, Cawley Career Education Center—Resumes and Cover Letters: http://careercenter.georgetown.edu/resumes-cover-letters
- Microsoft Office—Templates: Resumes and Cover Letters: https://templates.office.com/templates/Resumes%20and%20Cover%20Letters
- Purdue University Online Writing Lab: https://owl.english.purdue.edu/owl

References

American Nurses Credentialing Center. (2012). *Educational design process: 2013 mini manual.* Silver Spring, MD: Author.

American Psychological Association. (2009). *Publication manual of the American Psychological Association* (6th ed.). Washington, DC: Author.

Curriculum vitae. (n.d.). In *Merriam-Webster's online dictionary* (11th ed.). Retrieved from http://www.merriam-webster.com/dictionary/curriculum%20vitae

Feery, B., & Tierney, C.M. (2002). Résumés: The recruiter's perspective. In C.L. Saver (Ed.), *Nursing Spectrum student career fitness tool kit 2002–2003* (pp. 18–21). Hoffman Estates, IL: Nursing Spectrum.

Green, T. (2010). Putting relevance in your resume. *NASN School Nurse, 25*(1), 10.

Haseltine, D. (2013). Job-search basics: How to convert a CV into a resume. *Nature Immunology, 14,* 6–9.

Mathieu, J. (2010). Revamping your résumé for your specialty. *Journal of the American Dietetic Association, 110,* 353–360.

Purdue University Online Writing Lab. (n.d.). Résumé workshop presentation. Retrieved from https://owl.english.purdue.edu/owl/resource/719/06

Resume. (n.d.). In *Merriam-Webster's online dictionary* (11th ed.). Retrieved from http://www.merriam-webster.com/dictionary/resume

Welton, R.H. (2013). Writing an employer-focused resume for advanced practice nurses. *AACN Advanced Critical Care, 24,* 203–217.

CHAPTER 12

Promoting Nursing Research and Evidence-Based Practice in the Clinical Setting

A S an NPDS, it is important that you understand your role and responsibilities related to research, evidence-based practice (EBP), and quality improvement (QI) based on standards at your workplace and on a national level. It is also important to clarify your expected involvement in these activities not only as an educator, but also as a mentor for clinical nurses and others within your healthcare organization. Over time, practice changes at your workplace may modify your involvement in these activities (American Nurses Association [ANA] & National Nursing Staff Development Organization [NNSDO], 2010).

It is crucial that you create a professional development plan aimed to strengthen your research, EBP, and QI skills, especially in an ever-changing healthcare field. This chapter will focus on the role of the clinical nurse in research and EBP and the various strategies that you can use as an NPDS to help nurses in these initiatives.

Understanding Your Role in Research and Evidence-Based Practice

Research, EBP, and QI are three separate yet related activities that often confuse nurses. Shirey et al. (2011) offered a comprehensive review and comparison of these three important initiatives, giving examples of their application in clinical practice settings. Reading these types of publications is extremely helpful in developing professionally and strengthening competencies. Discussing similar articles through active dialogue with colleagues can provide you with an even deeper understanding of these topics.

According to Polit and Beck (2012), *research* consists of "systematic inquiry that uses orderly, disciplined methods to answer questions and solve problems" (p. 741). *EBP*, on the other hand, is a "clinical problem-solving strategy that emphasizes the integration of best available evidence from disciplined research with clinical expertise and patient preferences" (Polit & Beck, 2012, p. 727). The ultimate goal of EBP is quality patient care and health outcomes (Melnyk, Fineout-Overholt, Stillwell, & Williamson, 2009). In EBP, nurses are expected to translate evidence obtained through research, clinical expertise, and patient preferences to their daily practice rather than continuing to do things the way they have always been done (Melnyk et al., 2009). This national movement toward EBP in healthcare settings may require nurses to learn new concepts, develop new skills and competencies, or refine skills they had previously learned during their professional careers. Such skills may include learning how to conduct a literature search, evaluating the strengths of research reports, and applying research evidence appropriately in practice related to a specific clinical issue (Melnyk et al., 2009).

Chapter 2 presented the NPDS practice model (ANA & NNSDO, 2010). Contained within this model were two throughputs relevant to this chapter: research and scholarship, and EBP practice and practice-based evidence (ANA & NNSDO, 2010). The topics of scholarship related to writing for publication in peer-reviewed journals (see Chapter 8) and disseminating your scholarship to the healthcare community through professional abstracts, oral podium presentations, and poster displays (see Chapter 9) were discussed in previous chapters.

Performance expectations of NPDSs regarding research and EBP also are included in *Nursing Professional Development: Scope and Standards of Practice*, addressed within the specialist's Scope of Responsibility (under Program Management), Core Competencies (under Leadership), and Intertwined Elements (under Research and Consultant role) (ANA & NNSDO, 2010). Specifically, NPDSs are expected to exhibit an understanding of the research process and model the application of EBP. The NPDS's role in research and EBP may vary and can include "advisor, investigator, collaborator, translator, integrator, or evaluator" (ANA & NNSDO, 2010, p. 17).

Similarly, QI is a method used within a particular clinical setting, such as a clinical unit, with the goal of strengthening the outcomes of a system or process (Dearholt & Dang, 2012; Institute of Medicine [IOM] Committee on Assessing the System for Protecting Human Research Participants, 2002). Searching for and appraising research studies related to a particular clinical problem is an integral step of the EBP process (Melnyk, Fineout-Overholt, Stillwell, & Williamson, 2010). A research study may be initiated at a clinical setting if there is little or no evidence found regarding the problem. The QI process usually "includes a method of measuring a particular outcome, making changes to improve practice, and monitoring performance on an ongoing basis" (Dearholt & Dang, 2012, p. 5). Ideas for EPB projects often begin with QI processes that uncovered a clinical problem or nursing practice issue on the clinical unit (Dearholt & Dang, 2012).

Evaluating the Qualifications of Clinical Nurses and Understanding Their Roles in Research and Evidence-Based Practice

RNs at your organization likely differ in terms of their educational backgrounds and experiences. As a result, their understanding of research and EBP will vary depending on their prior academic preparation and participation in continuing education (CE) programs on these topics. Because their ability to actively participate in research and EBP efforts on their clinical units may greatly differ, it is important that you develop strategies tailored to their needs.

Research and EBP skills are influenced by nurses' exposure to these topics during their prelicensure RN academic programs, additional academic (graduate degree) preparation, or informal CE. For example, nurses who completed their bachelor of science in nursing (BSN) degree within the past five years would have been introduced to research and EBP through required courses. Classroom lectures, discussions, and projects would have been used to help them understand and apply the basic steps of the research process, recognize and retrieve published research articles from nursing journals, and understand the value of research findings in clinical nursing practice. Some students may have had practical experience in research by working with school of nursing faculty who were actively engaged in a research project.

Current curriculum standards related to research and EBP for BSN degree-granting programs can be found in *The Essentials of Baccalaureate Education for Professional Nursing Practice* under Essential III: Scholarship for Evidence-Based Practice (www.aacn.nche.edu/education-resources/BaccEssentials08.pdf) (American Association of Colleges of Nursing [AACN], 2008). Similar curriculum standards for recent diploma and associate degree in nursing graduates can be found at the National League for Nursing website (www.nln.org). Regardless of the initial educational preparation of RNs, most new graduates possess novice skills related to research and EBP when they accept their first nursing positions.

Following completion of their BSN, nurses who pursue a master of science in nursing (MSN) degree further develop their skills related to the research process and EBP through required courses and, in some instances, a hands-on research practicum with an experienced nurse researcher. While in school, some graduate students may work in paid positions as research assistants with school of nursing faculty on a specific research project. These students learn the key steps of the EBP process, including how to retrieve and critique published research studies focused on a particular clinical problem. Some schools of nursing require graduate students to plan and implement a small research project (thesis) under the direction of faculty with expertise in research and on the topic of the research. Students may be required to present their project as a formal presentation or poster. They also might be encouraged to write and submit an article with their results to a nursing journal. Curriculum standards related to EBP and research for graduates of MSN programs expect competencies at a higher level than those of BSN graduates. These skills can be found in *The Essentials of Master's Education in Nursing* (AACN, 2011) under Essential IV: Translating and Integrating Scholarship Into Practice (www.aacn.nche.edu/education-resources/MastersEssentials11.pdf) or at the National League for Nursing website (www.nln.org).

After graduation, nurses with an MSN can learn more about research and EBP through various informal education offerings. Some nurses are employed in settings where they are involved in clinical research "designed to generate knowledge to guide practice in nursing and healthcare fields" (Polit & Beck, 2012, p. 721). Some nurses may work in institutions where clinical trials are conducted, while others may participate in unit-based research and EBP activities that focus on a clinical problem, education, or leadership problems. Many of these opportunities will be discussed throughout this chapter.

Nurses who work in clinical settings possess strengths that make them excellent candidates to participate in clinical nursing research and EBP projects. Because nurses provide direct care to patients on a daily basis and develop close relationships with them, they are in a unique position to identify clinical issues or problems (Dearholt & Dang, 2012). Nurses, because of their clinical expertise, are also in a prime position to critically evaluate the clinical significance of research reports and determine if findings are appropriate to their practice. They can also design creative ways to incorporate research findings into their daily practice. Through involvement in research, clinical nurses can positively influence the lives of patients and their family members, the nursing profession, their workplaces, and other healthcare providers.

Nurses work in clinical environments that differ based on a variety of factors, including the patient acuity level (e.g., ambulatory care departments, intensive care units), clinical specialty (e.g., operating room, oncology, obstetrics, psychiatric unit), patients' developmental stage (e.g., newborn, adolescent, adult, geriatric), and type of health care provided (e.g., hospitals, long-term care, industry, home care, nurse-managed wellness center). These diverse work settings provide rich environments in which nurses, as primary caregivers, can design and implement a variety of research and EBP projects.

As an NPDS or unit-based educator, you should build upon nurses' foundational knowledge and skills in research and EBP and support their success by "igniting a spirit of inquiry"

(Melnyk et al., 2009, p. 49) within your organization that helps them realize the value of their participation. You can help them overcome obstacles by developing a plan to strengthen their competencies. Over time, your mentorship will not only contribute to the success of nurses on your clinical unit but also strengthen your own expertise—a win-win situation.

Benefits of Participating in Research and Evidence-Based Practice

Participation in nursing research and EBP benefits not only you but also various stakeholders, including patients and their families, nurses and other healthcare professionals, and healthcare organizations and their academic partners. The benefits to each of these groups will be discussed in the following section.

Positive Patient and Family Outcomes

Engaging in research and EBP on your clinical unit can positively influence patient health outcomes (IOM, 2001). Nursing care provided to patients and families should reflect current best practices and be based on sound evidence that results in positive outcomes. This process of applying published research, expert findings, and patient preferences to nursing interventions is the basis of EBP (Polit & Beck, 2012). Research-based modifications in practice can positively influence the quality of care that patients receive, improve their health status, and subsequently influence their recovery and healthcare outcomes. For example, findings that result from a unit-based clinical research study conducted on a head and neck surgical unit can help nurses develop the most effective way to prevent airway obstructions caused by mucus plugs in patients who have undergone a total laryngectomy. These research findings could result in development of a practice-based protocol. This protocol can be used by nurses caring for patients during hospitalization and has the potential to reduce a patient's risk of partial or complete airway obstruction caused by a mucus plug, minimize the anxiety and stress experienced by the patient during an airway obstruction, and minimize the expense of unnecessary interventions, supplies, and time (e.g., saline, suction catheters, nursing care).

It is important to realize that some nursing interventions continue to be based on customs or rituals and may lack scientific support. Some nurses may feel more comfortable doing things the way they always have done them, making it paramount to investigate these customs and rituals and their effectiveness on patient outcomes.

Nurses need to strengthen their research skills to accomplish the goal of EBP. They need to read and understand a research report to critically evaluate if results can be incorporated into daily nursing practice. Policies, procedures, standards of care, and clinical protocols used on clinical units should be grounded in evidence, including research findings. Therefore, nursing practice that is based on proof that is documented in research reports or other sources is referred to as EBP (Polit & Beck, 2012).

Professional Development

Participating in research and EBP initiatives is a professional responsibility outlined in professional nursing standards. Utilization of research and EBP is included in *Nursing: Scope and Standards of Practice* (ANA, 2015). According to Standard 13 of this document, RNs are expected to "integrate evidence and research findings into practice" (ANA, 2015, p. 77) and demonstrate specific competencies based on their educational preparation. For example, RNs are expected to use the "best available evidence from research findings" (O'Nan, 2011, p. 160) in guiding and initiating changes in their nursing practice (ANA, 2015). RNs are also expected to share these findings with colleagues and peers (ANA, 2015).

ANA places additional expectations on RNs prepared at the graduate level, such as oncology nurses with a clinical specialty or advanced practice nurses (e.g., nurse practitioners) (ANA, 2015). Graduate nurses are expected to contribute to EBP and research by "conducting or synthesizing research and other evidence" (ANA, 2015, p. 78) related to nursing practice, encouraging an environment of inquiry, and disseminating research results through "presentations, publications, consultation, and journal clubs" (ANA, 2015, p. 78).

In addition to these ANA standards, the Oncology Nursing Society (ONS) also emphasized EBP and research in *Statement on the Scope and Standards of Oncology Nursing Practice: Generalist and Advanced Practice* (Brant & Wickham, 2013). More specifically, oncology nurses are expected to contribute to "cancer nursing practice, education, management, quality improvement, and research" through various activities, such as "identifying clinical dilemmas and problems . . . , collecting data, critiquing existing research, and integrating relevant research into clinical practice to improve patient outcomes" (Brant & Wickham, 2013, p. 49). It is important for nurses to review appropriate scope and standards of nursing practice (e.g., scope and standards of care, certification, position statements) based on their clinical specialty to determine their professional organization's expectations.

IOM (2011) also advocates the expectation for nurses to understand and engage in research and EBP. In its landmark report *The Future of Nursing: Leading Change, Advancing Health*, IOM (2011) recommended that nurses continually "engage in lifelong learning" (p. 5) and lead "collaborative improvement efforts" (p. 2) that focus on the quality and safety of patient care. Skills and competencies in nursing research, EBP, and QI are among the key competencies that nurses need to develop and continually strengthen.

In response to IOM's early efforts to ensure quality and safe patient care (IOM, 2003), a national team of academic nurse leaders developed the Quality and Safety Education for Nurses (QSEN) project, which identified the knowledge, skills, and attitudes that prelicensure RN and graduate students need to attain prior to becoming practicing nurses (Cronenwett et al., 2007). These nurse leaders identified EBP and QI among a set of six quality and safety nurse competencies, which included patient-centered care, teamwork and collaboration, evidence-based practice, quality improvement, safety, and informatics (QSEN Institute, n.d.).

Although these six competencies were originally designed for use by faculty in academic programs, Barnsteiner et al. (2013) promoted the value of these tools for use by staff development educators in designing programs that strengthen quality, safe nursing care. Over time, the QSEN initiative expanded to include an academic clinical education model developed collaboratively between two Ohio facilities—Lourdes University College of Nursing, housed in a small Catholic university, and ProMedica, a large integrated healthcare system (Didion, Kozy, Koffel, & Oneail, 2013). This academic-clinical partnership involved revising an existing baccalaureate curriculum by adopting QSEN competencies as the conceptual framework and implementing a concept-based approach to curriculum development. Concepts congruent with the school's core values, such as "leadership, community, diversity, and value-based care," (p. 89) were also included in the curriculum. Clinical education also was reconceptualized as an integrated experience in which students actively engaged with clinical staff and remained at one clinical site to gain an overall understanding of patient safety and quality care from an integrated organizational perspective.

Similarly, Dolansky and Moore (2013) expanded upon the six core competencies in an effort to shift nurses' perspectives from that of an individual patient care situation to one that views patient safety and quality from a larger, systems-based view. The authors provided an example of a beginning EBP competency in which a nurse is able to discern between strong evidence versus opinion. This example progresses to a more advanced performance in which the nurse plays an active role in developing EBP standards of care in a patient setting (Dolansky & Moore, 2013).

Although participating in research is among the professional responsibilities of all nurses, your level of engagement may vary based on your educational preparation (ANA, 2015). Understand that findings generated from clinical research contribute to the knowledge base used to develop and change nursing practice (Polit & Beck, 2012). Research studies designed to clarify or answer problems that exist with patients and families in clinical practice attempt to minimize the gaps that currently exist in nursing practice. Publication of research reports contributes to nursing's body of knowledge and either support or challenge methods of patient care. This body of published work influences what you teach to both nursing students and practicing nurses. Without sound nursing research, few evidence-based advances can be made in nursing practice.

Personal and Professional Rewards

You can gain both personal and professional rewards by participating in research and EBP in your work setting. For example, you may receive a great deal of personal satisfaction in knowing that you played a key role in solving a clinical problem, making things on the clinical unit function more smoothly, or improving the quality of nursing care provided to patients and families. Some nurses note gaining personal rewards as they strengthen their beginning skills in nursing research and engage in research and EBP projects.

In addition to personal rewards, you can gain professional rewards, such as increased autonomy and job satisfaction, through active participation in research and EBP (Maljanian, Caramanica, Taylor, MacRae, & Beland, 2002). Advantages also can include expectations in a current position, plans for promotion, and long-term career goals. Review your current position description to understand your employer's expectations regarding research participation. Be sure to review the descriptions of positions above your current role and the requirements for promotion.

Recent research continues to support these favorable personal and professional rewards for nurses who engage in research and EBP projects. For example, oncology nurses (N = 12) who participated in an EBP project viewed their experience as a positive one that empowered them personally and professionally (Fridman & Frederickson, 2014). The authors of this phenomenological study also noted that the nurses perceived that patient outcomes improved as a result of their participation in such EBP efforts.

Nurses who develop their research skills, plan and implement unit-based clinical research projects, and apply evidence in their practice are great assets to employers. These nurses have the potential to assume leadership roles in changing nursing practice, thereby validating the significant role of professional nurses within their organizations.

If your career goal is to continue your formal education in clinical practice or obtain a faculty position in a school of nursing, strengthening your skills in nursing research and

EBP will support your advancement. Developing your research expertise also may help you obtain a research nurse position in settings that manage funded research studies, such as clinical trials.

Gains for Healthcare Organizations and Academic Partners

Healthcare organizations across the nation struggle to survive in today's market of financial constraints, regulations, nursing shortages, restructures, and competition. Employers are constantly pursuing ways to market themselves to attract potential patients and qualified nurses. One strategy that your employer may take is to emphasize the positive outcomes of its EBP and research-based patient care. Organizations with research and EBP environments can promote themselves as having the best practices, providing care that is cost-effective, cutting-edge, and evidence-based (Melnyk et al., 2009). Outcomes may include improvements on clinical issues, such as decreased length of hospital stays, effective management of treatment side effects following chemotherapy, fewer complication rates after hip replacements, or fewer medication administration errors. The use of EBP also positively influences reimbursements that healthcare organizations receive from insurers (Melnyk et al., 2009). Nurses need to be proactive and confront these healthcare challenges.

Cost-conscious healthcare environments suggest that nurses need to evaluate the influence of their nursing care on patient outcomes. This task can be accomplished through research. For example, studies can be designed to focus on alternative ways to perform nursing procedures, such as administering tube feedings that can result in quality patient outcomes with reduced expenditures on supplies and equipment. Money saved via innovative nursing practices supported through research can be redirected to other patient-centered needs.

As previously mentioned in Chapter 2, organizations seeking recognition through the American Nurses Credentialing Center (n.d.) Magnet Recognition Program® must provide evidence of "quality patient care, nursing excellence, and innovations in nursing practice" (para. 1). If your employer is seeking this designation, you will be expected to sharpen your research and EBP skills so that you can critically evaluate research findings and apply them to daily practice in your clinical setting.

Healthcare organizations that embrace research and EBP also offer ideal learning opportunities for their academic partners. These clinical settings allow nursing students to observe the professional behaviors of RNs and other healthcare role models and provide opportunities to apply research and EBP concepts in nursing practice. Research and EBP-rich healthcare organizations also offer faculty opportunities for professional development, consultation, and future research initiatives.

Barriers to Participating in Research and Evidence-Based Practice

Several barriers may prevent research and EBP activities from flourishing in clinical settings. The absence of research or the lack of quality research may provide you and other nurses with insufficient evidence to support EBP on some topics (Johnson, 2014; Polit & Beck, 2012). Other obstacles include nurses themselves (Johnson, 2014) and their employers (Polit & Beck, 2012). Each of these barriers will be discussed in more detail, along with suggestions to minimize them.

Lack of Time

How can I add research to my already busy day?

Lack of time may be a reason why you do not participate in nursing research and EBP projects (Johnson, 2014). Nurses focus most of their workday on providing nursing care to patients and families, organizing their day so they can complete patient assignments in a timely manner, and focusing on safely administering medications. Given these important priorities, some nurses may feel that little time remains for involvement in research and EBP projects.

One way to manage new responsibilities when you already have a tight schedule is to break them down into smaller, more manageable tasks. Try approaching research and EBP projects in a similar manner. For example, start by talking with your organization's librarian or a nursing faculty member who has students on your clinical unit and asking for help in retrieving nursing research articles on a clinical topic of interest, such as studies investigating how new nurses perceive their first clinical job, how nursing students feel about their clinical experiences, or common medication errors that occur on the clinical unit.

Read at least one article per week when you have a few free minutes. Keep a small collection of articles handy on your nightstand or on a table by your favorite chair. Try reading them during lunch or while waiting for an appointment. These strategies will help develop your research skills and pass the time. Consider the strength of each study and discuss them with coworkers or your manager to determine if they can be applied on your clinical unit. Over time, you will develop a better understanding of the latest research in a specific area, maybe even becoming your unit's resident expert on a clinical problem.

Lack of Knowledge

How and where do I begin?

Lack of knowledge and experience with the research or EBP processes may pose a barrier to you or other clinical nurses (Johnson, 2014; Melnyk & Fineout-Overholt, 2014). As mentioned at the beginning of this chapter, lack of knowledge may be an expected claim by nurses because of limited exposure to nursing research and EBP during their initial preparation as an RN. For some nurses, a lot of time may have passed since they first learned about research and practiced related skills.

Although employers do not expect newly hired nurses to be experts in nursing research and EBP, it is important to understand your responsibilities related to these activities. Meet with your supervisor and review your employer's guidelines for promotion to clarify these expectations and develop a plan.

Lack of Interest and Resistance

It is not my job!

Some nurses may feel that participating in research or EBP is not of value to them or part of their roles as professional nurses (Johnson, 2014). Others may not see the need to alter their nursing practice and will resist any change (Johnson, 2014; Polit & Beck, 2012). If these statements reflect your attitude, it is important to understand why you feel this way. Try to gain insight into your feelings. Perhaps your negative outlook regarding research is because you are not familiar with professional nursing standards or are unclear about your employer's expectations. Your feelings also may reflect your lack of knowledge or skills.

Regardless of the reasons, try to make the most of the situation. Start by reviewing the professional nursing standards and those of your specialty. Clarify your role with your supervisor to determine what expectations exist. For example, perhaps you envisioned an unrealistic goal of independently conducting a unit-based clinical study. Instead, you are expected to understand research studies and work with colleagues to integrate findings in your organization's standards of care, policies, or procedures.

Remember that it takes time to build your research and EBP skills. Your situation is not unique, as colleagues probably possess the same skill level in research as you do. What is important is that you begin to develop your skills and take advantage of opportunities to learn at work. This strategy can strengthen your nursing practice and enable you to make significant contributions.

Organizational Barriers

Although research and EBP offer organizations many benefits, factors within the workplace may hinder these activities. For example, employers should recognize that clinical nurses need dedicated time and resources to participate in research and EBP and develop their expertise (Polit & Beck, 2012). Leaders within the healthcare organization need to support efforts that foster EBP and influence patient outcomes (Polit & Beck, 2012).

Creating a Professional Development Plan for Your Research and Evidence-Based Practice Skills

Although some clinical nurses may be familiar with the research process and EBP from their formal academic preparation or participation in CE programs, it is unlikely that they have extensive experience designing and implementing these initiatives themselves. Rather than letting this challenge become an overwhelming one, it is important to take a positive approach, viewing this experience as a new opportunity. This approach can be accomplished in several ways, whether you are planning projects for your own professional development or are responsible for helping staff develop these skills as an NPDS or unit-based educator.

If engaging in nursing research and EBP projects is challenging for you, place this new experience in perspective by recalling how uncertain you felt in your role as a newly hired nurse or student nurse. Reflect how difficult it was to perfect your clinical nursing skills or to understand nursing concepts. After repeated practice, hours of studying, and guidance from your nursing instructors, you were able to master your skills and gain a higher level of understanding of nursing concepts. Mastering the steps of the research and EBP processes can be accomplished using similar strategies, such as gaining hands-on experience, completing additional studies, and seeking guidance from others who are more experienced.

Assessing Your Learning Needs

Remember that the research and EBP processes are not totally unfamiliar to nurses. Boost your confidence by comparing the steps of clinical research and EBP with other familiar processes. You may be surprised at what you already know. For example, examine the similarities of the research process with those of the nursing process outlined in *Nursing: Scope and Standards of Practice* (see Table 12-1) (ANA, 2015). A similar comparison can be made with EBP and the nursing process (Dearholt & Dang, 2012). Although you may not fully understand the research steps right now, examine how they align with the steps in the nursing process. The research process is also similar to QI activities that nurses conduct on the clinical unit. Results obtained through the nursing process, quality care activities, and research can lead to changes in nursing practice and healthcare systems (ANA, 2015).

Think about your past experiences with research projects and build upon these opportunities. For example, you may have been involved in recruiting patients on your clinical unit for studies conducted by others or collected blood samples or questionnaires based on a research protocol. Or, maybe you volunteered as a research participant and experienced the informed consent and data collection process. All of these experiences will help strengthen your research skills.

Read articles that report about projects conducted on familiar clinical issues. For example, Powers and Fortney (2014) described evidence that helped them arrive at their recommendation regarding standards for patient bed baths that aimed to decrease hospital-associated infections.

Creating a Realistic Plan to Strengthen Your Competencies

Before completing the research and EBP self-assessment activities in Figures 12-1 and 12-2, develop short-term and long-term goals based on a review of your employer's expectations of your current role. If you are an NPDS, develop goals that relate to you personally and meet staff needs. Build upon the strengths of your nursing staff and organization while minimizing potential barriers.

Keep these goals in mind as you develop a realistic plan to attain them over time. Start by prioritizing learning needs. For example, if you feel uncomfortable reading and understanding a research article, rank this activity among your top learning priorities. Similarly, you may choose to rank authoring a research journal article lower on your list, to be pursued after you have completed more preparation on this topic over the next two years.

Develop strategies to attain these goals by examining possible resources or opportunities. Be sure to inventory your personal and professional environment for resources, such as individuals who have expertise in nursing research and EBP, research and EBP literature, and educational offerings with content and hands-on experience from actual projects.

Table 12-1. Comparison of the Nursing Process and the Research Process

Nursing Process	Research Process
Assessment	Defining a research problem or clinical issue
Diagnosis	Clarifying the problem and its significance through review of the literature
Outcomes identification	Developing purpose, aims, and research questions or hypotheses
Planning	Developing a research proposal or plan
Implementation	Conducting the research study
Evaluation	Analyzing data and discussing findings

Note. Based on information from American Nurses Association, 2015.

Be flexible, take advantage of opportunities that may arise at a short notice, and reorganize your priorities if some were not part of your original plan. For example, you have a chance to learn how to collect data for a research project being conducted on your clinical unit. Although this research activity was not on your list for this year, you take advantage of the learning opportunity and revise your plan.

Allow yourself sufficient time to practice your skills before evaluating your progress at regular intervals, especially in advance of your annual performance review.

Nurses can assume a variety of roles in research and EBP projects based on their existing knowledge, skills, and experience. As a clinical nurse, you may choose to assume the role of a research participant or data collector for a project. Your role in these initiatives will be defined by your prior education, experience, and expectations of your current role.

Set aside time to list personal and professional reasons that may prevent you from attaining your goals and develop realistic strategies that will help you overcome these barriers. The next part of this chapter will offer strategies that clinical nurses can use to help them increase their knowledge and skills in research and EBP. Additional resources for strategies are listed in the Helpful Websites section at the end of this chapter.

Conducting a Self-Assessment

A systematic self-assessment of your talents will determine the research and EBP skills that you will need to learn, those you have already mastered, and those that you will need to further strengthen.

The self-assessment tool for research depicted in Figure 12-1 and a similar tool for EBP in Figure 12-2 can help determine your baseline competencies. The first column in both figures lists key research or EBP components that may be expected of clinical nurses. Using Benner's Stages of Clinical Competence (1984), indicate your perceived level of proficiency regarding each step: novice (1), advanced beginner (2), competent (3), proficient (4), and expert (5). This exercise will help you identify which research and EBP activities to include in your professional development plan. Remember that your educational background and prior experience in nursing will influence the results of your baseline assessment. You may find that you need to learn more about all the listed components. Modify the list of research and EBP activities according to your employer's expectations and adapt it to fit your professional and personal goals. Details about these steps will be explained later in this chapter.

Seeking Formal and Informal Education Offerings

Expand your research and EBP skills by participating in formal and informal learning opportunities. You could, for example, enroll in a face-to-face or online graduate-level course that addresses these topics. Consider course options like practicums or independent studies that offer flexibility and hands-on experience with a faculty member who can mentor you in a specific project.

Opportunities for learning more about research and EBP also exist through informal education offerings, such as in-service or CE programs sponsored by healthcare organizations and professional nursing organizations. For example, ONS offers web-based courses for nurses (e.g., Developing Skills for Evidence-Based Practice, Clinical Trials Nursing 101), with contact hours awarded upon successful completion.

Some colleges and universities offer workshops or certificate programs on research-related topics open to the nursing community. Many specialty professional nursing organi-

Figure 12-1. Self-Assessment of Research Activities

Research Activities	1	2	3	4	5
Conduct a literature review to retrieve nursing research.					
Identify nursing journals that publish research in your clinical specialty.					
Distinguish between a research and theory/practice article.					
Understand a published nursing research study.					
Evaluate (critique) the quality of a research report.					
Apply (utilize) research findings, as appropriate, in clinical practice.					
Participate in key aspects of a research project:					
• Identify a clinical problem to study.					
• Conduct and organize a literature review.					
• Draft a study's purpose and aims, research questions, and hypotheses.					
• Develop a research design.					
• Recruit participants.					
• Schedule participants for appointments.					
• Obtain informed consent from participants.					
• Collect data (e.g., instruments, samples, interviews, chart reviews, measurements, focus groups).					
• Administer a research intervention (e.g., educational program, counseling session, treatment).					
• Assist with data analysis or calculation of results.					
• Clarify study findings and discuss relevance to clinical practice.					
Actively participate in a research project as one of the following:					
• Participant					
• Project team member					
• Principal investigator (leader)					
Serve as member of a research review committee:					
• Review research proposals.					
• Review research abstracts.					
Participate as member of a committee related to research (e.g., professional nursing organization, shared governance council).					
Disseminate research findings to colleagues:					
• Submit an abstract.					
• Deliver a podium presentation.					
• Develop a poster presentation.					
• Publish in a peer-reviewed journal.					

Figure 12-2. Self-Assessment of Evidence-Based Practice Activities					
Evidence-Based Practice Activities	**1**	**2**	**3**	**4**	**5**
Step 0: Cultivate a spirit of inquiry.					
Step 1: Ask clinical questions in PICOT format.					
Step 2: Search for the best evidence.					
Step 3: Critically appraise the evidence.					
Step 4: Integrate the evidence with clinical expertise and patient preferences and values.					
Step 5: Evaluate the outcomes of the practice decisions or changes based on evidence.					
Step 6: Disseminate evidence-based practice results.					
Note. Based on information from Melnyk et al., 2010.					

zations sponsor instructional sessions on research and EBP as well as roundtables, forums, and reports on specific projects at national and local meetings. Some organizations offer membership in special interest groups or committees focused on nursing research and EBP. These subgroups usually sponsor education sessions prior to or during their national conferences. In the event that you cannot attend these sessions live, check to see whether they will be recorded or streamed. These multimedia sources can help you focus on particular topics and learn in a cost-effective, flexible manner. When listening to presentations, determine how they apply to your clinical setting. Think about the steps of the research and EBP processes and how they were addressed in the presentation. If research or EBP presentations are unavailable at your organization, suggest these topics to the education committee as a future program. Another option would be to experience the research process firsthand by volunteering as a participant in a research study, even if it involves simply completing a survey.

Accessing Print and Media Resources

Print and electronic publications, such as books and journals, along with other instructional media, such as audiotapes, videos, and Internet-based programs, are excellent resources to learn more about research and EBP. Basic nursing texts can be purchased through local college/university bookstores, advertisements in nursing journals and nursing conference proceedings, and through commercial websites. Many books provide a how-to approach to nursing research and EBP and vary in difficulty. Ask faculty with students on your clinical unit for advice in selecting the appropriate resources to meet your learning needs.

Many journals dedicate time to research and EBP content. For example, in November 2009 the *American Journal of Nursing* published a series of 12 articles on EBP authored by faculty from the Arizona State University College of Nursing and Health Innovation's Center for the Advancement of Evidence-Based Practice (Melnyk et al., 2009). These articles outlined EBP as a series of seven steps and included a clinical example that evolved with each issue and step. Readers were able to ask questions to the authors using a toll-free phone number at designated times throughout the series (Melnyk et al., 2009, 2010).

Similarly, some journals include a special feature in each issue dedicated to research or EBP information. For example, *MEDSURG Nursing* includes a "Research Corner" in which research topics are discussed. The Academy of Medical-Surgical Nurses also offers two independent modules in EBP (www.amsn.org/practice-resources/evidence-based-practice). In an *Oncology Nursing Forum* article, Berkey and Moore (2012) provided a detailed guide for nurse authors interested in preparing a research-based manuscript. The steps included in this article are helpful to authors regardless of their practice specialty.

Some specialty nursing organizations have taken EBP to a higher level by producing evidence-based clinical resources that nurses can use to bridge the gap between research and practice. For example, ONS's Putting Evidence Into Practice (PEP) resources provide evidence-based interventions for managing symptoms commonly experienced by cancer survivors (ONS, n.d.-a). Each topic outlines interventions reported to manage a symptom and the interventions' associated level of evidence. For example, fatigue is among the many symptoms that nurses can investigate using PEP (ONS, n.d.-b). The available interventions for fatigue are categorized according to their level of evidence and color-coded to guide users in their practice. Sources coded in green are Recommended for Practice or Likely to Be Effective; sources in yellow are Benefits Balanced With Harm or Effectiveness Not Established; and red color-coding indicates Effectiveness Unlikely or Not Recommended for Practice. Users can further locate the citation for each source of evidence per intervention. According to ONS, these resources can be helpful for planning "individual patient care, patient education, nursing education, quality improvement, and research" (ONS, n.d.-a, para. 1). NPDSs also should consider including PEP resources in educational offerings targeted to nurses who care for patients with cancer, such as orientation, continuing nursing education, and journal clubs).

Recognizing and Retrieving Research Articles

Making an effort to read research-based articles in professional nursing journals can help you become more familiar with the language and steps used in the process. Avoid getting overwhelmed with the abundance of content available by starting with research reports in clinical nursing journals (e.g., *American Journal of Nursing, Nursing*) or journals in your specialty (e.g., *AORN Journal, Oncology Nursing Forum*). The practical approach to research used in these journals often helps clinical nurses relate studies to nursing practice issues.

Although some nursing journals mainly publish research articles, other journals may include only a few research papers or none at all. The titles of some journals, such as *Nursing Research*, can give a hint as to whether they contain research-based articles. Author guidelines will help you determine if research articles are among the manuscripts considered for publication in specific journals. The list of nursing journals provided in Chapter 8 also can help you with this search.

Once you find an article, determine whether it is research based or discusses another topic, such as nursing theory, concept, or clinical practice issue. Some nursing journals, such as the *Oncology Nursing Forum*, use symbols (such as an "R") next to article titles in the table of contents to help readers recognize a research article. When in doubt, look for the main sections that should be included in a research article (see Table 12-2). Focus on any subheadings contained within the "Methods" section if you are still in doubt. Often, the title, abstract, or text of an article communicates that it is a research study. With experience, you will become familiar with the appearance of titles that indicate the article may be about a study.

Table 12-2. Key Sections and Components to Search in a Research Article

Section of Article	Components
Introduction	Purpose and specific aims (research questions/hypotheses) Background Significance Theoretical/conceptual framework (quantitative) Literature review
Methods	Design Sample/participants and setting Instruments Data collection procedures Protection of human participants Data analysis
Results (findings)	Values of statistical tests/content analysis Interpretation of significance
Discussion	Interpretation of results Limitations Implications for nursing practice Implications for future research

As your understanding of the research process increases, try reviewing research-based articles published within your clinical specialty. The knowledge you possess in your clinical area may help you better understand these studies and place them within the proper context of nursing practice. You can review recent print or electronic issues of these journals or conduct a literature search using key words on a topic of interest.

NPDSs need to understand the value of a literature review, especially when planning a research study or EBP and QI projects (Bernhofer, 2015). NPDSs also should be able to conduct a literature search themselves in order to properly mentor clinical nurses in this process. Understanding how research and EBP and QI projects differ is an important step before formally searching the literature.

If you have little experience in searching the literature, ask your organization's librarian for assistance in using appropriate databases (see Chapter 8) that focus on nursing, medicine, and healthcare topics. Search databases in other disciplines, such as psychology, sociology, and education, as needed. The Internet also can be a source of information for nursing research and EBP; however, be sure to evaluate the accuracy of the information you retrieve by reviewing its source.

Reading, Understanding, and Critiquing Research Articles

Learning to utilize different styles when reviewing journal articles will increase your comfort with reading, understanding, and critiquing them. Reading published articles also may help you discover opportunities to actively participate in the research process.

Begin this task by retrieving a recent research article published in a nursing journal focused on your clinical practice specialty or a topic of interest. For example, if your clinical specialty is adult health, try locating research articles in journals such as *MEDSURG Nursing*.

After determining a journal article, match your reading style with your general purpose for reading the article. Experts suggest using three different styles when reading a research article, with each increasing in complexity and time commitment.

On the lowest level, skim an article to determine if it is research based or to get a general sense about the project. This is an approach you may have used in school if you needed to read several pages in a limited time frame.

The second, more advanced style involves reading for comprehension to better understand the research content. Table 12-3 lists the key sections of a research article and their primary purpose. Identifying these parts in an article will provide you with important information about the study.

The highest reading level is an analytic approach. This third style is intended to critique the research study to determine its quality and evaluate whether its findings are applicable to your clinical situation. Critiquing a study is an advanced skill that you will need to develop over time. Be sure to include it as part of your career plan.

Table 12-3. Key Parts of a Research Article

Key Part	Purpose
Title	Provides key variables or concepts examined in the study; also may indicate population and setting under study and research design used
Abstract	Provides a general overview of the entire study, including problem studied, significance of study, purpose and aims, information about sample and setting, design, instruments, data collection and analysis used, results/findings, discussion, and implications for nursing
Introduction	Sets the stage for the research study; includes background information about the problem under study, significance (i.e., why it was important to conduct the study), purpose and specific objectives of the study (posed as research questions/hypotheses), review of related literature, and (if appropriate) theoretical/conceptual framework/model used to guide the study
Methods	Describes the details of the plan/blueprint for the actual study; includes an explanation of the design chosen to organize the study; description of the sample (participants), such as why they were included in the study and size; description of the setting in which the study was conducted; main variables/concepts under study and means to measure the concepts (e.g., instruments, interview guides, observations); procedures used to collect these data; how informed consent was obtained from subjects/participants; and procedures used to analyze the data collected
Results/Findings	Describes the results/findings according to the research questions/hypotheses posed in the introduction section of the article; includes which findings are significant and which are not meaningful; may include the results of statistical tests or content analysis procedures
Discussion	Provides possible explanations/interpretations for the results/findings of the study within the context of past published research on that topic or experience; includes limitations of the study that were beyond the control of the researcher; how the findings/results can be used by nurses in clinical practice, education, or administration roles; and possible ideas for future research studies on this topic
References	List of resources used by the researcher in developing the research article; provides the readers with other sources of past research that relate to this topic
Tables/Figures	Visuals that provide a ready reference for the primary data included in the study; summarize details of the study results/findings

Nursing organizations often contain helpful information for reading, understanding, and critiquing research articles. For example, ANA's NursingWorld website contains a Research Toolkit available to members only and holds a wealth of information about both research and EBP (www.nursingworld.org/Research-Toolkit). The site includes a guide that nurses can use to critique a nursing research article and evaluate a study regarding its level of evidence. This particular source can be accessed at http://nursingworld.org/research-toolkit/Critique -Research-Article.

Connecting With Experts

If possible, seek the advice and expertise of mentors who have experience in nursing research and EBP, especially nurses who have earned an MSN or doctoral degree in nurs- ing research or clinical practice. Identify possible experts employed within your work setting, such as advanced practice nurses, clinical nurse specialists, other NPDSs, or nurse researchers. If your agency has academic partners, try approaching nursing faculty who bring students to your unit for their clinical experience. Students enrolled in degree-granting programs in nurs- ing are also good sources.

Expand your search for experts through professional nursing organizations, such as spe- cialty and nursing alumni organizations, or through research teams led by nursing faculty in schools of nursing. Consider accessing unique web-based resources, such as the Center for Transdisciplinary Evidence-Based Practice (https://ctep-ebp.com), an enterprise that supports EBP across disciplines and focuses on improving health outcomes for patients and their fami- lies by assisting educators, clinicians, and healthcare leaders.

Be sure to communicate your interest in becoming involved in a research project with the appropriate people, such as your supervisor, mentor, other NPDSs, or colleagues. If these learning opportunities do not currently exist, suggest the development of a mentorship pro- gram in research through the local chapter of your professional nursing organization.

Resources in Professional Nursing Organizations

Professional nursing organizations can offer excellent resources to help you learn about nursing research through educational offerings; print, electronic, and multimedia resources; and experts in research and EBP. If research is your focus, select organizations that identify research activities in their mission statements. Take advantage of the support of these organi- zations by joining their research committees on the local, regional, national, or international level. For example, the ONS website offers "Resources for Researchers" (www.ons.org/practice -resources/role-specific-resources/researchers), where you can obtain essential ONS resources, such as information on funding, research agendas and priorities, and experts' opinions to help you with your research and evidence-based project questions. Chapter 7 provides a list of other professional nursing organizations from which you can choose.

Another organization to consult is Sigma Theta Tau International Honor Society of Nursing (n.d.), which offers nurses grants, resources, and learning opportunities at the international, national, and regional levels, as well as local chapters affiliated at university-based schools of nursing.

Seeking Hands-On Experience

Having hands-on experience with research and EBP projects will help you gain a better understanding of these processes. Let project managers know about your interest in assuming a leadership role on your unit regarding these initiatives. Ask for guidance in creating a plan that can help you develop your role and gain experience by spending time with staff in your organization's nursing education and research center. If your hospital has a shared governance structure, express your interest in serving as a member on the nursing research or professional development council.

Fostering Research and Evidence-Based Practice in Clinical Settings

As an NPDS, it is important to plan strategies to foster research and EBP within your health-care organization. One way to begin this process is by organizing a brainstorming session with coworkers who want to be involved in unit-based clinical research and EBP. As appropriate, invite nurses and other healthcare professionals, such as pharmacists, physical therapists, and social workers. It is important to let everyone have an opportunity to participate. The follow-ing section will provide you with strategies to enhance your research and EBP skills both as an individual and as a coordinator of unit-based initiatives.

Developing a Strategic Plan

To create a unit-based environment that is conducive to nursing research and EBP, draft a strategic plan with staff based on ideas generated from brainstorming sessions and feedback from assessments. Search the nursing literature for creative ways to help nurses on your unit learn more about the research process and play an active role in EBP. Prioritize specific goals or outcomes for your unit that deal with these topics, making sure they are harmonious with those of your unit and healthcare organization. Depending on the staff's abilities and available resources, goals may range from helping them learn how to read and understand research arti-cles to teaching them how to implement unit-based research or EBP projects.

Set a realistic timeline for these unit-based efforts and anticipate possible barriers that may result in staff's initial hesitation to play an active role. Be prepared to help them realize the potential influence that these efforts can play in their professional and personal lives. Keep activities open to staff who may choose to become involved at a later time. Schedule sessions on your unit for nurses to discuss their concerns about being involved in research and EBP.

Evidence-Based Models and Learning Needs

An important step in creating a work environment that supports EBP is to carefully review and adopt an EBP model that will help guide your efforts (Dearholt & Dang, 2012; Schaffer, Sandau, & Diedrick, 2012). In selecting an EBP activity, consider its congruence with your organization's culture and its users, such as clinical staff, academic partners, and resources. For example, Schaffer et al. (2012) conducted a review of six common EBP models: ACE Star Model of Knowledge Transformation, Advancing Research and Clinical Practice Through Close Collaboration [ARCC], the Iowa Model, the Johns Hopkins Nursing Evidence-Based Practice Model [JHNEBP], Promoting Action on Research Implementation in Health Ser-vices Framework [PARIHS], and the Stetler Model. The authors offered recommendations for users based on their practical applications. Schaffer et al. (2012) cited three models that orga-nizations may prefer because of their focus on decision making: PARIHS, ARCC, and the Iowa Model. The JHNEBP model was recommended for educators because of its focus on "finding and evaluating evidence" (Schaffer et al., 2012, p. 1197).

As an additional resource, Figure 12-2 outlines the steps included in the EBP model reported by Melnyk et al. (2010). After creating an environment at your workplace that fosters interest in EBP (step 0), step 1 of this model advises nurses to identify a clinical problem that they have experienced in patient care. They need to state the problem as a "PICOT" question that addresses patient population of interest (P), intervention or area of interest (I), comparison intervention or group (C), outcome (O), and time (T) (Melnyk et al., 2010).

In step 2, nurses should be able to recognize different types of research (i.e., qualitative and quantitative methods), understand common research terms included in published studies (see Table 12-2), and conduct a literature search appropriate for the PICOT question.

Step 3 requires nurses to evaluate the research and nonresearch evidence they retrieved and judge the level of evidence of each. Several models of evidence are available for nurses to use in this step, including Melnyk's Hierarchy of Evidence (Melnyk & Fineout-Overholt, 2014).

In step 4, nurses need to be able to make recommendations related to the clinical problem after careful review of the evidence, expertise, and patient preferences.

The learning needs of nurses associated with evaluating the outcomes of practice decisions or changes based on evidence (step 5) will be discussed at the end of this chapter. Skills and competencies needed by nurses to disseminate EBP results (step 6) was discussed in detail in Chapters 9 and 10.

Mobilizing Support and Resources

Once you have developed a plan for your clinical units, seek support systems to assist with these endeavors. Obtain support from your supervisor to maximize your success for programs and projects, especially in allotting resources such as time and financial support.

Consider using resources within your healthcare organization, such as the librarian, the nursing research department, or the nursing research council (if your workplace has a shared governance structure). Krom, Batten, and Bautista (2010) described how a clinical nurse specialist, health science librarian, and staff nurse collaborated to implement an EBP education program targeted to clinical nurses. Each of these EBP leaders brought their particular strengths to this initiative, resulting in increased knowledge and awareness for nurses in EBP. Similarly, an advanced practice nurse and medical librarian teamed with a hospital's nursing research team to implement a mobile library initiative aimed at increasing clinical nurses' awareness of the team and of unit-based online databases (Ryan & Joseph, 2013). A computer-on-wheels and library resources were used to demonstrate search techniques for nurses to conduct EBP projects.

Expand your collaboration and include other healthcare professionals and workers who have a vested interest in the clinical problem. Bohnenkamp, Pelton, Rishel, and Kurtin (2014a, 2014b) reported their success using an interprofessional team on an EBP project that focused on increasing compliance with sequential compression device use in a high-risk cancer group. The project was implemented in a gynecologic oncology surgical unit located in a hospital that held Magnet recognition. Besides staff nurses and charge nurses, nearly 15 other stakeholders made up a team of physicians, legal representatives, patient care technicians, housekeeping, central supply, unit educators, a patient and the patient's family, and a shared leadership council. Positive project outcomes reflected the efforts of the interprofessional team, which was committed to this practice change and improved patient care.

In addition to seeking colleagues within your organization, explore academic partnerships that your organization holds with schools of nursing or other agencies. These contacts may be valuable resources and sources of support for fostering nursing research and EBP on your clinical unit. For example, Wittmann-Price, Celia, and Dunn (2013) described a collaboration between professional development educators and an academic nurse researcher to strengthen research and QI projects at a healthcare organization. As a result of their efforts, the organization received Magnet recognition. According to the authors, NPDSs are instrumental in leading such initiatives, as opposed to external nurse researchers, because they have familiarity with the organization's culture and potential to succeed.

Similarly, Moore and Stichler (2015) reported a creative continuing education program they implemented to help advanced clinical nurses understand QI and EBP projects. The nurses, all employed on a short-stay unit at Sharp Memorial Hospital in San Diego, managed change projects guided by the Six Sigma DMAIC (Define, Measure, Analyze, Improve, Control) Change Acceleration Process (Arthur, 2011) and facilitated through classroom presentations and individual mentoring. This project resulted in a change in the unit's culture regarding the value of QI and EBP and dissemination of change project results through poster presentations.

Another successful academic-practice partnership was reported by McConnell, Lekan, Hebert, and Leatherwood (2007), who implemented an EBP improvement process focused on developing a sustainable oral hygiene protocol for older adult residents housed in a long-term care setting. This partnership benefited all stakeholders by facilitating the translation of research to clinical practice. The program created a practice setting conducive to student placements at the facility, and residents received quality oral hygiene based on current evidence.

Jamerson, Fish, and Frandsen (2011) described a successful nursing student research assistant program coordinated between St. Louis Children's Hospital, a pediatric facility with Magnet status, and two schools of nursing, the University of Missouri and Maryville University. In an effort to enhance the research capacity of clinicians at the hospital and to also help students learn about clinical research, hospital nurses and school faculty collaborated in a nursing research council to create a nursing research assistant program. Initially, the authors recruited students from undergraduate and graduate programs at the two schools and matched them with hospital clinicians to support their research studies. As the program progressed, this academic-clinician collaboration expanded to include students from six schools of nursing. Students and clinicians benefited from this unique collaboration. The researchers were able to complete their studies in a more timely fashion with the help of the assistants. The clinicians also gained a sense of pride and were eager to disseminate their results. Students appreciated the opportunity to apply what they learned about the research process to clinical practice by working directly with nurse researchers at the hospital.

Gradually Implementing and Addressing Diverse Learning Needs

As with introducing any new change, start by implementing small projects and ones that pose the least threat. Once your nursing staff develops their skills and confidence, gradually proceed to more advanced unit-based projects. Implement these initiatives slowly and integrate them into daily work schedules and activities as much as possible. Again, search the literature (evidence) for successful and creative approaches that have been previously used to support research and EBP.

Beginning a Unit-Based Journal Club

Consider starting a journal club on your clinical unit. A journal club consists of a group of nurses who meet on a regular basis to review and critique nursing research articles on a particular clinical topic of interest (Polit & Beck, 2012). Members of a journal club also may discuss whether study findings can be applied to their clinical settings.

Although some nursing research journal clubs may be organized through a hospital's shared governance practice and education council (Gloeckner & Robinson, 2010), consider beginning one on your own clinical unit. Select a research article that is of interest to the staff on your unit, ask everyone to read the article, and then meet up and discuss it. Provide staff with questions for reflection before the meeting. Be cognizant of the knowledge levels of the nurses who attend the journal club, as staff nurses on your unit may vary in their understanding of the research process. Be sensitive to scheduling the sessions at times that will accommodate shift schedules. Consider beginning discussions about the research steps addressed in the study followed by the study's quality and applicability to patients in your clinical setting. Brainstorm possible ways that the study could be replicated on your unit and discuss what the next step should investigate. Have staff take turns retrieving research articles, developing questions, and leading the group discussion. Gradually advance to reviewing several articles that investigate a common topic, then critique their methods and compare their findings.

Consider implementing a virtual journal club for nurses on your unit, as described by Berger, Hardin, and Topp (2011). This journal club was sponsored by the nursing research council of the hospital and implemented using its intranet portal and blog features. The council began the journal club by first identifying a clinical topic based on problem areas on the units. Next, a council nurse searched the literature to locate a relevant research study and drafted a critique that was reviewed by a research consultant prior to being posted. Finally, the council nurse added discussion questions for nurses to comment on in the blog and oversaw the review process and staff comments.

The virtual journal club resulted in numerous benefits, including allowing nurses to participate regardless of their schedule, enabling staff with diverse research skills to comfortably engage in discussions, and increasing staff nurses' interest and skills in nursing research. Depending on their participation, nurses were awarded CE credits or credits toward advancement in their career ladders (Berger et al., 2011).

Sharing Experiences

Ask staff to share their research and EBP experiences with each other during unit-based programs. Sometimes hearing someone else's reflections about an experience may help nurses develop their career plans and allay anticipated fears. For example, discussions may include their perspectives on research or EBP projects presented at a regional nursing conference they just attended. Invite faculty from academic partnerships to join the group to share perspectives that might complement the staff's clinical interests.

Exploring Research and Evidence-Based Practice Roles

As mentioned earlier in this chapter, if you want to be more involved in research and EBP, seek possible opportunities at your workplace or any academic partnerships that can provide you with hands-on experiences, such as recruiting participants, collecting data, or conducting literature reviews as a member of a research team. Work with your manager or personnel from a nursing education and research department, as they can connect you with others who can help. Share your interests with faculty from affiliated schools of nursing who have students on your clinical unit. Faculty members often seek nurses who can help them with their research or projects on a part-time or full-time basis. Meet with your manager to explore possibilities for your clinical unit to serve as the setting for future research or EBP projects.

Consider developing a research internship program for staff nurses at your workplace. Clancey (2009), an education and development specialist, created a program to address barriers that nurses faced in conducting research. In this study, interns attended a course on basic nursing research and the steps of the EBP process. Then, the educator mentored the interns as they completed 72 hours of paid time over six months dedicated to their research. The program was successful in minimizing barriers related to lack of time, support, and knowledge reported by nurses. It also increased staff nurses' interest in research and involvement in clinical research projects.

Similarly, Green et al. (2014) implemented an evidence-based practice academy in which select clinical nurses completed a six-month educational program aimed at building capacity for EBP within a hospital. The academy consisted of classroom instruction on EBP, practical application under the direction of an experienced mentor (a former graduate of the academy), and protected time to complete a unit-based EBP project. Results included positive outcomes related to completed projects and a team of EBP graduates prepared to sustain future efforts.

Some healthcare organizations have focused efforts on training a team of nurses to lead EBP initiatives. For example, Beinlich and Meehan (2014) described a resource nurse program in which unit-based RNs were tasked with helping colleagues use evidence-based strategies to prevent, assess, and treat pressure ulcers in patients admitted to their clinical settings. They were also responsible for conducting unit-based educational programs and journal clubs, assessing the status of patient ulcers with staff on the unit, participating in key meetings and rounds, and engaging in ongoing QI initiatives. Outcomes captured over a three-year period revealed decreased pressure ulcer prevalence, occurrence, and associated costs.

Integrating Topics Into Your Unit's Education Plan

Include research and EBP topics in your unit's education plan. Invite nurse researchers to talk about their research projects with staff. In addition to focusing on the project itself, ask speakers to describe how the idea originated and how the findings influenced nursing practice. Start a special research series of unit-based in-service programs that focus on the research process. For example, topics may include identifying a clinical problem to study, determining types of research designs, sampling techniques, and protecting human participants. Consider reviewing the basics of a research critique using a research article familiar to staff. Refer to Table 12-3 for more ideas, or ask nursing staff to take turns developing a 30-minute presentation or poster on each topic (see Chapter 9).

Try to incorporate research and EBP in all of your unit-based programs. For example, when conducting clinically oriented in-service programs, such as managing nausea and vomiting experienced by patients following chemotherapy, include one or two recent research articles on this topic. Discuss research findings as they apply to the standards of care for managing these symptoms in patients on your unit.

McCurry (2014) updated a classic teaching approach called the "Great American Cookie Experiment," which has been used and modified for nearly three decades to introduce both nursing students and hospital-based staff nurses to the research process (Hudson-Barr, Weeks, & Watters, 2000; Long & Reider, 1995; Thiel, 1987). This project, originally conceived by Thiel (1987), simulated the steps of the research process by having students judge the quality of and preference for two chocolate chip cookies, both prepared using different ingredients. McCurry (2014) updated the approach for millennial learners by using technology to capture responses, analyze data, and report results. The project was successful in helping participants understand nursing research in light of their active involvement. Similarly, Sternberger (2002) recreated Thiel's experiment using music samples (rather than cookies) as the study purpose for students enrolled in an online research course.

Also consider using some of the active teaching strategies that Spiers, Paul, Jennings, and Weaver (2012) described to help undergraduate nursing students learn how to read and use qualitative research. Their creative teaching-learning methods included the use of research-based crossword puzzles and games that enabled students to build upon what they already mastered when learning new research concepts.

As you review the literature on research and EBP, think about designing strategies based on evidence. Be sure to recognize the varied learning needs of staff nurses and disseminate your initiatives so others can continue to build upon your successes. For example, Weitzel and Robinson (2011) described a study in which 11 staff nurses, who were members of a hospital-based nursing research council, relied on the evidence gleaned from the nursing literature to design and sponsor a week aimed at increasing nurses' awareness, knowledge, and participation in nursing research. The council wanted nurse attendees to recognize their role and ability to change nursing practice at their organization, understand the many resources available to them to accomplish this goal, and become aware of EBP projects currently in progress. Council members consulted with expert researchers who were advanced practice nurses on the hospital's nursing research advisory group and members of their local chapter of Sigma Theta Tau International Honor Society of Nursing. Daily sessions, scheduled during National Nurses Week, were designed to meet the wide-ranging learning needs of participants who were prepared in various prelicensure RN programs (Weitzel & Robinson, 2011). Programs included a research conference day with informative breakout sessions of varying levels, poster displays of ongoing and completed EBP projects, networking opportunities with the nursing research council members, active participation in the aforementioned cookie experiment, and a session that disseminated the results of the cookie experiment. The authors reported favorable outcomes, received helpful input for future topics, and listened to requests to expand the week using an interprofessional perspective.

To help clinical nurses strengthen their understanding of statistics used in sources of evidence, consider developing strategies similar to those reported by Granger et al. (2013). These authors created a toolbox for NPDSs to use when teaching clinical nurses how to interpret the language of data and their associated symbols in analysis. The toolbox also was intended to help nurses incorporate the language of data in their work settings. Various teaching strategies that aligned with adult learning principles were discussed as possible delivery methods.

Piloting a Unit-Based Project

As mentioned earlier in this chapter, one way for clinical nurses to understand the process and value of nursing research and EBP is by participating in these endeavors. NPDSs play an important role in recruiting and supporting nurses in their involvement. Once their confidence and understanding of the research and EBP processes increase, challenge their skills by involving interested nurses in a unit-based research or EBP project.

In planning a unit-based clinical research project, be sure to seek the expertise of an experienced nurse researcher or advanced practice nurse who can guide and mentor interested staff nurses in designing and implementing the study. The research project should address a problem that exists on the clinical unit. Findings have the potential to be incorporated into patient care. Results can be shared with other nurses through unit-based in-service or CE programs and disseminated through oral or poster presentations and publications in peer-reviewed nursing journals.

Mentors usually are prepared in nursing at the master's or doctoral level and employed at your healthcare organization or by an academic partner. They may hold positions such as an NPDS, clinical nurse specialist, or nurse researcher. Faculty employed at an affiliated university or college-based school of nursing also can serve as excellent research mentors. Regardless of the source, the research mentor needs to understand the knowledge, skills, and time constraints faced by clinical nurses involved in a research project and provide support.

Under the direction and guidance of this research mentor, determine how interested staff can participate in the study. Consider inviting other members of the healthcare team to join the project, such as social workers, nutritionists, and physical therapists. The project's chance for success can be maximized by allowing staff to have ownership of it.

Implementing a research study on a clinical unit can be a challenge, so suggest ways that interested nursing staff can participate. Use Figure 12-1 to carefully match the research skills of each participant with the tasks that need to be accomplished. Plan a schedule of research team meetings in advance and identify an effective means that can be used to foster ongoing communication among team members, especially in light of conflicting work schedules. Consider using email, a secure intranet system, or dedicated project software for communication among team members.

Before you begin your project, work with a research mentor in identifying resources, such as the services of a health science librarian or statistician, to successfully plan and complete the project. These individuals can help with the literature review, access to a library database to retrieve and duplicate references, payment of fees charged to use instruments, and assistance with data analysis. Some of these services are available to employers of healthcare organizations at no charge; check with your supervisor.

Gaining support for this project from your employer is essential for the project to succeed. Start by discussing the study with your supervisor before your begin the planning phase. Your employer may be able to help you obtain financial and other resources. For example, your supervisor may allow you to dedicate a portion of your daily work schedule to the project. Regular discussions and open communication with your supervisor about the project can serve as a source of encouragement for both you and the research team.

Think about choosing a problem of interest that may be fairly easy to complete. Consider designing a pilot study or replicating a previously published study before you decide to implement an original research project. Once you have a list of possible research ideas, ask the staff to prioritize them. Consider selecting a topic that is on the top of the list for most staff, is critical to quality patient care, causes the most distress for staff, or is the least costly to implement. Because of their close involvement in patient care, clinical nurses can be extremely helpful in identifying a clinical problem to study and clarifying the purpose and specific aims of a research project. Continue to develop the remaining steps of your research proposal—your plan for conducting the study.

After developing your proposal, submit it to the appropriate institutional review board at your organization. This is a group of individuals that will review the ethical implications of the study. Your supervisor or research mentor can help you determine if other committees at your agency are required to review your proposal and provide approval. Following approval from these groups, implement the project. Continue to meet regularly as a research team to monitor the progress of the study and to discuss concerns or issues that arise.

Following completion of your study, meet as a team to evaluate this new experience and prepare final reports. Carefully examine the results of your study and compare them to similar past studies. Determine whether the results of your study should be used to investigate patient care on your unit or be incorporated into clinical documents, such as policies, procedures, or standards of care. The research team should develop plans for the next unit-based research project, considering comments obtained from the evaluation meeting.

Develop a plan to disseminate study results with others through peer-reviewed journal publications and formal oral or poster presentations (see Chapters 8 and 9). Use a variety of approaches in disseminating your research findings in a timely manner so that they can reach nurses who can understand and best use the findings in their practice. In addition to journal publications, consider sharing information about your project in your organization's newsletter or through a poster on your unit. Think about your target audience when submitting your abstract for presentation at professional nursing conferences. Be sure to include your study results in unit-based in-service programs as part of your dissemination plan.

Recognize and celebrate the efforts of your research team. Talk with your supervisor about awarding certificates of recognition or providing other means of acknowledgment. Consider planning these awards during National Nurses Week or at an annual nursing research event.

Evaluating Outcomes and Considering Sustainability

As an NPDS, you have developed a plan to involve nurses in research and EBP projects on your clinical unit, gathered a group of interested nurse leaders and academic partners, and implemented several educational programs aimed to strengthen the skills and competencies of clinical nurses. After EBP projects are implemented, it is important to not only evaluate the results of these projects related to the clinical problem but to also consider ways to sustain these advancements over time (Melnyk, Fineout-Overholt, Gallagher-Ford, & Stillwell, 2011).

As indicated in step 5 of Figure 12-2, Melnyk et al. (2010) encouraged nurses to carefully review project outcomes to determine what changes were successful or not successful and to consider appropriate revisions as follow-up. This step of EBP aligns with the NPDS's role related to problem-based evidence (see Chapter 2) (ANA & NNSDO, 2010).

The final step of Melnyk's EBP process is to share the results of your efforts with unit staff and appropriate individuals within your healthcare organization through newsletters, posters, and other available communication venues.

Summary

As an NPDS, it is important that you understand your roles and responsibilities related to research, EBP, and QI based on standards at your workplace and on a national level. In addition to strengthening your own competencies in these areas, you may also be responsible for developing and implementing unit-based initiatives with clinical nurses to strengthen their research and EBP skills. Consider strategies to help staff nurses overcome potential barriers to participating in these initiatives. Methods to develop EBP skills include reading and understanding research studies, critiquing evidence, using research in practice, and disseminating findings. NPDSs need to evaluate the results of these initiatives and develop strategies to sustain research and EBP advances within their organizations.

Helpful Websites

- Academy of Medical-Surgical Nurses—Evidence-Based Practice: www.amsn.org/practice-resources/evidence-based-practice
- Agency for Healthcare Research and Quality: www.ahrq.gov

- American Nurses Association
  - Appraising the Evidence: www.nursingworld.org/Research-Toolkit/Appraising-the-Evidence
  - Critique a Research Article: www.nursingworld.org/research-toolkit/Critique-Research -Article
  - Research Toolkit (members only): www.nursingworld.org/MainMenuCategories/The PracticeofProfessionalNursing/Improving-Your-Practice/Research-Toolkit/default.aspx
- Center for Transdisciplinary Evidence-Based Practice: https://ctep-ebp.com
- Duke University Medical Center Library and the Health Sciences Library at the University of North Carolina at Chapel Hill—Introduction to Evidence-Based Practice Tutorial: http:// guides.mclibrary.duke.edu/c.php?g=158201&p=1036002
- National League for Nursing: www.nln.org
- Oncology Nursing Society
  - Levels of Evidence: www.ons.org/practice-resources/pep/evaluation-process
  - PEP Rating System Overview: www.ons.org/practice-resources/pep
  - Resources for Researchers: www.ons.org/practice-resources/role-specific-resources/ researchers
- Oregon Health and Science University—Evidence-Based Practice Toolkit for Nursing: What Is EBP?: http://libguides.ohsu.edu/ebptoolkit

References

American Association of Colleges of Nursing. (2008). *The essentials of baccalaureate education for professional nursing practice.* Washington, DC: Author.

American Association of Colleges of Nursing. (2011). *The essentials of master's education in nursing.* Washington, DC: Author.

American Nurses Association. (2015). *Nursing: Scope and standards of practice* (3rd ed.). Silver Spring, MD: Author.

American Nurses Association & National Nursing Staff Development Organization. (2010). *Nursing professional development: Scope and standards of practice.* Silver Spring, MD: American Nurses Association.

American Nurses Credentialing Center. (n.d.). ANCC Magnet Recognition Program®. Retrieved from http://www. nursecredentialing.org/magnet.aspx

Arthur, J. (2011). *Lean Six Sigma for hospitals: Simple steps to fast, affordable, and flawless healthcare.* New York, NY: McGraw-Hill.

Barnsteiner, J., Disch, J., Johnson, J., McGuinn, K., Chappell, K., & Swartwout, E. (2013). Diffusing QSEN competencies across schools of nursing: The AACN/RWJF Faculty Development Institutes. *Journal of Professional Nursing, 29,* 68–74. doi:10.1016/j.profnurs.2012.12.003

Beinlich, N., & Meehan, A. (2014). Resource nurse program: A nurse-initiated, evidence-based program to eliminate hospital-acquired pressure ulcers. *Journal of Wound, Ostomy and Continence Nursing, 41,* 136–141. doi:10.1097/ WON.0000000000000001

Benner, P. (1984). *From novice to expert: Excellence and power in clinical nursing practice.* Menlo Park, NJ: Addison-Wesley.

Berger, J., Hardin, H.K., & Topp, R. (2011). Implementing a virtual journal club in a clinical nursing setting. *Journal for Nurses in Staff Development, 27,* 116–120. doi:10.1097/NND.0b013e318217b3bc

Berkey, B.S., & Moore, S. (2012). Preparing research manuscripts for publication: A guide for authors. *Oncology Nursing Forum, 39,* 433–435. doi:10.1188/12.ONF.433-435

Bernhofer, E.I. (2015). Reviewing the literature: Essential first step in research, quality improvement, and implementation of evidence-based practice. *Journal for Nurses in Professional Development, 31,* 191–196.

Bohnenkamp, S., Pelton, N., Rishel, C.J., & Kurtin, S. (2014a). Implementing evidence-based practice using an interprofessional team approach. *Oncology Nursing Forum, 41,* 434–437. doi:10.1188/14.ONF.434-437

Bohnenkamp, S., Pelton, N., Rishel, C.J., & Kurtin, S. (2014b). Implementing evidence-based practice using an interprofessional team approach: Part two. *Oncology Nursing Forum, 41,* 548–550. doi:10.1188/14.ONF.548-550

Brant, J.M., & Wickham, R. (Eds.). (2013). *Statement on the scope and standards of oncology nursing practice: Generalist and advanced practice.* Pittsburgh, PA: Oncology Nursing Society.

Clancey, J.K. (2009). Nurse research internship program: A unique mentoring program. *Journal of Neuroscience Nursing, 41*(6), E1–E6. doi:10.1097/JNN.0b013e3181bb68d2

Cronenwett, L., Sherwood, G., Barnsteiner, J., Disch, J., Johnson, J., Mitchell, P., … Warren, J. (2007). Quality and safety education for nurses. *Nursing Outlook, 55,* 122–131. doi:10.1016/j.outlook.2007.02.006

Dearholt, S.L., & Dang, D. (2012). *Johns Hopkins nursing evidence-based practice: Models and guidelines* (2nd ed.). Indianapolis, IN: Sigma Theta Tau.

Didion, J., Kozy, M.A., Koffel, C., & Oneail, K. (2013). Academic/clinical partnership and collaboration in quality and safety education for nurses education. *Journal of Professional Nursing, 29,* 88–94. doi:10.1016/j.profnurs.2012.12.004

Dolansky, M.A., & Moore, S.M. (2013). Quality and Safety Education for Nurses (QSEN): The key is systems thinking. *Online Journal of Issues in Nursing, 18*(3). doi:10.3912/OJIN.Vol18No03Man01

Fridman, M., & Frederickson, K. (2014). Oncology nurses and the experience of participation in an evidence-based practice project. *Oncology Nursing Forum, 41,* 382–388. doi:10.1188/14.ONF.382-388

Gloeckner, M.B., & Robinson, C.B. (2010). A nursing journal club thrives through shared governance. *Journal for Nurses in Staff Development, 26,* 267–270. doi:10.1097/NND.0b013e3181fc0445

Granger, B.B., Zhao, Y., Rogers, J., Miller, C., Gilliss, C.L., & Champagne, M. (2013). The language of data: Tools to translate evidence for nurses in clinical practice. *Journal for Nurses in Staff Development, 29,* 294–300. doi:10.1097/NND.0000000000000011

Green, A., Jeffs, D., Huett, A., Jones, L.R., Schmid, B., Scott, A.R., & Walker, L. (2014). Increasing capacity for evidence-based practice through the Evidence-Based Practice Academy. *Journal of Continuing Education in Nursing, 45,* 83–90. doi:10.3928/00220124-20140124-20

Hudson-Barr, D., Weeks, S.K., & Watters, C. (2002). Introducing the staff nurse to nursing research through the Great American Cookie Experiment. *Journal of Nursing Administration, 32,* 440–443. doi:10.1097/00005110-200209000-00004

Institute of Medicine. (2001). *Crossing the quality chasm: A new health system for the 21st century.* Washington, DC: National Academies Press.

Institute of Medicine. (2003). *Health professions education: A bridge to quality.* Washington, DC: National Academies Press.

Institute of Medicine. (2011). *The future of nursing: Leading change, advancing health.* Washington, DC: National Academies Press.

Institute of Medicine Committee on Assessing the System for Protecting Human Research Participants. (2002). *Responsible research: A systems approach to protecting human research participants.* Washington, DC: National Academies Press.

Jamerson, P.A., Fish, A.F., & Frandsen, G. (2011). Nursing student research assistant program: A strategy to enhance nursing research capacity building in a Magnet status pediatric hospital. *Applied Nursing Research, 24,* 110–113. doi:10.1016/j.apnr.2009.08.004

Johnson, J.A. (2014). Why are nurses so reluctant to implement changes based on evidence and what can we do to help? *Journal for Nurses in Professional Development, 30*(10), 45–46.

Krom, Z.R., Batten, J., & Bautista, C. (2010). A unique collaborative nursing evidence-based practice initiative using the Iowa model: A clinical nurse specialist, a health science librarian, and a staff nurse's success story. *Clinical Nurse Specialist, 24,* 54–59. doi:10.1097/NUR.0b013e3181cf5537

Long, C.M., & Reider, J.A. (1995). Research reflections: The cookie experiment revisited. *Nurse Educator, 20*(3), 13.

Maljanian, R., Caramanica, L., Taylor, S.K., MacRae, J.B., & Beland, D.K. (2002). Evidence-based nursing practice, Part 2: Building skills through research roundtables. *Journal of Nursing Administration, 32,* 85–90. doi:10.1097/00005110-200202000-00006

McConnell, E.S., Lekan, D., Hebert, C., & Leatherwood, L. (2007). Academic-practice partnerships to promote evidence-based practice in long-term care: Oral hygiene care practices as an exemplar. *Nursing Outlook, 55,* 95–105. doi:10.1016/j.outlook.2006.12.003

McCurry, M.K. (2014). The Great American Cookie Experiment updated for the millennial learner. *Journal of Nursing Education, 53,* 180. doi:10.3928/01484834-20140220-11

Melnyk, B.M., & Fineout-Overholt, E. (2014). *Evidence-based practice in nursing and healthcare: A guide to best practice* (3rd ed.). Philadelphia, PA: Wolters Kluwer Health/Lippincott Williams & Wilkins.

Melnyk, B.M., Fineout-Overholt, E., Gallagher-Ford, L., & Stillwell, S.B. (2011). Evidence-based practice through organizational policies and an innovative model. *American Journal of Nursing, 111*(9), 57–60.

Melnyk, B.M., Fineout-Overholt, E., Stillwell, S.B., & Williamson, K.M. (2009). Evidence-based practice: Step by step: Igniting a spirit of inquiry. *American Journal of Nursing, 109*(11), 49–52. doi:10.1097/01.NAJ.0000363354.53883.58

Melnyk, B.M., Fineout-Overholt, E., Stillwell, S.B., & Williamson, K.M. (2010). Evidence-based practice: Step by step: The seven steps of evidence-based practice. *American Journal of Nursing, 110*(1), 51–53. doi:10.1097/01.NAJ.0000366056.06605.d2

Moore, S., & Stichler, J.J. (2015). Engaging clinical nurses in quality improvement projects. *Journal of Continuing Education in Nursing, 46*(10), 470–476.

O'Nan, C.L. (2011). The effect of a journal club on perceived barriers to the utilization of nursing research in a practice setting. *Journal for Nurses in Staff Development, 27*, 160–164. doi:10.1097/NND.0b013e31822365f6

Oncology Nursing Society. (n.d.-a). PEP rating system overview. Retrieved from https://www.ons.org/practice-resources/pep

Oncology Nursing Society. (n.d.-b). Putting Evidence Into Practice: Fatigue. Retrieved from https://www.ons.org/practice-resources/pep/fatigue

Polit, D.F., & Beck, C.T. (2012). *Nursing research: Generating and assessing evidence for nursing practice* (9th ed.). Philadelphia, PA: Wolters Kluwer Health/Lippincott Williams & Wilkins.

Powers, J., & Fortney, S. (2014). Bed baths: Much more than a basic nursing task. *Nursing, 44*(10), 67–68.

Quality and Safety Education for Nurses Institute. (n.d.). QSEN. Retrieved from http://qsen.org/about-qsen

Ryan, M., & Joseph, C.B. (2013). A mobile medical library initiative: Promoting nurses' professional development and information-searching skills for evidence-based practice. *MEDSURG Nursing, 22*, 57–59.

Schaffer, M.A., Sandau, K.E., & Diedrick, L. (2012). Evidence-based practice models for organizational change: Overview and practical applications. *Journal of Advanced Nursing, 69*, 1197–1209.

Shirey, M.R., Hauck, S.L., Embree, J.L., Kinner, T.J., Schaar, G.L., Phillips, L.A., … McCool, I.A. (2011). Showcasing differences between quality improvement, evidence-based practice, and research. *Journal of Continuing Education in Nursing, 42*, 57–68. doi:10.3928/00220124-20100701-01

Sigma Theta Tau International Honor Society of Nursing. (n.d.). About STTI. Retrieved from http://www.nursingsociety.org/about-stti

Spiers, J.A., Paul, P., Jennings, D., & Weaver, K. (2012). Strategies for engaging undergraduate nursing students in reading and using qualitative research. *Qualitative Report, 17*(48), 1–22. Retrieved from http://nsuworks.nova.edu/tqr/vol17/iss24/2

Sternberger, C. (2002). The great music experiment: Taking the cookie experiment to the web. *Nurse Educator, 27*, 106–108. doi:10.1097/00006223-200205000-00004

Thiel, C. (1987). Views on research: The cookie experiment: A creative teaching strategy. *Nurse Educator, 12*(3), 8–10. doi:10.1097/00006223-198705000-00004

Weitzel, T., & Robinson, S. (2011). Nursing Research Week: Promoting staff nurse awareness of research activities through a week-long celebration. *Journal for Nurses in Staff Development, 27*, 280–284. doi:10.1097/NND.0b013e3181b1ba29

Wittmann-Price, R., Celia, L., & Dunn, R. (2013). Successful implementation of evidence-based nursing practice: The indispensable role of staff development. *Journal for Nurses in Professional Development, 29*, 202–204. doi:10.1097/NND.0b013e31829b2212

CHAPTER 13

Meeting the Learning Needs and Marketing the Talents of Clinical Nurses Through Continuing Education Programs

A S mentioned in Chapter 2, continuing education (CE) is among the key throughputs included in the NPDS practice model described in *Nursing Professional Development: Scope and Standards of Practice* (American Nurses Association [ANA] & National Nursing Staff Development Organization [NNSDO], 2010). NPDSs often assume a leadership role in CE activities and may be expected to "create, manage, implement, coordinate, and evaluate" (ANA & NNSDO, 2010, p. 6) CE initiatives within their work settings. Although CE exists as a separate entity within the model, portions of it often overlap with other throughput domains, supporting an updated focus on the "dissemination and use of evidence-based practice" (ANA & NNSDO, 2010, p. 2).

ANA (2000) defined CE as the "systematic professional learning experiences designed to augment the knowledge, skills, and attitudes of nurses" (ANA, 2000, p. 43). CE activities are intended to not only help nurses provide safe, quality care to patients but also to assist them in attaining professional goals identified in their career plans. Therefore, CE activities focus on nurses' continuing competence and lifelong learning regardless of their work setting or employer (ANA, 2000). In this respect, these programs differ from most staff development activities (e.g., in-service, orientation) designed to improve nurses' performance in their roles within specific work settings. Staff development activities are labeled as being employer-specific, facility-specific, or organization-specific content (American Nurses Credentialing Center [ANCC], 2012a). However, ANCC (2012a) stated that in-service education offerings that provide "new content knowledge that would be transferable to other job settings" (p. 3) may be eligible for contact hours.

All professional nurses are expected to actively participate as learners in CE activities, regardless if they are NPDSs, clinical nurses, nurse faculty, unit managers, or unit-based educators. In addition to assuming the role of learner in CE, your responsibilities as an NPDS may include designing, coordinating, or presenting CE offerings for clinical nurses within your organization. If you are a unit-based educator, you also may help guide clinical nurses in seeking CE activities inside and outside your healthcare organization. In addition to implementing these activities at your workplace, you may be involved in developing CE programs through your own professional nursing organization as part of your service and professional development.

Regardless of your responsibilities related to CE, it is important to understand the process involved in sponsoring CE activities and be aware of the various opportunities that exist for clinical nurses. You also need to learn how to develop a CE program within your employer's expectations. This chapter will discuss possible features of these programs.

Professional Standards for Continuing Education Programs

ANCC, a subsidiary of ANA, is responsible for implementing credentialing programs, such as the accreditation of CE activities developed and sponsored for nurses (ANA, 2000). Serving in this capacity since 1991, ANCC, through its Commission on Accreditation, establishes standards and guidelines for organizations to follow as they design and implement CE activities. It also oversees many specialty practice certifications for nurses, the Magnet Recognition Program®, and nursing skills competency programs (ANCC, n.d.). The latter two were detailed in Chapters 1 and 3.

Professional organizations can apply to ANCC (n.d.) to be recognized as providers of CE (www.nursecredentialing.org). An ANCC-approved provider can be from any country in the world. Any organization interested in sponsoring nursing CE offerings must submit an application fee to obtain one of following CE provider categories: accredited provider through ANCC; approved provider through a constituent member association, such as a state nurses association; or an ANCC approver for a specific educational offering. An ANCC approver is any organization in the United States that approves providers of CE activities and ensures they follow ANCC criteria (ANCC, n.d.).

Organizations that are granted provider status by ANCC have the authority to conduct and award CE programs with oversight by their accredited approvers. For example, a school of nursing in Pennsylvania may choose to become an approved provider of CE through the Pennsylvania State Nurses Association (PSNA), an accredited approver through ANCC's Commission on Accreditation.

ANCC also offers a joint accreditation option for nursing, medicine, and pharmacy (ANCC, 2012a). This innovative initiative not only helps these three professions sponsor quality interprofessional CE offerings together as a healthcare team but also enables them to process CE applications using one review process (ANCC, n.d.). CE programs are awarded through each profession's respective accrediting organization: Accreditation Council for Continuing Medical Education (ACCME) for medicine, Accreditation Council for Pharmacy Education (ACPE) for pharmacy, and ANCC for nursing.

Provider organizations are expected to follow specific guidelines outlined in provider accreditation and approval program manuals. These manuals present an overview of the accreditation program and include relevant policies, procedures, and criteria to follow when developing CE programs, submitting application forms, and undergoing review. In the example presented in this chapter, the school of nursing in Pennsylvania would follow the policies outlined in PSNA's (2013) *Continuing Education Approval Program Manual*, published by the school's CE approver and congruent with ANCC criteria.

As an NPDS, you will need to understand the accreditation process and your specific responsibilities associated with CE program planning. It is important to investigate how CE programs are processed at your healthcare organization or professional nursing organization. Prior to developing your own CE offering, review these requirements with a nurse who is experienced in developing CE programs and can mentor you in this process.

Because the amount of time that nurses directly participate in CE activities determines the number of contact hours they are awarded, educators need to carefully consider this when planning a CE event, scheduling speakers, and verifying attendance. One contact hour of CE is awarded to participants for every 60 minutes of organized programming they attend (ANCC, 2012a). Participants receive a document, such as a certificate, at the conclusion of the CE event that serves as an official record of contact hours awarded.

Sources of Continuing Education Activities for Nurses

In the past, CE activities were described as being either traditional or independent (ANA, 2000). Traditional CE activities were those educational offerings paced by the provider and requiring nurses to be physically present at the learning activity. Conversely, independent CE activities were designed for completion independently by learners at their own pace. Advances in technology over the past decade have transformed not only where learning can occur but also who are included as learners (ANA & NNSDO, 2010). For example, distance learning technologies can enable nurses around the world to participate in the same CE activity.

According to ANCC, CE offerings for nurses can currently be categorized as being "provider directed, provider paced; provider directed, learner paced; or learner directed, learner paced" (ANCC, 2012a, pp. 20–21). Regardless of the approach, CE activities need to incorporate adult learning principles in their design and teaching-learning strategies (ANCC, 2012a). Strategies for providing these CE programs will be discussed later in this chapter.

Provider-Directed Continuing Education

In provider-directed CE, the provider is responsible for regulating all components of the activity, such as the learning objectives, content, and methods of delivery and evaluation (ANCC, 2012a). Provider-directed CE is further defined as being either provider paced, where the provider controls the timing of the learning activity, or learner paced, where participants control their own learning rates.

Nurses can participate in provider-directed CE offerings by attending workshops, programs, or provider-directed conferences sponsored by their workplace, professional nursing organizations, commercial companies, colleges and universities, or other community agencies and groups. Although some of these offerings take place in a classroom setting, distance learning options exist as well. For example, some CE offerings are available using satellite video conferencing, the Internet, or audio conferencing techniques.

Although many employers sponsor CE programs for their nursing staff, some organizations allow their nurses to attend programs sponsored by outside sources, such as professional nursing groups, schools of nursing, or independent firms. The employer may or may not cover travel and time costs.

If your employer provides this benefit to staff, it is important for you, as a unit-based educator, to develop ways that all nurses can benefit from a CE program, even if they are unable to attend. For example, ask nurses who attend outside CE programs to present key points of these programs in a unit-based in-service program, post a one-page report on the unit's bulletin board or on the organization's intranet site, or send a brief email to colleagues. Be sure to include these external CE programs in developing your unit's education plan, as identified in Chapter 6.

Nurses can participate in provider-directed, learner-paced CE activities through a variety of options, such as feature articles printed in nursing journals or accessed through the Internet. To receive contact hours, nurses read the offering, answer a series of questions that pertain to the topic, complete an evaluation form, and submit (e.g., mail, fax, email) the completed test and evaluation to the provider. A certificate for a specified number of contact hours is provided if the nurse attains a passing score. CE opportunities often require a minimal processing fee. Many journals, such as *Oncology Nursing Forum*, *American Journal of Nursing*, *Nursing*, *AORN Journal*, and *Journal of Continuing Education in Nursing*, sponsor independent home study or online options for nurses.

Suppose, for example, that you are interested in learning more about chronic pain management in adults. A provider-directed, provider-paced CE activity would involve attending a one-hour face-to-face session or viewing a one-hour webinar. This activity could be coordinated by your hospital (e.g., by the nursing education and research department).

Maybe you want to learn about this topic at your own pace (provider directed, learner paced), as your tight schedule prevents you from attending courses face-to-face. You decide to use a CE feature article from an oncology nursing journal to accomplish this goal. You read the article at your own pace, complete and submit the required paperwork (e.g., quiz, evaluation form), and pay a fee (if applicable) to receive a certificate that validates the predesignated contact hours. Alternative options to CE articles include an online course, e-books, self-learning modules, and independent studies (ANCC, 2012a).

Learner-Directed Continuing Education

Learner-directed CE activities also exist and are considered learner-paced activities (ANCC, 2012a). For example, let's say that you identified a learning need focused on managing pain experienced by adults. You would first establish your learning goals, collect and review needed resources, and evaluate specific outcomes related to your goals. You control not only the amount of time that you will need to learn but also the time that you will need before you are ready to demonstrate your proposed learning outcomes.

Reasons for Continuing Education for Nurses

According to the Standards of Professional Performance outlined in *Nursing: Scope and Standards of Practice* (ANA, 2015), RNs are expected to attain "knowledge and competence that reflects current nursing practice" (p. 5). Continuing education provides opportunities for nurses to fulfill their expectations for lifelong learning, continuing professional competence, and role performance (ANA, 2015). Chapter 2 discussed the NPDS's role in facilitating CE for other nurses, with the ultimate goals (outputs) of learning, change, and professional role competence and growth (ANA, 2015). Similarly, NPDSs must be cognizant of their own CE needs to maintain competence in their professional roles (Dickerson, 2010).

Evidence of successful completion of CE activities is a requirement for RNs in particular situations. For example, states with mandatory CE stipulations in their nurse practice act require nurses licensed within the state to obtain a defined number of contact hours for relicensure. The overall goal of states that support this legislation is to assure the public that RNs remain current in their nursing practice. According to ANCC (2014), approximately 36 states required mandatory CE for their RNs to maintain licenses. The number of required contact hours varies by state and ranges from 5 to 15 hours per year, with most states requiring a maximum of 15. For example, nurses requesting license renewals in Pennsylvania and California must complete a minimum of 30 contact hours every two years, while RNs in Rhode Island and Massachusetts must complete an average of 5 and 7.5 hours each year, respectively (i.e., 10 and 15 contact hours over a two-year period) (ANCC, 2014).

Nurses need a particular number of contact hours in specified areas to maintain specialty certifications and any other professional development requirements. The American Board of Nursing Specialties (n.d.) defines certification as the "formal recognition of the specialized knowledge, skills, and experience demonstrated by the achievement of standards identified by a nursing specialty to promote optimal health outcomes" (para. 1).

When nurses are *certified*, it means that a professional nursing organization or agency has recognized them for their knowledge in a general or specialty practice area. After meeting certain eligibility criteria and clinical practice requirements, the nurses passed an examination to validate their abilities and received initial certification. For nurses to maintain this credential, these certification organizations offer various options in addition to retesting, such as evidence of participation in specific CE programs with contact hours awarded.

For example, the Oncology Nursing Certification Corporation (ONCC) developed the Individual Learning Needs Assessment (ILNA) for nurses seeking renewal in oncology nursing certification (ONCC, 2012). This method begins with nurses taking a self-assessment to identify subject areas in which they need to strengthen and then allows nurses to earn points by submitting various sources as evidence of their professional development in these areas, including CE programs. The number of points required for renewal varies based on each nurse's assessment results, but all candidates are required to earn at least 25 points. ONCC publishes how many ILNA points can be earned through continuing nursing education, continuing medical education, academic education, publications, and presentations (ONCC, 2012).

Developing a Continuing Education Program

As an NPDS or unit-based educator, you may have the opportunity to participate in a CE program planning committee or assume a leadership role as a nurse planner (ANCC, 2012a). Regardless of the role you play, it is important to understand the steps involved in assessing, planning, implementing, and evaluating CE programs according to current published ANCC criteria. These steps should be familiar, because they reflect those involved in presenting an in-service educational program (see Chapter 6). Each step will be discussed in detail in the section that follows. You can also find detailed guidelines online for designing education programs in various ANCC publications (see www.nursecredentialing.org/Accreditation/ResourcesServices).

What to Do Before the Continuing Education Program

Careful assessment and planning are essential skills for you to use when developing a CE program. Both skills require your attention to several steps when preparing each CE activity.

Assessing Target Learners, Specific Learning Needs, and Gaps

In the first step of creating your CE program, you will need to determine who the potential participants will be and their specific educational needs. Clarify if your CE offerings are limited only to nurses who are employed by your organization, nurses from the local community, or both. Similarly, determine what format you will use for the program (e.g., face-to-face, Internet-based distance learning approach). Understanding the boundaries of your target audience will influence the what, where, when, why, who, and how aspects of your learning needs assessment.

Next, identify the learning needs of your target audience using evidence collected not only from the learners but also from appropriate experts (ANCC, 2012a). For example, nurse managers, quality improvement and nursing research department staff, unit-based educators, and other clinical staff can provide you with diverse perspectives on the learning needs of the nurses within your setting.

Rather than depend solely on the traditional annual needs assessment survey completed by learners, investigate sources of evidence that will help you zero in on nurses' learning needs. It is essential to deliver CE activities designed to "close a gap between what learners currently know or do in practice and what they should know or do" (DeSilets, Dickerson, & Lavin, 2013, p. 433). This gap analysis will help you design an appropriate CE program for a group of nurses and evaluate changes in their knowledge, skills, and practice over time.

Dickerson (2014) emphasized that nurse planners need to consider the intended outcome of an educational activity and answer the "why" questions rather than focusing on the "what." Such evidence should support the development of required knowledge, skills, and practices.

Review aggregated results from ongoing organizational initiatives for ideas, such as quality improvement projects, performance improvement reviews, feedback from prior CE programs, and other organizational outcome data (ANCC, 2012a). Current trends and issues in nursing and health care also can provide you with sources of evidence for learning.

Be creative yet efficient when collecting and analyzing evidence needed to develop a comprehensive learning needs assessment. Technological advances, such as electronic surveys and research databases, enable NPDSs to complete surveys and literature reviews with ease in a timely manner. Consider other approaches to collect meaningful data, such as face-to-face focus groups, email messages, telephone calls, or distance education assessment tools (e.g., wikis). DeSilets et al. (2013) suggested developing assessment questions that allow nurses to reflect on specific problems or issues that they encounter in their daily nursing practice. Regardless of the assessment method, it is important to be able to "identify and validate a gap in knowledge, skills, or practice that the educational activity is designed to improve or meet" (ANCC, 2012a, p. 8). Logically speaking, the more specific you are in identifying a learning gap (e.g., "50% of the electronic health records reviewed on the surgical oncology units in the hospital on July 1 . . ."), the easier it will be for you to assess the influence that a CE program had on improving that gap over both a short-term and long-term basis.

Confirming Criteria for Approved Continuing Education Activity

After you have identified a unique learning need for your target audience of nurses, verify that the proposed program content meets ANCC requirements and therefore is eligible for contact hours. According to ANCC (2012a), the content of the proposed program should be as evidence based as possible, presented beyond the nurses' basic knowledge level, generalizable to other work settings, and able to "enhance professional development or performance of the nurse" (p. 6).

Sometimes, awarding CE credit depends on the nurse learners and whether they had previously participated in the same program (ANCC, 2012b). For example, perhaps nurses at your hospital are required to attend a three-hour CE program on IV therapy as part of their annual review. This year, nurses on unit 3B attended the course and received three credit hours. Next year, these same nurses can only be awarded credit hours on the new content added to the program. If the content remained the same from the previous year, then the program would be considered a staff development offering for these nurses and not a CE activity with credit hours. However, any newly hired nurses from unit 3B would be eligible to receive credit hours for this program, as it would be their first time participating. When in doubt, contact your designated approver with any questions to decide if your educational activity meets the criteria of a CE program.

For example, according to the needs assessment you recently conducted for your clinical units, it is evident that staff nurses need to develop their skills in serving as preceptors for newly hired staff nurses. The nurses on the units also expressed this need and asked for your assistance. You also know that a local school of nursing plans to recruit staff nurses from your units to precept junior nursing students in a summer internship program. In response, you decide to plan a one-day CE program on preceptor development. Although about 30% of nurses on your four clinical units are experienced preceptors, nurses hired over the past two years possess novice-level preceptor skills, at best. You plan to repeat this program over the next year, because all of the nurses on the clinical unit cannot attend the program at the same time.

Developing a Detailed Plan

After you have identified learners and assessed their needs, develop a detailed project plan for your CE program. This plan will help you organize the tasks you need to accomplish, keep you on track, and communicate needs to others involved in the project. Include specific tasks, due dates, and the people responsible for each task.

Organizing and Orienting a Planning Committee

The next step involves organizing a committee to develop your program. According to ANCC (2012a), a planning committee includes a nurse planner and at least one other person with expertise in the topic to determine the qualifications of the potential presenters. Recruit individuals who have expressed an interest in participating in this activity and have the talents to make the project a success. Lubejko and Dickerson (2014) recommended that, before recruiting members for a CE planning committee, you first determine the knowledge and skills needed to plan and implement a successful program. Then, invite members who possess these characteristics. For example, in addition to yourself, you decided to have four nurses on your planning committee. You included two experienced preceptors as members of your CE planning committee and one nurse with experience in leading similar CE projects.

Once you have gathered the members of the CE planning committee, explain the committee's charge. Review any expectations you have of them, such as attending meetings and meeting deadlines. Designate specific roles and responsibilities for each member and establish an effective communication method, such as email, so that information can be shared among members in a timely manner. Establish the dates, times, and locations of future planning meetings, starting with the target date for the CE program and working backward. Spend some time helping committee members get acquainted with each other and understand your requirements in regularly orienting and updating the committee.

Consider using creative ways to orient your committee members to their ongoing roles in planning, documenting, implementing, and evaluating CE activities. For example, Losko (2009) described how the Ohio State University Wexner Medical Center reframed its traditional workshops to orient or update more than 100 nurses concerning their roles and responsibilities. They created an annual workshop called "The Re-View," which was modeled after *The View*, a popular daytime television program. Evaluation data provided by participants were quite positive and met program objectives in an entertaining manner.

Determining Key Project Tasks

After orienting the members of your planning committee, make a list of key tasks that need to be accomplished before the date of the CE program and assign due dates for each. Figure 13-1 lists examples of activities that need to be included among your tasks for your entire program, along with the names of the committee members responsible for accomplishing each task and the due dates for each task.

Verifying the Date, Time, Location, and Facilities

After determining tasks, establish the date, time, and location of your program. Be sure to verify the availability of any classroom location if it is a face-to-face offering. Allow yourself

Figure 13-1. Checklist for Organizing a Continuing Education Program		
Task	**Due Date**	**People Responsible**
Before the Program		
Assess learners and learning needs gap.		
Determine available resources.		
Develop a detailed plan.		
Organize and orient a planning committee.		
Determine key tasks of the project.		
Verify the date, time, location, and facilities.		
Estimate audience size and special needs.		
Determine the purpose and objectives.		
Determine key content.		
Recruit and confirm speakers and materials, including duplicating and organizing handouts.		
Develop a brochure/announcement for the program.		
Establish a method for verifying participation and successful completion.		
Determine a method of evaluation.		
Submit continuing education program application.		
Day of the Program		
Check accommodations.		
Set up the registration table.		
Greet participants and speakers.		
Introduce speakers.		
Maintain time schedule.		
Orient participants and review evaluation.		
Award certificates.		
After the Program		
Analyze and review evaluations.		
Make revisions for future programs.		
Complete the budget process.		
Write thank-you letters and provide feedback to speakers and planning committee.		
File documents in a secure location.		

sufficient time to plan this event, scheduling at least several months in advance to secure large conference rooms within your organization. Choose a location and room that will provide a good learning environment for the type of program you are planning and that is accessible to all participants and appropriate for the teaching strategies that will be used (e.g., small group work). The learning environment also should be a comfortable size for the program's anticipated number of participants. Consider access to tables that will allow participants to have a writing surface for note-taking or program activities.

Be sure to make arrangements for the physical layout of the classroom, such as the seating pattern and speaker facilities. Consider a room for vendor exhibits, if you choose this option. If you are unfamiliar with the room, visit it beforehand.

Investigate if special services, such as access to food services and audiovisual equipment, are readily available for this room. Speak with the appropriate representatives from food and technical services to plan for these needs in advance. Determine if assistance with audiovisual equipment is available or if you need to assign this task to a member of the planning committee.

Another thing to consider is the approximate length of your program. Discuss with nurse managers about staffing issues and budget constraints that may influence this decision.

Determine the number of participants you will invite to the CE program. Consider a variety of factors when making this decision, such as budget constraints and the need for providing adequate staffing to remain on the clinical units to care for patients. Anticipate if participants will need special accommodations because of physical limitations, such as accessing the room using a wheelchair.

Determining Available Resources

As you plan your CE program, identify specific resources available, such as finances, typing and duplication of documents, human resources (e.g., expert speakers, media experts), and physical resources (e.g., conference rooms, audiovisual equipment). List the resources you do not have and will need for the project, including time and staff support. Keep track of the cost of each task as you move through the planning process. Discuss your need for unavailable resources with your supervisor well in advance to explore funding opportunities.

ANCC emphasized that CE programs must be presented without "promotion or bias" (ANCC, 2012a, p. 6). Therefore, the nurse planner and the planning committee must closely adhere to ANCC guidelines regarding sources of sponsorship and commercial support related to CE programs (ANCC, 2012a). More specifically, *commercial support* is defined by ANCC (2012a) as "financial or in-kind contributions given by a commercial interest that are used to pay for all or part of the costs" (p. 28) of a CE activity. Conversely, individuals or groups that provide such contributions but do not meet ANCC's definition of being a source of commercial support are referred to as *sponsors* (ANCC, 2012a). It is important to remember that individuals or groups defined as commercial support or sponsors cannot serve as providers or co-providers of your CE offerings. When in doubt, contact your approver organization.

Determining Purpose and Objectives

At this point in the process, you will need to develop your program's overall purpose. Using the previous example in this chapter, the planning committee and speakers have decided the program's purpose will be "to assist staff nurses to effectively function as a preceptor on the clinical unit for newly hired nurses and/or nursing students."

After confirming the program's purpose, develop specific educational objectives or outcomes in the form of "knowledge, skills, and/or practice changes" (p. 10) that you expect from nurses attending the program (ANCC, 2012a). Ensure that each objective is learner focused, limited to one measurable verb, and details what learners "will be able to know or do" (ANCC, 2012a, p. 10). While the number of objectives depends on the purpose of the CE offering, some sources recommend focusing on one or two per hour (PSNA, 2013).

Determining Content, Teaching-Learning Strategies, and Contact Hours

After you have determined the purpose and objectives for your CE program, identify the key content that should be included with the help of experts or speakers. Content should match objectives, enable participants to achieve these objectives, and be based on the best evidence available, such as "literature/peer-reviewed journals, clinical guidelines, best practices, and content experts/expert opinion" (ANCC, 2012a, p. 10). This evidence is validated using a hierarchy model (ANCC, 2012b), such as the Melnyk Pyramid, which distributes evidence on seven levels from the lowest (7) to highest (1) (Melnyk & Fineout-Overholt, 2014). In this model, the lowest level consists of expert opinion, whereas the highest level includes reports such as systematic reviews and meta-analysis of randomized controlled trials. Using the previous example of a CE program on precepting, you ask staff nurses at your hospital who are experienced preceptors to serve as content reviewers to help you identify topics. The committee also works with the hospital librarian to review, evaluate, and prioritize recent evidence on preceptors (ANCC, 2012a). As you refine the program's content, refer to your needs assessment to ensure that it is developed at a level that learners have not yet mastered. After listing content topics, assign an approximate time limit for each to determine the number of eligible contact hours.

Once you have determined the program content, select appropriate teaching-learning strategies that will enable learners to attain objectives. Strategies should align with educational objectives, encourage learners' active participation, and be appropriate for the time allotted and the size of the audience. When calculating contact hours, be aware that the program must last at least 30 minutes, and any time calculations for partial hours should be "rounded down to the nearest 1/10th or 1/100th" (ANCC, 2012a, p. 11). CE offerings available to nurses in print or formats other than face-to-face rely on different mechanisms, such as pilot testing, to estimate the contact hours (ANCC, 2012a).

For example, after reviewing the literature on preceptor programs, you decide that learning how to provide constructive feedback to student nurses about their daily clinical performance should be one of the topics. Given the time allotted for the program, you assign a 60-minute time limit to this topic and plan to involve participants using role-play with an audience volunteer. You continue to assign time limits to each topic on your list until you have developed a tentative schedule for the entire program. You will use this information later when designing a marketing brochure for your program.

Recruiting Speakers and Materials

After designing the format of your program, recruit appropriate speakers for the topics. Speakers who participate in CE offerings should possess expertise on the topic, its learners, and its teaching-learning strategies (ANCC, 2012a). Nurses are expected to participate in the planning of the educational activity (PSNA, 2013).

Consider inviting nurses within your organization to be speakers, if appropriate. This strategy is an effective way to market your talents and those of colleagues and helps everyone in their professional development.

When communicating with speakers, provide the proposed description of the program, its purpose, and objectives. Invite their suggestions for refining these aspects. Provide them with a brochure of the program, if available, and include information on its date, time, location, and audience. Remind them of the audiovisuals available and confirm their needs. Keep in contact with the speakers up until the time of the event. Consider purchasing small gifts to give to your speakers for their efforts.

Presenters, content reviewers, experts, and planners must complete biographical and conflict of interest forms as part of the required application process (ANCC, 2012a). Information provided on a biographical form allows committee validation of qualifications related to the CE topic. The conflict of interest data help a committee determine any "affiliation or relationship of a financial nature with a Commercial Interest Organization that might bias a person's ability to objectively participate in the planning, implementation, or review of a learning activity" (ANCC, 2012a, p. 28). The nurse planner must ensure the program is free of bias by resolving any actual or potential conflicts of interest for anyone involved in its planning or presentation (e.g., the planning committee, speakers, content experts).

The planning committee also needs to ensure that a written education plan is prepared and reviewed prior to submitting a CE application. This plan describes the program's overall purpose and educational objectives with an associated content outline, time allotted to each portion, the presenters, and teaching-learning strategies or resources (PSNA, 2013). Chapter 6 provided an example of how to develop a lesson plan.

Provide speakers with the appropriate forms to complete these tasks, using those designed by the representatives at your organization who will submit the CE application for approval. Encourage speakers to use active learning strategies in their presentations and include realistic examples, such as case studies, that will pique the interest of participants.

Ask speakers to provide information that you can use to introduce them as well as a copy of any handouts they will need duplicated for participants. Request these materials well in advance of the CE program so that you have sufficient time to organize them into packets or an electronic format.

After compiling the handouts and brochures for your program, organize them in a packet that can be distributed to participants on the day of the CE program or electronically before the event. Include other essential documents, such as evaluation forms. Consider including a list of participants and speakers in the packets, along with contact information participants can use to network with each other. Include name tags that participants can wear during the conference. If lunch is not available on site, include suggested restaurants that participants can visit.

Advertising the Continuing Education Program

If appropriate, develop a brochure or announcement to market your program. Work with representatives from your organization's public relations or media services department to accomplish this task. If an official brochure is not needed for your program, you can provide program information in another manner, such as a handout. Use samples of past brochures in developing one for your program, including key information about the program, objectives, content, and speakers, as well as logistical information regarding registration, contact hours, sponsors, breaks, and lunch. Consider distributing the brochure via email to invite nurses both inside and outside of your organization.

Establishing a Method for Verifying Participation and Successful Completion

The planning committee is responsible for developing a method for verifying participation in CE programs and determining successful completion (ANCC, 2012a). For example, some places rely on sign-in sheets or self-reports to verify attendance. Regardless of the method, be sure that it complies with requirements for gaining approval for CE programs and record keeping. Also, decide if partial credit for the CE program will be provided and share this information with participants (ANCC, 2012a).

Successful completion of the CE activity should be determined by the planning committee on a case-by-case basis and clearly communicated to participants before the start of the program (ANCC, 2012a). Although some programs require submitting a completed evaluation form, others have participants pass a post-test or execute a return demonstration. Consider how participants will be given appropriate feedback either during or after program completion.

Check with CE representatives regarding documents or certificates of completion awarded to participants after successful completion of program requirements (ANCC, 2012a). Such documents must contain the participant's name; number of contact hours awarded; name and address of the provider (or website); the title, date, and location of the program; and the accreditation/approval statement according to the guidelines provided by the CE approval organization (ANCC, 2012a). The following statement is an example: "Duquesne University School of Nursing is an approved provider of continuing nursing education by the Pennsylvania State Nurses Association, an accredited approver by the American Nurses Credentialing Center's Commission on Accreditation." The signature of the person administratively responsible for the event is often included with this statement.

Determining a Method of Evaluation

During the planning phase for the CE program, you will need to determine the methods you will use to evaluate whether objectives were met. Learners will also have an opportunity to evaluate the effectiveness of speakers, their teaching strategies, and the learning environment (ANCC, 2012a). The evaluation form should include feedback from learners regarding their ability to attain stated objectives, the knowledge and skills they gained, and their "anticipated change in practice" (ANCC, 2012a, p. 12). Participants usually are asked to supply suggestions for future programs, which will assist you in validating future learning needs. If appropriate evaluation forms are unavailable, you will need to develop them. Sample forms may be available through your CE representative and can be adapted to reflect your specific program.

In addition to using short-term evaluation methods (e.g., post-tests, return demonstration, evaluation forms), it is important that the planning committee also tracks the long-term influence of a CE activity (ANCC, 2012a). Using the preceptor example presented throughout this chapter, you may decide to conduct a follow-up study with nurses who attended the program at six months and one year after program completion to assess their self-reported changes in practice. You also can obtain feedback from the new graduates and nursing students mentored by these nurse preceptors. Other methods of assessment can include observation of performance and collection of quality outcome measures (ANCC, 2012a).

Submitting the Continuing Education Application

After you have obtained the aforementioned information during the planning phase, work with your CE representative to prepare your program's application and other required documents, such as the educational plan, all biographical or conflict of interest forms, disclosures, and advertisements. Be sure to do this well in advance of the actual event, per your approved provider guidelines, so that certificates can be available to participants following the program.

What to Do the Day of the Continuing Education Program

Your careful planning should pay off when the day of your CE program arrives. Members of your planning committee can help oversee the day's events by greeting speakers and participants, providing them with packets, and guiding them accordingly. They also can acquaint speakers to the requested audiovisual equipment and introduce them to any available technicians. At this point, be sure to make a last-minute check on details, such as food services and room setup.

Start the program by introducing the planning committee and sponsors and thanking them for their assistance. Orient the participants to information provided in their packets and provide them with logistic information, such as evaluation forms, the schedule for the day, and facilities. Using a prepared script, be sure to make required disclosures to participants before the program begins, such as the number of contact hours that will be awarded; criteria for successful program completion; any conflicts of interest for the nurse planner, planning committee, speakers, and content experts; and the program's accreditation/approval statement (ANCC, 2012a). Participants also need to know the program's purpose and objectives and any sources of commercial support or sponsorship (ANCC, 2012a).

As the day progresses, anticipate potential problems and be ready to manage them. Keep the program on schedule by providing speakers with cues. Consider using small time cards to signal speakers regarding their status within the allotted time frame.

Provide participants with certificates as they return completed evaluation forms to the registration desk. Thank participants, speakers, and vendors for attending the CE program. Be sure to extend your personal appreciation to members of the CE planning committee.

What to Do After the Continuing Education Program

After completing your CE program, convene a meeting of the planning committee to analyze and review a summative evaluation based on feedback provided by participants on their evaluation forms. Review the planning process that was used in developing the CE events. Develop suggestions for future programs based on this feedback and start planning the next program, incorporating these suggestions.

Be sure to send thank-you notes to the speakers, sponsors, vendors, and planning members involved with the program. Provide speakers with feedback about their individual presentations based on the summative evaluation.

Organize and file essential documents that resulted from this event. Be sure to maintain the records of the CE offerings and course participants for six years, unless guided otherwise by your approver (PSNA, 2013). Make sure these documents are confidential and archived in a place where they can easily be retrieved.

Review the final budget that was allocated for your CE program. Ensure that all receipts have been accounted for and submitted to the appropriate person.

Evaluate the long-term influence of your CE program using the methods you created during project planning, such as tracking the performance of nurses who attended the program as they precept new nurses. These data also will help you revise future CE programs on the topic.

According to Dickerson (2013), communicating the outcomes of CE programs is an expectation of the NPDS's role related to collegiality, research, and leadership standards, as discussed in *Nursing Professional Development: Scope and Standards of Practice* (ANA & NNSDO, 2010). In fact, Dickerson (2013) referred to this responsibility as "making your voice heard" (p. 101). Share the outcomes of your CE program and projects with peers through your organization's newsletter, an abstract or podium presentation at a professional nursing conference (see Chapter 9), or a manuscript describing the outcomes to a nursing journal (see Chapter 8).

Summary

NPDSs often assume responsibility for planning CE programs targeted to nurses at their healthcare organization and those who work in the community. CE programs can help nurses develop new competencies, strengthen previously acquired knowledge and skills, and market their expertise to the professional community. NPDSs need to understand published standards and guidelines for CE programs when designing both provider- and learner-centered CE programs for nurses. Multiple steps need to be accomplished before, during, and after the CE event, from assessing the learning needs of targeted learners, to evaluating and disseminating the outcomes of CE programs. Finally, NPDSs should also track the long-term influence of CE programs and use these results when designing future programs.

Helpful Websites

- American Nurses Association—Nursing Legislative Issues and Trends: http://nursingworld .org/MainMenuCategories/Policy-Advocacy/State/Legislative-Agenda-Reports
- ANCC
  - Accreditation: www.nursecredentialing.org/Accreditation.aspx
  - Resource Center: www.nursecredentialing.org/Accreditation/ResourcesServices
- Oncology Nursing Society—Approver Unit: www.ons.org/education/approver-unit
- University of Michigan Library Research Guides—Nursing: Melnyk Pyramids: http://guides .lib.umich.edu/c.php?g=282802&p=1888246

References

American Board of Nursing Specialties. (n.d.). Frequently asked questions. Retrieved from http://www .nursingcertification.org/questions.html

American Nurses Association. (2000). *Scope and standards of practice for nursing professional development.* Washington, DC: Author.

American Nurses Association. (2015). *Nursing: Scope and standards of practice* (3rd ed.). Silver Spring, MD: Author.

American Nurses Association & National Nursing Staff Development Organization. (2010). *Nursing professional development: Scope and standards of practice.* Silver Spring, MD: American Nurses Association.

American Nurses Credentialing Center. (n.d.). ANCC accreditation. Retrieved from http://www.nursecredentialing. org/Accreditation.aspx

American Nurses Credentialing Center. (2012a). *Educational design process: 2013 mini manual.* Silver Spring, MD: Author.

American Nurses Credentialing Center. (2012b). *2013 primary accreditation application manual for providers and approvers: Approver unit webinars questions and answers.* Retrieved from http://nursecredentialing.org/ Documents/Accreditation/AccredVideo-FaqSheets/2013ManualWebinarFAQ-Approver.pdf

American Nurses Credentialing Center. (2014). State boards of nursing CE renewal requirements. Retrieved from http://www.nursecredentialing.org/StateCERequirements

DeSilets, L.R., Dickerson, P.S., & Lavin, S. (2013). More on gap analysis. *Journal of Continuing Education in Nursing, 44,* 433–434. doi:10.3928/00220124-20130925-17

Dickerson, P.S. (2010). Continuing nursing education: Enhancing professional development. *Journal of Continuing Education in Nursing, 41,* 100–101. doi:10.3928/00220124-20100224-07

Dickerson, P.S. (2013). Making your voice heard: Sharing outcomes of continuing nursing education. *Journal of Continuing Education in Nursing, 44,* 101–102. doi:10.3928/00220124-20130222-02

Dickerson, P.S. (2014). Needs assessment: Collecting the evidence. *Journal of Continuing Education in Nursing, 45,* 104–105. doi:10.3928/00220124-20140224-11

Losko, H.A. (2009). Educating nurse planners: Taking continuing nursing education on the talk show circuit. *Journal of Continuing Education in Nursing, 40,* 389–390. doi:10.3928/00220124-20090824-08

Lubejko, B.G., & Dickerson, P.S. (2014). The planning team—Who belongs? *Journal of Continuing Education in Nursing, 45,* 244–245. doi:10.3928/00220124-20140527-11

Melnyk, B., & Fineout-Overholt, E. (2014). *Evidence-based practice in nursing and healthcare: A guide to best nursing practice.* Philadelphia, PA: Lippincott Williams & Wilkins.

Oncology Nursing Certification Corporation. (2012, January). Individual Learning Needs Assessment. Retrieved from http://www.oncc.org/files/ilnabrochure.pdf

Pennsylvania State Nurses Association. (2013). *Continuing education approval program manual* (R-2013 ed.). Harrisburg, PA: Author.

CHAPTER 14

Developing a Career Plan as a Proactive Approach for the Future

YOU have accomplished your goal of becoming an NPDS or unit-based educator on your clinical unit. Although your current energies are likely focused on helping nursing staff provide safe and quality patient care, you also may be responsible for their professional career development. Learn more about this process by reflecting on your own professional goals and developing a career plan for yourself. This first-hand experience will help you mentor others as they create their career plans.

Understanding a Career Plan

A career plan is a personal blueprint designed to help you shape the direction of your professional career. Although a written version of your career plan can be thought of as a tool or worksheet, this document is really the result of an organized and systematic decision-making process called *career planning*. This process can be conceptualized into six key components: assessment, diagnosis, outcomes (goals), planning, implementation, and evaluation.

Career planning is a familiar concept to most nurses, as its components are similar to those of the nursing process (standards of care) outlined in *Nursing: Scope and Standards of Practice* (American Nurses Association [ANA], 2015). However, in this case, you are both the planner and the focus of the plan. This process also resembles the steps used in developing an education plan for unit-based in-service programs (see Chapter 6). Table 14-1 compares the components of the nursing process with key steps used in developing a career plan.

Table 14-1. Comparison of the Nursing Process and a Career Plan

Nursing Process	Career Plan
Assessment	Gather data about yourself, past/current positions, and the market for future roles.
Diagnosis	Analyze assessment data and make judgments.
Outcomes identification	Define short- and long-term goals.
Planning	Develop interventions and due dates for each goal.
Implementation	Accomplish interventions listed in the plan.
Evaluation	Evaluate progress on the plan and revise as needed.

Note. Based on information from American Nurses Association, 2015.

Some healthcare organizations have partnered with academic institutions to provide career coaching services to clinical nurses interested in advancing their education (Fowler, 2014). Be sure to explore whether your employer has similar academic-practice partnerships. If such partnerships do not exist at your workplace, assume a leadership role in further investigating this option and suggesting it to the proper personnel.

Purpose of a Career Plan

According to ANA (2015), nurses should demonstrate their ongoing commitment to the nursing profession through "continuous learning and strengthening individual practice within varied healthcare settings" (p. 11). You can develop a career plan to facilitate this learning process. A career plan can help organize your career development and aid any role transitions you may experience throughout your career (ANA & National Nursing Staff Development Organization, 2010). This is true whether your goals relate directly to your current nursing position or to future opportunities.

As previously mentioned, a career plan helps you identify and direct your career goals in a timely, systematic fashion. Because a career plan contains target dates matched with goals and interventions (strategies), it also minimizes distractions along the way. This process enables you to focus your everyday professional decisions toward reaching your professional goals. It also assists you in determining the knowledge, skills, and experiences needed to attain these goals. Suppose, for example, that you are a staff nurse on an adult medical-surgical unit. Despite your enthusiasm in caring for patients, you feel your professional life does not have focus. You lack a sense of identity compared to nurses who work on other specialty units. You regularly volunteer for projects at your workplace and within the community but are unsure you are making the best professional decisions in selecting these projects. You enjoy medical-surgical nursing and would like to strengthen your knowledge and skills in this clinical area. Developing a career plan can help you clarify your professional goals and guide your daily decisions related to this specialty field.

A career plan also can assist you in meeting or even exceeding expectations at your current position. It may even allow you to develop the complex behaviors and skills required for promotion at your workplace. For example, suppose you recently assumed a Staff Nurse I position at your local community hospital. You want to be the best nurse possible, but you feel a bit overwhelmed, as this is your first professional nursing job. Each day poses a challenge, as you focus on providing safe, quality patient care in a timely, organized manner. You are still having trouble organizing your day and prioritizing your patient care activities. Regardless, you are determined to meet your employer's expectations at your upcoming performance evaluation. You also want to exceed your unit manager's expectations in some areas. Developing a career plan that contains goals that mirror key components of your position description can minimize your concerns and keep you on target professionally.

A career plan can increase your marketability as a professional nurse. Given the current and future shortage of nurses in the United States (American Association of Colleges of Nursing [AACN], 2014), opportunities exist to refocus your professional interests toward another specialty or to a new role that fills a gap in patient services. These opportunities for professional growth may exist at your current workplace or through other healthcare or community agencies. Be creative in developing your career goals, and match them with healthcare and nursing marketing projections, if possible.

For example, suppose your clinical unit has experienced an extremely low census rate over the past year and is scheduled to merge with another unit within your organization. You will be expected to provide competent nursing care not only for patients who traditionally were admitted to your unit but also for new patients with urologic conditions. You are unfamiliar with caring for patients with these needs. Although you know that you will be learning about the nursing care for these patients in the near future, you want to get a head start, especially because some of these new patients have already been admitted to your unit. Develop a career plan that will help you gain the in-depth knowledge and skills you will need to provide safe, quality care to urology patients. You may also design this plan to allow you to refocus your career if you choose to transfer to a clinical unit with a different specialty.

Finally, a career plan can serve as an effective tool to communicate your career goals and learning needs to those who can support your plan, such as your immediate supervisor, a faculty member in your school of nursing, the clinical specialist or educator assigned to your unit, a colleague, or a family member. Sharing your plan with these individuals can help them better understand your goals and learning needs. They may be able to provide you with emotional support or resources (e.g., time, finances, learning opportunities) that will help you attain your goals. Because your career plan provides the impression of you being a self-directed, focused, and organized individual, consider placing a copy of it in your professional portfolio (see Chapter 10).

Regardless of your nursing experience or educational background, now is the best time for you to develop your career plan. Remember, a career plan can change over time, so be sure that it is dynamic and constantly evolving to meet ever-changing professional goals and healthcare trends. For example, suppose an unexpected opportunity to serve as a preceptor for an undergraduate nursing student arises on your clinical unit. Although this role was not part of your original career plan, you decide to take it. You realize your employer will require you to be a preceptor for promotion in the future, so you decide to volunteer now and learn in advance. You also would like to determine if teaching other nurses is a role you may want to pursue in the future. You make these changes and modify your career plan accordingly.

Developing a Career Plan

As previously mentioned, the process of developing a career plan is similar to the steps involved in the nursing process. The actual plan can merely be a draft created with pencil and paper, saved on a smartphone, or typed in a word-processing document. Regardless of what method you choose to record your career plan, it needs to be easily accessible and revisable. The information that follows will walk you through the step-by-step process of developing a career plan and also will provide you with a case study for clarification.

Conduct a Self-Assessment

The first step in developing a career plan is to conduct a self-assessment. Start your assessment by conducting a self-inventory, including your educational background, community involvement, awards, certifications, experiences, knowledge, and skills. Use your professional portfolio (see Chapter 10) and résumé (see Chapter 11) to assist with this step. Make a list of your personal and professional strengths, along with areas that need further improvement.

Include feedback from others who know you well, such as your supervisor, peers, and faculty, to gain their perspectives on your strengths and weaknesses. Recall patient and family comments that speak to your knowledge and skills as a professional nurse.

In addition to collecting data about your current qualities, gather information about the qualifications you will need to attain your future dreams. Start by asking yourself, *What would I like to be doing in the future?* Think about your future as two different time spans: short-term, which can be conceived as up to three years from the present, and long-term, which can be three to five years from now. Talk with nurses who hold desirable positions, and ask for their personal suggestions about qualifications you should acquire to secure a similar position. Obtain the position descriptions of these desirable jobs, and familiarize yourself with the functions, qualifications, and responsibilities of these roles.

If your healthcare facility has a career center, meet with counselors to explore their self-assessment tools and any other resources that can help you. Remember to contact your alma mater and investigate what career services are available to you as an alumnus.

Work with your local librarian to retrieve current reports that describe trends in the nursing profession and healthcare marketplace. Be sure to investigate the strategic plan of your current healthcare organization and include key points in your assessment.

Analyze Your Assessment Data

After you have conducted a thorough self-assessment, organize the data, looking for patterns or trends. Attempt to form some judgments (or diagnoses) about your strengths, weaknesses, professional and personal interests, needed qualifications, and nursing and healthcare trends. Your judgments will help you progress toward the next two steps of career planning: determining your goals (outcomes) and developing interventions (strategies) to attain these goals.

Develop and Prioritize Your Goals (Outcomes)

Use your analysis of the assessment data to develop goals or outcomes that will direct your professional career. These goals should be measurable, challenging, and realistic. They should also be tailored to your specific situation and based on your assessment data and the resources available to you, such as time and money. Identify both short-term and long-term goals, and develop a rationale for goal selection. You can accomplish this by determining a goal's importance to you and why you should be doing it.

Although goals need to reflect what and where you want to be in your professional life, consider matching them with the goals of your clinical unit and healthcare organization. If you plan on changing jobs in the future, review the goals of potential future employers. Reflecting on organizational goals when preparing your career plan will help you become a valued employee with a unique niche in an organization.

Remember to keep your personal goals in mind when developing professional goals. Your professional life does not function in isolation from your personal life. Planned or unplanned personal life events can alter any career plan. Anticipate personal changes, such as marriage, birth of a child, relocation to another state, or a family illness. Rather than viewing these life events as barriers to your career goals, be proactive by integrating them with your career goals. In fact, personal goals may change your career plan to a different but equally exciting focus.

After you have identified your professional goals, set a target date for attaining each goal. Whereas a target date for a long-term goal can be expressed by a year, short-term goal dates should include both a month and year. If you can be more specific, include an exact date. Prioritize your goals in order of time and importance, starting with short-term goals.

Develop a Plan

After you have established your goals, start working toward accomplishing the first goal on your list. Develop a list of interventions, a "to-do list," that you will need to complete to help you reach that goal. Keep each goal's target date in mind as you assign a due date for each intervention. Reorganize your interventions according to their due date, starting with the closest one. Repeat this procedure for each subsequent goal.

Interventions may vary in their complexity and in the time needed to complete each one. Some interventions may take little time, such as joining a professional nursing organization, while others may take much longer, such as completing a formal nursing degree. Interventions may overlap across more than one goal.

Seek a Nursing Degree

Some perceive pursuing a nursing degree as a difficult process. By breaking this process down into logical steps, you can make this endeavor manageable. You will need to make two key decisions: the type of degree you want and where you will pursue it.

Start by exploring available degrees of interest and deciding which one you will pursue. Rely on feedback from your assessment data to help you make this decision. Be sure to include information from mentors, literature reviews, and career counselors. Determine the educational preparation (degree) that is required for you to reach your career goal and that best prepares you to accomplish the responsibilities of your aspired position.

Next, identify universities or colleges that offer the degree you desire. You can obtain a list of accredited schools of nursing through the Accreditation Commission for Education in Nursing (formerly known as the National League for Nursing Accreditation Commission) (www.acenursing.org) and the Commission on Collegiate Nursing Education (www.aacn .nche.edu/ccne-accreditation). Check both sites, as the two lists differ depending on which agency granted accreditation status. You also could obtain this information from the websites of individual schools of nursing. See the Helpful Websites section of this chapter for additional information regarding schools of nursing and accreditation.

After locating accredited schools of nursing that offer your desired degree, retrieve and review information about each school through their websites or by calling a nurse recruiter from each school. School websites offer valuable information about programs, including unique recognitions the school has attained, such as rankings in distance education offerings, centers of excellence in nursing education, and social media. Use the tool presented in Figure 14-1 to examine the features of each school, determine their match with your interests, and narrow down your choices.

Finally, visit the schools that interest you the most, if possible. Speak with faculty, current students, and alumni. Use this information in making your final decision.

If you already have an advanced degree in nursing, consider enrolling in a post-master's certificate program at a college or university. These programs allow nurses with master's degrees

Figure 14-1. Rating Scale for Evaluating a School of Nursing

Directions: Review the following features of a school of nursing listed in the left column. Rate your personal preference for each feature in selecting a school. Use a scale from 1–3 to conduct this rating, with 1 indicating the least amount of importance to you and 3 indicating the highest amount of importance. Use the results to evaluate schools on an individual basis.

Feature	Rating
University and school of nursing:	
Mission and philosophy matches my values.	
Private or public institution matches my needs.	
School is accredited by university and nursing accrediting bodies.	
School has a good reputation, locally and nationally.	
Leadership of the university and school has a good reputation.	
School places value on quality teaching and research.	
Administration, faculty, and staff are friendly and accessible.	
Interesting community partnerships exist.	
Organization offers unique opportunities (international nursing, research, nursing centers).	
Academic program:	
Program offers degrees that reflect my interest.	
Program offers undergraduate and graduate programs.	
Program offers certificate programs of interest to me.	
Admission requirements are clear and attainable.	
Advanced standing for previous course work and experience is valued and available.	
Prerequisites are easily attainable.	
Program of study (curriculum) is interesting, innovative, challenging, and current.	
Courses can be completed full-time or part-time.	
Required credit hours are reasonable to attain in a timely manner.	
Opportunities exist for accelerating course work.	
Courses include opportunities to pursue my interests and flexibility and interdisciplinary focus.	
Exit examinations (comprehensive examination) and final projects (thesis or dissertation) are required for graduation.	
The first-time licensure examination pass rate of undergraduates is acceptable.	
Program includes international nursing opportunities.	

(Continued on next page)

Figure 14-1. Rating Scale for Evaluating a School of Nursing *(Continued)*

Feature	Rating
Student services:	
School offers support with services such as advisement, registration, and orientation.	
School offers various student activities.	
School provides opportunities for tutors.	
Effective communication flow exists between faculty and students.	
Financial resources:	
Opportunities for financial aid, such as loans, scholarships, awards, and graduate assistant positions, are available.	
Tuition is affordable to me.	
Physical facilities:	
Campus is conducive to foster my learning, including classrooms, computer laboratories, and skill laboratories.	
Class size is appropriate for my learning needs.	
Parking is available at a reasonable cost.	
Clinical experience:	
Clinical opportunities are appropriate to my needs and career interest.	
Size of clinical groups (faculty-to-student ratio) is acceptable.	
Opportunities to experience innovative community-based events (e.g., nurse-managed wellness centers) are available.	
Faculty:	
Faculty are excellent teachers and researchers.	
Faculty have an excellent reputation regionally and nationally.	
Faculty have a record of publishing in refereed publications and conducting research in my areas of interest.	
Faculty use active learning strategies in courses.	
Faculty are accessible and friendly.	
Faculty mentor students.	
Students/alumni:	
Student demographics reflect my needs, including cultural diversity.	
Students/alumni express positive comments about their learning experiences.	
Outcomes of graduates (accomplishments and competencies) are positive.	

(Continued on next page)

Figure 14-1. Rating Scale for Evaluating a School of Nursing *(Continued)*	
Feature	**Rating**
Employers value graduates of this school and seek them for employment.	
Alumni association is active and contributes to the school.	
Student organizations are supported and valued.	
Technology:	
Latest technology is used in teaching.	
Distance learning opportunities exist.	
If courses are offered through distance learning, campus visits are required.	
Students have access to computers and software.	
Students have access to state-of-the-art technology.	
Various methods of communication are available (e.g., email, voice mail, office hours, newsletters).	
School's website is informative and inviting.	
Other resources:	
Library facilities are adequate and accessible on site and at a distance.	
Career planning services are available.	
Counseling, test-taking, and writing assistance is available.	
Recreational and social activities are available.	
Books required for courses are easily accessible print or electronic forms.	
Opportunities exist for international study and service initiatives.	

to build upon their current knowledge and clinical skills by expanding their expertise in a new area of study, such as nursing education, nursing administration/leadership, forensic nursing, or advanced nursing practice (AACN, n.d.). Certificate programs require a formal application process and a minimum number of formal academic credits for completion. If you plan to pursue a research-focused (PhD/DNS) or practice-focused (DNP) doctorate in nursing, compare the options using the helpful guide published by AACN (2014).

Implement Your Career Plan

After you have developed your goals and target dates, implement your interventions as listed, starting with the first item. Continue to implement your plan, making decisions along the way as scheduled. Even though a career plan is intended to serve as a guide, try to stay on schedule. As mentioned earlier, you should have developed your career plan with enough flexibility to easily make changes. Remember that it is not unusual for your career plan to change because of unexpected opportunities or events. As you complete the interventions, document your accomplishments in your professional portfolio (see Chapter 10) and update your résumé (see Chapter 11).

Evaluate and Revise Your Career Plan

Evaluation is an integral part of developing a career plan. Monitor your career plan regularly to determine if you are on track. Conduct a more involved evaluation of your plan at least yearly. A good time to do this is when you are scheduled for your annual performance review. If your plan is not helping you meet your goals, then reevaluate it and make changes as needed. If it is taking you more time than expected to complete your interventions, rethink your goals, target dates, and interventions.

In addition to evaluating your career plan, be sure to update it annually so that it always reflects a five-year span. Think about your next set of goals as you accomplish existing ones. Consider developing an alternative career plan in the event that you lose your job or need to change your career path immediately. This will help you survive financially and emotionally.

Case Study

You are an RN who graduated from a bachelor's nursing program and has worked for the past two years as a Staff Nurse I on a medical oncology unit. You want to make oncology nursing part of your career goals. Your self-assessment reveals that you demonstrate excellent communication skills with patients and families, especially those patients experiencing end-of-life situations. Peer evaluations from a unit-based in-service program you presented on bereavement were extremely positive. You enjoy caring for these patients and families and helping staff learn new skills.

After talking with a mentor, you decide that you will need at least a master's degree in nursing to attain your dream job. You also will need to develop your knowledge and skills in oncology nursing, participate in professional nursing organizations, and volunteer in the community. Other skills you need to develop include presenting at conferences or meetings and engaging in various types of scholarship (e.g., publishing, quality improvement, evidence-based practice, and research). It is also important for you to regularly review articles in key oncology nursing journals.

During your review of your organization's strategic plan, you see that it will expand its services in cancer care by opening an outpatient chemotherapy unit within the next two years. Your employer values certification for employees and considers this credential in promotions to advanced clinical nursing positions. A literature review describes not only a nursing shortage but also a current and impending shortage of nursing faculty (AACN, 2015). You remember your days as a student nurse and the excellent clinical instructors who mentored you. The dream of teaching in a school of nursing comes back to you now.

You identify and prioritize two short-term goals and one long-term goal. You assign a target date and rationale for each goal. Figure 14-2 illustrates an example of your goals, target dates, and a rationale for each entry.

You examine your first short-term goal and develop a list of interventions that need to be accomplished to reach this goal. You assign realistic due dates for each intervention. Next, you reorganize your interventions by dates. You repeat this process with your next two goals. Figure 14-3 provides a detailed example of interventions based on your first short-term goal.

Figure 14-2. Example of Short- and Long-Term Goals, Target Dates, and Rationale in a Career Plan

Short-term goal #1: Obtain certification in oncology (OCN®) (July 2016).
Rationale: You, your employer, and the nursing profession value certification. It involves an increase in pay and professional recognition. Certification is preferred for advancement within your organization and would make you competitive in acquiring a position on the chemotherapy unit in the future.

Short-term goal #2: Obtain promotion to a staff nurse II position on an oncology unit, preferably on the outpatient chemotherapy unit (July 2017).
Rationale: Seeking promotion to the next level is an obvious step in your career and results in more prestige and an increase in pay. This is a minimal requirement for nurses in a chemotherapy unit.

Long-term goal #1: Obtain a full-time faculty position in a school of nursing (2020).
Rationale: Teaching in a school of nursing has always been a dream of yours. Your self-assessment and analysis revealed that you possess many strengths as a teacher, such as oral communication skills, working with students, and teaching skills. Trend literature has identified a shortage of nursing faculty in the future, so the market seems good. You notice many ads for nurse faculty positions in your local community.

After discussing your choices with colleagues, family, and other important individuals, you decide to pursue a master's of science in nursing at your local university. After speaking with faculty, you choose to apply to the university's nursing education program. With their assistance, you develop a program of study that allows you to still focus on clinical projects in oncology nursing while gaining expertise in nursing education. The school's distance learning program will provide you with the flexibility you need in light of your busy work schedule and

---

Figure 14-3. Example of Interventions Matched With Short-Term Goal #1 in a Career Plan

Short-term goal #1: Obtain certification in oncology (OCN®) (July 2016).
• Obtain information for OCN® testing from the Oncology Nursing Certification Corporation website (June 2015).
• Review OCN® eligibility criteria* (June 2015):
  – A current, active, unencumbered license as an RN in the United States, its territories, or Canada at the time of application and examination (done)
  – A minimum of one year (12 months) of experience as an RN within three years (36 months) prior to application (done)
  – A minimum of 1,000 hours of adult oncology nursing practice within the two-and-one-half years (30 months) prior to application (done)
  – Completed a minimum of 10 contact hours of continuing nursing education in oncology or an academic elective in oncology nursing within the three years (36 months) prior to application. The contact hours must have been provided or formally approved by an accredited provider or approver of continuing nursing education. A maximum of 5 of the 10 required contact hours in oncology may be continuing medical education in oncology. (done)
• Seek support for testing fee from employer or the Oncology Nursing Society (July 2015).
• Obtain study materials (e.g., references, study guides, sample examinations) (August 2015).
• Develop a study plan based on the resources (August 2015)
• Develop an OCN® study group on your unit (September 2015).
• Take an OCN® review course and revise your study plan as needed (fall 2015 or spring 2016).
• Submit application form with payment (before April 20, 2016).
• Take OCN® exam (July 20, 2016).

* Certification criteria are from Oncology Nursing Certification Corporation, n.d.

personal responsibilities. You access the application through the school's website and plan to complete the admission requirements. You are excited and look forward to this major step in your professional career.

A year goes by and you have been able to accomplish the interventions of your career plan in a timely manner, despite an unexpected family illness. Your workplace recently developed an academic partnership with a local school of nursing. This change has enabled you to be a guest speaker on oncology nursing to junior students enrolled in an undergraduate nursing course. You volunteered to be a preceptor for a senior nursing student who is completing an independent study on your clinical unit in oncology nursing over the summer. You decide that these activities, although not in your original plan, can be easily added to it and will significantly contribute to helping you attain your goals.

Prior to your annual performance evaluation, you conduct a formal assessment of your career plan. You feel that no major changes are needed at this time. You feel pleased that you have been successful in accomplishing the interventions you identified in your career plan to help you attain your goals. You share your success with your manager and other nurses on your clinical unit.

Summary

NPDSs may be responsible for helping clinical staff develop their professional career plans. Creating your own personalized career plan based on realistic short-term and long-terms goals can be an effective way to first experience the process in order to mentor others. A career plan helps you assess and direct your career goals in a timely and organized way. Begin the process by conducting a self-assessment, analyzing your assessment data, and developing and prioritizing your goals. Be sure to evaluate and revise your career plan on an ongoing basis after implementing it. Use what you have learned during this process to mentor clinical staff at your healthcare organization.

Helpful Websites

- AllNursingSchools: www.allnursingschools.com
- American Association of Colleges of Nursing—Your Nursing Career: www.aacn.nche.edu/students/your-nursing-career
- American Nurses Association—NursingWorld: www.nursingworld.org
- GradSchools.com: www.gradschools.com
- Johnson & Johnson: Discover Nursing—Campaign for Nursing's Future: www.discovernursing.com
- Nurse Journal: http://nursejournal.org
- Peterson's: www.petersons.com
- U.S. News and World Report: www.usnews.com

References

American Association of Colleges of Nursing. (n.d.). *Your guide to graduate nursing programs.* Retrieved from http://www.aacn.nche.edu/student/news/2011/grad-brochure

American Association of Colleges of Nursing. (2014). Nursing shortage fact sheet. Retrieved from http://www.aacn.nche.edu/media-relations/NrsgShortageFS.pdf

American Association of Colleges of Nursing. (2015). Nursing faculty shortage fact sheet. Retrieved from http://www.aacn.nche.edu/media-relations/fact-sheets/nursing-faculty-shortage

American Nurses Association. (2015). *Nursing: Scope and standards of practice* (3rd ed.). Silver Spring, MD: Author.

American Nurses Association & National Nursing Staff Development Organization. (2010). *Nursing professional development: Scope and standards of practice.* Silver Spring, MD: Author.

Fowler, D.L. (2014). Career coaching: Innovative academic-practice partnership for professional development. *Journal of Continuing Education in Nursing, 45,* 205–209. doi:10.3928/00220124-20140417-02

Oncology Nursing Certification Corporation. (n.d.). Testing and renewal. Retrieved from http://www.oncc.org/resource-center/testing-and-renewal#e-new

Index

The letter *f* after a page number indicates that relevant content appears in a figure; the letter *t*, in a table.

A

abstract
  importance of, 220
  of presentation, 232–234, 233*t*
  word count limit for, 220
academic partnerships, 21, 29
  gains from engaging in
      research and evidence-
      based practice by, 287
  for research and evidence-
      based practice, 299–300
accountability, 23
accreditation, of healthcare orga-
    nizations, 27–28
accreditation agencies
  in continuing competence, 56
  in identification of core compe-
    tencies, 61–63
accreditation programs, 46–47
accreditation standards, 56
admission to school, résumé
    for, 265
adult learning
  fostering, 71–73
  principles of, 72–73
  familiarizing unit staff with, 93
advertising
  for continuing education activ-
    ity, 319
  for in-service educational pro-
    gram, 168
affective objectives for in-service
    educational program, 171,
    173, 173*t*
aggregate competence data,
    70–71
American Academy for Preceptor
    Advancement (AAPA), 129
American College of Surgeons
    Commission on Cancer
    (ACS CoC), 3

American Nurses Association
    (ANA)
  joining, 194
  on nursing professional devel-
    opment, 17–18
  on research and evidence-
    based practice, 284–285
  on standards of practice, 27
American Nurses Credentialing
    Center (ANCC)
  and continuing education, 310
  Magnet Recognition Program
    of, 8, 28, 125
  Nursing Skills Competency
    Program of, 62–63
andragogy, 72–73
anecdotes, 94
assistive personnel (AP), learn-
    ing needs of, 77–79
Association for Nursing Pro-
    fessional Development
    (ANPD), 18, 45, 194
attendance record for in-ser-
    vice educational program,
    178, 179*f*
audiovisuals
  for in-service educational pro-
    gram, 175, 176*t*
  for presentation, 237–238
author guidelines, 213
authorship of manuscript, 211
awards
  in portfolio, 257*t*, 259
  and résumé, 265, 271

B

benchmarking, 8
  of preceptor programs,
    128–129
Bloom's taxonomy for in-service
    educational program, 170–171

brochure for continuing educa-
    tion activity, 319

C

Cancer Program Standards 2012:
    Ensuring Patient-Centered
    Care (ACS CoC), 3
career development, 21
career goals
  in portfolio, 250, 258*t*, 261
  on résumé, 267
career plan, 325–336
  case study on, 333–335, 334*f*
  defined, 325
  development of, 327–332
    analyzing assessment data
      in, 328
    conducting self-assessment
      in, 327–328
    developing and prioritiz-
      ing goals (outcomes) in,
      328–329
    developing plan in, 329
    seeking nursing degree in,
      329–332, 330*f*–332*f*
  evaluating and revising of, 333
  helpful websites on, 335
  implementing, 332–333
  nursing process vs., 325, 325*f*
  purpose of, 326–327
  understanding, 325–326, 325*f*
career planning, 325
casual staff, learning needs of, 76
CBO. *See* competency-based ori-
    entation (CBO)
CE. *See* continuing education
    (CE)
certificates
  in portfolio, 257*t*, 259
  on résumé, 268
certification(s), 47